D1084793

STUTTERING
AND
PERSONALITY DYNAMICS

Play Therapy, Projective Therapy, and Counseling

ALBERT T. MURPHY
Co-Director, Speech and Hearing Center
Boston University

and

RUTH M. FITZSIMONS
Head Speech and Hearing Therapist
Warwick (R.I.) Public Schools

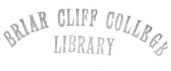
THE RONALD PRESS COMPANY　　·　　NEW YORK

This book is dedicated to the families in which there is a stuttering child, and to our own respective families—Terry, Mark, and Steven Murphy, and Leo and Helen FitzSimons

Preface

This book presents a psychodynamic, interpersonal approach to the problem of stuttering. We are convinced that stuttering speech is a symptom of deep-seated personal difficulties and that it is only by understanding the individual stutterer that we can deal successfully with his speech problem. The self-process concept of stuttering presented in this book combines the rich insights of clinical counseling and educational psychology with those of psychiatry and speech pathology. We believe it offers the most promising approach to diagnosis and treatment of stuttering behavior.

The first two parts of this book deal in some detail with the etiology of stuttering behavior. These chapters show that stuttering, like all psychogenic speech problems, is a disorder symptom whose roots lie in disturbed interpersonal relationships and the stutterer's fractured self-image. They also try to make clear the significance of both early and contemporary interpersonal experiences upon speech adjustment, and particularly the effects of disrupted *non*speech developmental tasks upon speech behavior. But the major part of the book is devoted to diagnostic and therapeutic techniques. There are detailed analyses of the basic concepts, goals, and methods in individual and group play therapy, role playing, projective techniques, creative dramatics, and client-centered counseling. To us, the goal structure and aim of all these forms of dynamic speech therapy is the development of greater personal and speech comfort in the stutterer through increased self-awareness and reduction of anxiety. Accordingly, in all these approaches the focus is on the clinician-stutterer relationship, for its warm, acceptant, permissive content is the key to effective therapy. Thus we have also stressed the personal qualities of the clinician, the effect of his own personality on diagnosis and therapeutic efficiency. In a very real sense, we think of the skilled clinician as an artist. Pliability, creativity, and sensitive intuition are precious therapeutic aids when combined with rigorous study and training. Finally, to enable the reader to share these therapeutic experiences more intimately, we have included many transcriptions of actual therapy sessions with stutterers, parents, and teachers.

We recognize that much remains to be learned about stuttering. The present volume is an attempt to share our experience in working with stuttering persons in schools and in clinical and hospital settings. It is an outgrowth of a decade of action, trial and error, success and failure in trying to help individuals who stutter to find for themselves more satisfying and productive lives as persons as well as speakers. We know that reading a book is only the beginning of wisdom, that it is only through serious study, practical experience, and thoughtful experimentation and self-searching that deep understanding can come. But reading a book, especially one written from a psychodynamic point of view, should provide the reader of whatever orientation with the opportunity to re-examine his own beliefs in the light of the convictions presented. This is all to the good. For the effective clinician is the worker who believes strongly in his therapeutic approach and who is able to create a therapeutic relationship that is secure and, thereby, productive.

Finally, we would like to express our appreciation to those publishers who have permitted us to quote from their materials, and to Mr. R. K. Smith for his photographic contributions. The insight and stimulation that we have received from those who stutter and from the students with whom we have worked has been of very great value. The wise counsel of Dr. R. Corbin Pennington during the early stages of the book did much to improve the quality of this work. And to our typists, Mrs. Doris Adams and Mrs. Ruth Pampel, go our thanks.

ALBERT T. MURPHY
RUTH M. FITZSIMONS

September, 1960

Contents

Part I

Introduction

Chapter **1**

Stuttering: The Disorder and the Challenge

> *You start a question and it's like starting a stone. You sit quietly on the top of a hill; and away the stone goes, starting others.*——Robert Louis Stevenson

I rose at seven o'clock. It is going to be a hot day. My father's voice awakens me. Another day of work lies before me. Can I handle it? It would be so much easier to lie here in this soft bed than to go into town and do one's best only to be laughed at. Today I am supposed to answer phone calls. Can I speak smoothly enough to handle it? Will they laugh at my speech on the phone? I hate the phone— would that it never were invented! I hate the twentieth century with its modern gadgets which have so complicated the life of man and made him forget the simple virtues of our forefathers. If I were only a shepherd in Abraham's time, minding my flock with a loyal wife to succor me, how happy I should be!

I'm dressed and shaved. I go to the breakfast table. Obstinately I refuse conversation with Father, addressing only a few words to Mother. The challenge of the car lies before me. Will I hit someone on the short drive to the station? Of course not. It's foolish to think so! Still, one never can tell. How I hate this prattle of my parents about baseball and business.

I'm in the train station. I read snatches of *The Case of Sergeant Grischa*. Good book. Would willingly exchange places with Grischa, escaped Russian war prisoner, strong, virile, simple, resourceful. Reminder: Will have as little talk as possible with Mary at the office today. I'll make believe I'm the resourceful Sergeant Grischa. I'll talk to everyone with a loud sigh, short sentences, skip lightly over unimportant words. I know everything about speech except how to talk. Damn!!! Look at all these fools. No sense or sensibility, but they can talk when, with whom, and about whatever they please.

3

How cruel that I, with all my potentialities, cannot. The crowd is watching a construction crew working—the wonders of modern progress. Blast modern progress! It's engulfing you, people, but you don't know it. It will chew you up, piece by piece. Here comes the train. Sometimes I'd like to throw myself in front of it, but no will power. Besides, it would be exhibitionistic.

On the train. Could read. No, Dad said it might permanently injure my vision, reading on a jiggling train. Smoke? No. Might interfere with my breathing. I've got to talk on the phone today. Oh, if only the train were going a long, long way—Malibu, Timbuktu, Zanzibar, Madagascar, Bali, pineapples, mangoes. . . . I get off. Tramp, tramp, tramp. There's Alan Green. He speaks to me when there is no one around to speak to. Not now. I'm not important enough. Girl tagging along at his elbow and two other young businessmen with him. What if he did ask me to join them? Could I hold up my end of the conversation, make myself interesting? There's a bum on the street. I'd change places with you, Bud.

Into the elevator. Good morning to the elevator woman. Would like to say more but better not. I wonder if Mary is up there already. Yes, she is. She's having an argument on the phone with her latest boy friend. I sit down. She comes over, touches me lightly on the shoulder. "I'm free now. I'm all through with him." This doesn't affect me. Hope it makes her unhappy. I don't care. But I am lonely. Wouldn't want to marry her. But she is pretty. Maybe I could ask her to lunch. If she did go, I'd show her I was attractive; I'll bide my time. Morning becomes more pleasant though, but a voice keeps repeating, "She is not for you." I need some water to wet the tape. I ask Helen if there is a fountain. Fountain pen? No, w-w-w-w-water f-f-f-fount-t-t-tain. "You can get the water in the sandwich shop next door." No, I think I'll bring the whole thing upstairs. She asks me if I want her to ask at the sandwich shop for a glass of water. No thanks. What does she think I am—a spineless coward? I could ask if I wanted to!

Mary had asked me to lunch with her at 12 o'clock. Now she calls up John. In beautiful, smooth, sweet tones asks him to meet her for lunch. So that's it. That simple-minded, fair-haired stock clerk. Him over me! What's he got—carefree, word talker, empty-headed. Is that what she wants? She's intelligent; surely not—but yes. I go to lunch. I try to read *Sergeant Grischa*. Can't. I think of them. I'm a failure with the girls. Still, she's not the kind of girl I want. I don't care for her, don't like her. Can't stand her, abominate her. She's nothing to me. I get back to Grischa. Can't. Yes, I can read. I love books. But do they take me away from girls? Could I be happy except for this reading habit? No, it's my speech. I go back to the office. Mr. Brown comes in. I ask him to read my report. He says it's good, a few spots ragged. I want to answer some of his criticisms. I can't find the words. I meekly assent to them. Perhaps they are just, anyway. She's back. I must get some answer. I don't care for her but must get to first base. Prove my manhood. Get her to go out. My speech is a big drawback. I write a note. Want a final answer. "Tell me if you don't want to have anything further to do with me." "Aren't you ashamed to write anything like that?" she asks. Why? "Do I have to spell it out?" She doesn't want anything further to do with me. My speech. If I could only talk! I ask her what's wrong with me. She says she won't answer 'cause I'll get mad. Says I get mad too easily, resented my not talking to her. I apologize. She says just be agreeable to her in the office. Be a good boy, she means. Treats me with contempt. Five o'clock, off. I walk down town amid thoughts of my weaknesses. I am weak, weak, weak. Humiliated. Ashamed. I want to go home and cry. Why? Don't know. They don't understand. It would make Mom sick. But I've got to. Feel better. Maybe they can sooth, calm me. Mom's not home. I'll wait for her. I hate life. I don't care for that girl. Not at all. I've humiliated myself for someone I don't care for.

The young man who expressed these thoughts reveals to us a glimpse of a single day of frustration. Although we get an inkling of his aspirations, fears, doubts, conflicts, and defenses, no small sampling of his thoughts can reveal adequately the scope and depth of this individual's feeling of futility. Yet, he is but one of a million people in our country who speak in broken words.

STUTTERING: IN RETROSPECT

Stuttering, of interest throughout history, has been one of mankind's great puzzles. It is only in the last few decades, however, that the possibility of a solution to the puzzle has come within reach, as the characteristics and impact of the individual pieces become identified and linked to reveal greater meaning in the complex stuttering mosaic. Even as recently as 1931, there were only a few books dealing with speech disorders, and these were comparatively limited in coverage. Then in that year appeared the first comprehensive, scientific text on speech and hearing disorders, *Speech Pathology,* by Lee Edward Travis. This book may be considered the dividing line between the pre-experimental and the experimental period in speech therapy, as well as the culmination of what may be thought of as the first epoch in speech pathology.

The beginnings of the new era may be traced to the work of Carl Emil Seashore and his associates at the State University of Iowa. In 1922 Seashore and his Iowa colleagues began a training program that was to prepare a new kind of specialist in the area of speech and hearing disorders. The first graduate of this program was Lee Travis, who, in 1924, was appointed Director of the University of Iowa Speech Clinic. He and his associates, utilizing principles and methodologies from education, psychology, psychiatry, and neurology, performed extensive laboratory research in speech pathology, especially in the area of stuttering, and produced scores of publications in a wide variety of professional journals, culminating in the important 1931 book, *Speech Pathology*. For a full account of the origin and development of the University of Iowa Speech Clinic, the reader should consult *Stuttering in Children and Adults: Thirty Years of Research at the University of Iowa* (Johnson and Leutenegger, 1955). For all speech therapy students as well as for all persons who are working with speech- and hearing-handicapped people, the book's foreword should be required reading. The material is a vital part of every speech clinician's professional legacy, for the early Iowa story, still continuing in strength and creativity, comprises an important chapter in the history of speech and hearing pathology.

The psychologist Ebbinghaus once observed that psychology had a long past but a short history. The field of speech pathology can be so described. Professor Edwin Boring of Harvard, speaking of the experimental psychologist, said that he "needs historical sophistication within his own sphere of expertness. Without such knowledge, he sees the present in distorted perspective; he mistakes old facts and old views for new ones; and he remains unable to evaluate the significance of new movements and new methods. . . . A sophistication that contains no component of historical orientation seems to me to be no orientation at all" (Boring, 1929, p. vii). Perhaps speech pathology is still too youthful a discipline to have its history written, but some day soon, some person will undertake the task, and all workers in the field will profit in the reading of it.

STUTTERING: IN PRESENT PERSPECTIVE

With speech pathology's scientific awakening at Iowa and elsewhere, stuttering persons were beginning to be evaluated and guided more effectively. Gradually the specialization of speech therapy came to occupy a respected place in the course offerings of large numbers of colleges and universities. The literature on stuttering alone has become voluminous. Now most states have laws recognizing the needs of speech-handicapped children. The number of speech defectives that flows into our schools, clinics, and hospitals has been increasing annually; and the demands for services and workers outreach the supply. The progress of the profession has been noteworthy. Today it is clear that the science of speech pathology has been making and will continue to make significant contributions to human welfare. Speech pathology is a recognized discipline, one very unlike the speech field of earlier days, not merely in relation to its great fund of knowledge but also in relation to its methods and basic principles.

But speech pathology, like every other embryonic discipline, has experienced many growing pains. Functions and philosophies of persons who have worked to help stuttering individuals have varied widely. Sometimes it has appeared that workers have played almost as many roles as there were stutterers referred to them. Many clinicians, for example, have worked within conceptual frameworks which emanated from the thinking of teachers whose early training had been largely in the fields of drama and the speech arts: discussion, debate, and public speaking.

Gestalt psychology has emphasized that human behavior is more than an aggregate of parts and that it is more pro-

ductively studied as a function of a total organism. Thus
the study of the speech mechanism (part) does not give us
an understanding of the total human system (whole). Rather,
the part can be understood only after we uncover the meaning of the whole. Workers have recognized the necessity of
understanding structural and functional relationships and of
searching for broader webs of experience patterns which
constitute the entire life of the stuttering person. Certainly
there can be no clear separations among such components
of the human system as emotion, speech, intellect, social- and
self-perceptions, and stresses. The task is to try to understand the stuttering individual's previous and present life
experiences as they affect his present functioning; to observe
him as he struggles to maintain a personal equilibrium in
his social setting; to observe through a period of time the
effects of his emotions on his intellectual and speech-expressive capabilities; and to recognize and take account of his
associated adjustment deviations. The focus of attention
goes beyond the speech component. It centers on the individual as a thinking, feeling human being who must continually adjust to an ever-changing environment. The person's speech is but *one indicator* of the success of his attempts
to make a harmonious adjustment of self with environment.

Whether it is realized or not, speech specialists come very
close *per force* to being practitioners of clinical psychology,
even with individuals in public speaking classes. Much of
the past therapeutic success of speech clinicians with stutterers can be attributed to the undefined emotional relationship that existed between clinician and stutterer, rather than
to the specific speech-correction techniques employed. Stated
differently, the intermittent success of some well-known devices and mechanical manipulations in the stutterer's total
adjustment probably was due mainly to: (1) an accepting,
supportive attitude by the clinician toward the stutterer; and
(2) a resolution of stresses within the stutterer (because of
the developmental personal relationship accompanying the
speech procedures). The importance of such psychological

considerations is something which has been overlooked at times.

Workers who are inclined toward strict experimentation believe that objectively measurable behavior is the only aspect of the person that can be analyzed. From this point of view we can record what a person does, writes, and speaks. Thus, if a person is unable to talk, we must assume that we are less able to know what his feelings are or what is "on his mind." If, in addition, the person is not able to write or move his muscles, as in some cases of aphasia or schizophrenia or even stuttering, we may very well not know at all what this person is feeling or thinking. Behavioristic speech pathologists feel that two factors in the stutterer's behavior can be observed and measured, viz., stimulus and response. But one crucial question is left unanswered: What about the *motives* behind the behavior? Is it enough to say that disordered speech means we are less able to understand the thoughts and feelings of the stutterer? May we not assume that if a person cannot talk, it may well be that, unconsciously, he is motivated to keep people from knowing his true feelings? This critical area concerning the determinants of the person's disordered speech has not been tapped in much of the speech pathology research. Sometimes it seems as though the implicit pledge of allegiance to scientific objectivity has served as a barrier and possibly a deterrent to the analytical, synthesizing, creative, and intuitive insight of the clinician. Therapists of stutterers encounter the problem of distinguishing overt, observable behavior from subjective, implicit behavior. It does not seem possible to deny or skirt subjective experiences in any discussion of the stuttering disorder. Such experiences quite possibly function in closely approximate accordance with the laws operant in the experience of neuromotor responses, even though the problem of conceptualizing and measuring such experiences is considerably greater. Verbal behavior (especially the disruption or lack of such behavior) as an indicator of subjective experiences is of enormous importance to our understanding, not only of oral communication breakdown in stutterers but of all human beings as well. Unfortunately, such implied behavior on the part of either client or clinician is often decried or perhaps dismissed as "clinical." It is possible that some productive ideas in speech therapy have been rejected because they are clinically rather than experimentally derived. This is exactly the situation Freudian psychology encountered in its infancy, although much systematic experimentation has shown psychoanalytic theories to be more rather than less accurate (Hilgard, 1956, pp. 297–306). Likewise, in speech therapy, psychological notions have not always taken root easily.

[some] . . . speech counselors try to adopt a more client-centered approach, but because of lack of training or experience, or due to a basic feeling of doubt concerning the client's capacity to grow and achieve better adjustment abilities if given certain emotional or expressive freedoms in an atmosphere of reintegration, or because of a personal feeling of discomfort in trying to maintain a relationship they are unable to "control" according to rigidly pre-set attitudes, therapy structures, and goals, gradually assume a more comfortable role of therapy *director*. In any case, such persons sincerely feel that this is the best approach to the situation; no doubt, often it is, but perhaps often it is just the only thing they are able to do (Murphy, 1955, p. 260).

Unfortunately, from some points of view, and fortunately from others, attitudes about etiology and therapy of stuttering are countless, although all workers are dedicated in their own way to the understanding and improvement of this behavior disorder. An additional hurdle for the student is the level of language usage and terminology pertaining to stuttering. Neurological, psychological, psychoanalytic, educational, and semantic systems and vocabularies await the unsuspecting adventurer into the field. Wendell Johnson's classical capsule autobiography of the diagnostic and therapeutic odyssey of a person who has stuttered gives an amusing but deadly accurate view of the research highways and the treatment byways a person so affected could travel.

In working with personality cases, I am somewhat like the surgeon who remembers his own appendectomy each time he enters the operating room. Some day I hope to write "The Memoirs of a White Rat."

As a severe stutterer, with the adjustment problems that go with stuttering, I have been examined, diagnosed, tested and treated, checked up on, drilled, observed, and charted; I have been psychoanalyzed; I have written my autobiography and changed my handedness. In the laboratory my reflexes have been checked, my eye movements have been photographed, my breathing has been recorded on yards and yards of smoked paper; my blood has been analyzed, my blood pressure measured, my pulse palpated and I have been hyperventilated; my phi phenomena have been examined and so has my chronaxie; I have sat in cold water while my tremors were recorded; I have taken sodium amytal and hashish and described the resulting sensations to a laboratory stenographer; I have sat for electrocardiograms, audiograms, and electroencephalograms; my intelligence has been estimated, my body build classified, my voice recorded, my basal metabolic rate determined, my emotions rated, my nerve impulses graphed; and I have been asked whether I liked my mother better than my father and whether I find it hard to get rid of a salesman. I have talked with pebbles in my mouth, with my teeth together, while breathing with diaphragm and in time to a metronome. I have relaxed, gone on and off diets, sung the scale and stuttered on purpose (Johnson, 1946, p. 391).

The fact that more research, more writings, and more convention hours have been devoted to stuttering than to any other speech handicap is another indication of the disorder's complexity. Van Riper (1954) presents an excellent introductory survey of stuttering theories along with an extensive annotated bibliography which the beginning student will find extremely helpful. Hahn (1956) has edited a detailed review of old and new stuttering theories. Berry and Eisenson's (1956) review is short but cogent. An enlightening comparison and practical amalgamation of points of view has been made by Ainsworth (1945). More recently, an exposition of the theories of six leading practitioners has appeared (Eisenson et al., 1958).

A POINT OF VIEW IN STUTTERING

Although the general philosophy of stuttering and therapy will be revealed as the book unfolds, at this point the reader well may ask, "Whose viewpoint do you support? Johnson? Travis? Van Riper?" That we support much of the thinking of all these men will become evident. In addition, we support many of the ideas of such thinkers as Freud, Carl Rogers, Harry Stack Sullivan, and O. H. Mowrer, among others. It is not practicality or a mere eclectic convenience that allows us to accept or be stimulated by the views of these men. This book attempts to seine out fertile thoughts and methods which psychology, psychiatry, and speech therapy offer and to weave them into an ever-increasingly meaningful whole. This selective realignment and integration of ideas from various sources is an effort to perceive undistortedly the deepest wisdom of numerous mentors. With these perceptions we have merged our own ideas and experiences to form productive, practical, and personal foundations for therapy in order to serve stuttering individuals better.

Regardless of the "approach" followed, any explanation of stuttering, in respect to the individual stutterer or to stutterers generally, is but a series of hypothetical formulations more than an accurate record of facts. Indeed, a complete record of facts would be so massive as to be unmanageable. The clinician or theorist bases his diagnosis and therapeutic choice on *samplings* of the individual or group behavior, and he accepts the analysis of these samplings as indicative of the person's life story.

To repeat, it is impossible to recognize all those who have influenced the thinking of this book, but the stimulation has emanated primarily from the following disciplines: speech pathology, clinical psychology, learning theory, psychiatry, psychoanalysis, and sociology. In speech pathology, the outstanding influence stems from Lee Travis, while the great body of literature on speech disorders has served as constant stimulant and valuable checkmate. There has been no single identifiable influence in clinical psychology, although the authors have utilized the principles and methods of the subareas of projective psychology, perception, and anxiety theory. The philosophy and practices of Carl Rogers form a substantial portion of the basis for much of our thinking. The brilliance of O. H. Mowrer, John Dollard, and Neal E. Miller has illuminated our thinking about learning theory.

Our psychoanalytic foundations derive from Freud's writings and from personal utilization of many Freudian principles in theory and therapy. The influence of Harry Stack Sullivan's interpersonal theory of psychiatry has been very considerable.

There is a permeating nucleus of basic dynamics interwoven throughout the book, a few of which will be only named at this point. It will become clear to the reader that in our discussions of oral communication disruption, strong emphasis is shown to considerations of (1) early socialization experiences, especially in relation to the early mother-child relationship; (2) the impress of perceptual, motor, conceptual, and allied "developmental tasks" on verbal functioning; (3) the effects of nonverbal functions and learning on verbal behavior; (4) *anxiety*, its origins and effects; and (5) the self-process, including acceptance and rejection of self, self-differentiation and integration, and self-defensive processes.

However, the pervading least common denominator which serves as undercurrent and overtone throughout the book is the *clinical approach*. The clinical method as employed herein is applicable in school settings as well as in "clinics." By clinical approach we refer to the application of dynamic speech and psychological principles and procedures to the speech-social adjustment of the individual stutterer. The emphasis is on the individual. In this light, speech therapy may be regarded as a form of applied or clinical psychology whose scope comprises two fundamental goals: (1) the diagnosis of present and past behavior characteristics and capacities through measurement, observation, and analysis; and (2) recommendations, based on the integrated findings and allied case history data, for obtaining improved social-speech adjustment of the stutterer. Differentiating between diagnostic and treatment findings is not always simple. In fact, the treatment process is always "diagnostic therapy." The clinician must continually assess and reassess the "raw data," which in this case refers to the constantly fluctuating behavior of the stutterer as he strives for psychological and speech equilibrium and comfort in his therapeutic, social, or educational milieu. In relation to diagnosis, we note that most persons designedly or unwittingly make diagnostic inferences about stuttering, and they tend to react to the stutterer in the light of their diagnosis—be it accurate or distorted. One of the stutterer's most severe problems is the fear of or the actual misperception by the listener and viewer of "what he really is." Perhaps of equal or greater importance, however, is the *diagnosis of the stutterer made by the stutterer himself.* The stutterer, though reacting to his surroundings, is constantly reacting to self; his problem is to make an adequate (realistic and developmental) perception and reaction to self and surroundings (others) at the same time.

Play therapy, creative dramatics, or the counseling interview can give diagnostic insights as well as therapeutic gains. Conversely, many speech, personality, and even intelligence tests which are considered to be diagnostic may trigger within a stutterer a greater self-awareness, a common ingredient and goal of many therapies. In such cases, referring to the diagnostic procedure as "therapeutic diagnosis" is not an altogether extreme notion. Distinguishing between diagnostic and therapeutic events is not always possible or necessary, but the clinician's readiness to *attempt* to differentiate and the *ability* to differentiate are always desirable.

In traditional speech therapy, the stuttering person's present behavior has sometimes been evaluated primarily on the basis of oral diagnostics. That is, the worker's attention and interests have centered primarily on what the speech mechanism is doing. If the speech is severely nonfluent, the person may be described as a "severe stutterer"; if the speech deviations consist of mild blockings, he may be termed a "mild stutterer." Sometimes breathing patterns are analyzed; the rate of movement or degree of alacrity of parts of the speech mechanism are evaluated; mouth or facial grimaces, tremors, or tension points are described or rated. The average number of repetitions per word and the average duration of prolongations may be computed, along with the measuring of such items as the use of starters and postponement devices.

There is indeed a great variety of testing procedures and instruments.

However, the requirements of diagnosis in stuttering go beyond the cumulation of speech scores. Two decades ago one writer made the following statement concerning the goals of diagnosis in speech disorders:

Our main concern is with interrelations. . . . All techniques are set up to answer the following questions. (1) What sort of an organism is involved; (2) what environmental factors have played and are playing upon the organism to precipitate certain reactions; (3) exactly what are the expressions of the interaction between the organism and its environment . . . we wish to know all that has happened to the individual since conception and specifically what situational elements are impinging upon him at the moment . . . we want to know the symptoms expressive of the speech defect, the precise pathological expressions and pathophysiological processes (Travis, 1938, pp. 28–30).

Speech scores alone are but measurements or judgments of the outward manifestation of an inner disequilibrium, mild or severe. Because the stutterer's speech behavior is affected by emotional factors, by the dynamics of his personality constellation, by his attitudinal shifts which accompany situational changes, by his unique reaction patterns, and by his rigid, distorted, or realistic levels of aspiration or self-perception, these factors need analysis as much as or more than do the oral characteristics. Psychodynamic speech therapy is concerned with the total situation, the fusion or confusion of the stutterer's inner drive and outer reality.

It is not possible to classify stutterers according to a particular physiological or psychological pattern. Stutterers' attitudes and reaction patterns are not readily subjected to statistical analyses. The lives of different stutterers cover too wide and too variable an emotional gamut to allow it. Because present personal problems are inextricably interwoven with past life experiences, they are less accessible to metrical evaluation. Because of this intricacy, stuttering dynamics can be most meaningfully understood by the individual case study approach. Though, as a group, stutterers reveal certain similar behavior patterns, individual stutterers *may* reveal *any* degree of personal adjustment or physical health from normal to inferior. Stutterers are not creatures from a strange land. They are people from any street in any town. As a group, they are not uniquely different from other humans. Compared to nonstutterers, most stutterers are more *like* than different. The flux and flow of emotions which are experienced by stutterers are found in nonstutterers also. It is a matter of pattern and degree, not kind. Berry and Eisenson summarize an array of points of view as an indication of the varying attitudes about the social adjustment of stutterers. According to these writers, different clinicians are apt to make the following differing statements:

1. Stutterers, as a group, are perfectly normal persons who happen to have speech handicaps. If they have maladjustments, it is because stutterers are human beings and as such may have maladjustments.
2. Stutterers are maladjusted persons for whom stuttering is a manifestation of maladjustment.
3. Stutterers, because of their stuttering, tend to become maladjusted.
4. Stutterers are anxiety-ridden persons who concretize their anxieties and insecurities in their speech.
5. Stutterers are infantile persons who revert to infantile oral behavior because of their anxieties and insecurities.
6. Stutterers are severely maladjusted, passive, schizoid persons, who require psychoanalytic therapy if they are to recover (Berry and Eisenson, 1956, pp. 255–56).

As Berry and Eisenson state, it is possible that each of the generalizations holds for some stutterers and none for all stutterers. It is also possible that the generalizations may be flavored by a given clinician's particular professional and philosophical propensities and training. Also, the disparate findings might originate from biased samplings of particular workers. The possibility that the personalities of stutterers may be ranged along a broad continuum, from well-adjusted to poorly adjusted, is one deserving of more extensive consideration. Chapters 5 and 6 include an enlargement of this consideration.

The authors' conception of stuttering may be stated briefly at this point. Chapters 3 through 6 will be devoted to a detailed consideration of what is stated or implied in this section. First, stuttering behavior is primarily a psychogenically motivated symptom which manifests itself most discernibly in oral functions. However, the entire dynamic equilibrium of the individual may be affected in varying degrees. Not only his verbal but also his nonverbal behavior may be deviant. His perception of his current environment and the people and objects in it may be distorted. His attitudes toward, and reaction patterns to, that environment may be atypical. Quite often stuttering is a manifestation of underlying confusions, doubts, anxieties, and feelings of inadequacy. It is originally an emotional response to parental or environmental pressures, the result of conflicts in interpersonal relationships. In short, stuttering speech is like a theater marquee sign: It tells us something is going on, but in order to know what is happening, we usually have to go "inside" to find out.

Clinical support for these statements may be found by considering observations such as the following: (1) when the stutterer's general anxiety or feeling of discomfort increases, the stuttering symptom tends to increase; (2) the greater the uncertainty or feeling of hesitancy experienced by the stutterer, the greater the tendency to stutter more severely; (3) the more unrealistic his general attitude or perception of the world around him and of himself, the more unmanageable does he find his stuttering to be; (4) the more self-critical he is, the worse his stuttering tends to become; (5) the more chronically rigid his over-all behavior, the more severe the stuttering is likely to be; (6) the more withdrawn socially the stutterer is, the more severe his stuttering is likely to be; (7) the more intolerant he is of the actions of others, of his own actions, and especially of his own basic impulses, the worse the stuttering is likely to be; (8) the more dependent the stutterer is, the more severe the stuttering is likely to be.

Many other factors may be considered. For example, in general, the more persistently inconsistent, prejudiced, judgmental, and "intellect-bound" the stutterer is, the worse the stuttering seems to become.

Oppositely we observe in regard to stutterers in general, that the stuttering speech tends to *decrease* as a function of the following processes: (1) diminishing general or specific anxiety and fear—or increasing comfort; (2) increasing self-confidence and feeling of personal worth; (3) realistic perception or appraisal and acceptance of self and surroundings; (4) greater emphasis on abilities rather than disabilities; (5) increasing social interactions; (6) greater tolerance of behavior of others and own basic feelings; (7) increasing independence, pliability, consistency, and affectuality.

However, it is important to realize that a given stutterer of any age may be functioning anywhere along a rather broad range of speech and general adjustment. Among individuals who stutter, there are some with very few significant allied or specific behavioral deviations. There are also stutterers who have a great many allied or accompanying personosocial disabilities—defensiveness, withdrawal, general immaturity, extreme overdependency, eating problems, gastrointestinal disturbances, and dermatological symptoms. In such instances, the stuttering symptom is only one manifestation of a diffused personality fractionation.

Obviously it becomes important to estimate (to the extent that our experience, training, maturity, and working conditions will allow) approximately where Johnny Green is functioning on the adjustment continuum, if we are to structure our rehabilitation program appropriately. We see immediately how importantly the clinician's conception of stuttering will affect his choice of therapeutic approach. Thinking of Johnny's emotional problems as minimal would lead to a more formal speech therapy program. For the complex disorder, formal speech drill alone would be fallacious; if a child has a fever, we do not place him in an icebox. Therapy designed to moderate the emotional determinants is needed. For given cases, then, the indicated treatment procedure may range from formal speech therapy (speech drills, assignments) combined with some degree of counseling, to speech counseling (including such procedures as modified play therapy and role playing), to psychotherapy (nonspeech-specific), to psychiatry.

In summary, where there is no emotional subsoil connected with the speech symptom, a more direct, informational, formal speech therapy program is indicated. The focus is on the symptom. However, to the degree that the stuttering is motivated by psychological stresses, to that degree must speech therapy become *more* of a two-way client-clinician relationship involving varying degrees of catharsis, support, reflection, and insight-development. The focus is not on the speech symptom as such or as much, but upon the individual and the development of more effective general (thus, speech) improvement through the gathering of greater understanding concerning the relationships between the speech disorder and the underlying or associated behavior dynamics. Hence we may conclude that: *Stuttering is one pattern of adjustment. It is the most effective adjustment possible for the individual at a given moment.* It is deeply purposive.

THE CHOICE OF THERAPY

Whether procedures in helping stutterers make better adjustments are called re-education, correction, counseling, guidance, rehabilitation, or therapy is of little consequence. The purpose of all such activities is the same—to produce more self- and socially-developmental behavior. Therapy methods are numerous; hence each practitioner must be ever receptive to the possible contributions of others who are looking for the same "answers" to the stuttering enigma along slightly different pathways.

Although the greater portion of this book is devoted to a discussion of principles and actual practices of speech therapy and counseling with stuttering individuals, a few prefatory words are indicated at this point. What form of therapy finally is chosen depends on the clinician, on his training, his experience, and his personality. Some clinicians will focus more attention on the speech, the stuttering itself. Others will be concerned more with the underlying psychosocial factors which they feel motivate the speech; to them, stuttering is symptomatic behavior. Finally, clinicians may use different blends of these two orientations. Regarded in simple terms, an individual clinician may function at any point along a therapy-approach continuum:

Cause centered	Combination (cause-speech) centered	Speech centered

Choice of therapeutic approaches is dependent also on whether the clinician concentrates on the stuttering person, his environment, or some combination of the two. Placed in the form of another continuum:

Focus on the environment	Combined focus	Focus on the person

Combining these continua allows us to arrange a schematic representation of the many therapeutic structure arrangements possible in working with stuttering persons.

In Fig. 1, vector (1) represents therapy focused more or less exclusively on the stuttering person. Therapy is structured so as to alter the emotional life of the individual on the basis of the following assumptions: (1) that underlying dynamic forces are producing the stuttering behavior and (2) that resolution of these emotional motivants will produce modification or cessation of the deviant speech behavior. In this approach there is no attention to, or direct attempt to modify, the speech behavior as such.

Vector (2) represents a structure in which the basic assumptions are those in (1), but in addition to working with the person, the clinician counsels the parents, teachers, or perhaps the spouse concerning the impress of their own reaction patterns and attitudes upon the stuttering person's behavior. Here, again, there is no direct attention to the speech as such.

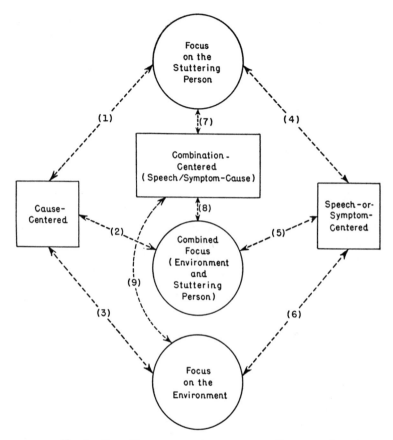

FIG. 1. BASIC THERAPEUTIC APPROACHES TO STUTTERING.

Vector (3) includes the assumptions of (1) and (2) except that the clinician establishes a working relationship, not with the stuttering person but with important elders in his environment—usually parents, relatives, or teachers; the stuttering individual receives aid by virtue of attitudinal changes within these elders.

Vector (4) represents a structure wherein the clinician works with only the stuttering person in a situation which focuses attention upon speech behavior. Therapy's purpose is to control or modify the stuttering by the use of speech exercises, drills, and possibly breathing techniques, as well as by direct discussions of speech and speech situations.

Vector (5) represents the approach of (4), except that the aid of important elders, usually parents or teachers, is enlisted to implement and reinforce the speech techniques.

Vector (6) differs only in its emphasis upon the elders; the stuttering person receives help from them, the focus being speech; instructions to parents concerning speech exercises to be used at home with their preschool stuttering child who is not seen for treatment represents one form of this approach.

Vector (7) signifies that the clinician is working with the stuttering person only, not with related persons in his environment, and that in addition to being concerned with the speech behavior *per se* and its modifications through practices and discussions of speech, there is at the same time a concern with emotional and social factors which may be affecting the general and speech behavior.

Vector (8) represents a similar orientation except that, in addition, the clinician works directly to improve environmental conditions.

Finally, vector (9), the clinician may confer intermittently with the parents about their stuttering child, but the child himself does not receive therapy. This therapeutic program is geared not only to a discussion of the speech deviation and parental ways of dealing directly with the speech behavior but also to a consideration (through advice giving, suggestions, counseling interaction, or other means) of the effects of the attitudes of persons on the child and to the child's own attitudes and basic emotional needs.

Therapeutic approaches may embrace any gradation or combination of approach components. In addition, given clinicians will tend to use different vectors with different stuttering persons. Finally, the clinician may use one or any number of "vectors" with a given stutterer. For example, the parents of Jimmy, a preschool stuttering child, are interviewed regarding their son's stuttering behavior. The clinician provides general counseling to the parents for several sessions—vector (3), or V-3. Later, Jimmy is assigned to therapy which is essentially a continuing diagnostic play therapy. The parents continue in general counseling (V-2). As Jimmy's underlying tensions are released and resolved, and as the parental attitudes improve, the therapist gradually introduces a more speech-oriented structure in both therapy with Jimmy and counseling with parents (V-8); toward the end of therapy, the clinician's focus may be almost entirely on speech as such in both the therapy sessions with Jimmy and the counseling sessions with the parents (V-5); for a while, only Jimmy may be seen (V-4), prior to cessation of therapy and a final consultation with the parents.

Clearly, the clinician's evaluative inclinations, basic philosophy, training, experience, and working conditions serve as determinants of the therapy approach. Environmental emphasis, i.e., the changing of parental attitudes and behavior, is to be used more frequently in cases of younger stuttering persons, especially those of pre- and elementary-school age. The older the child, the more must therapy's emphasis be placed on the stuttering individual, until by late adolescence or adulthood there is real doubt as to whether work with the parents is effective at all in improving the stuttering person's life adjustment.

THE PERSON WHO IS THE CLINICIAN

The critical importance of the clinician, not only his training and experience but also his own need system, constantly recurs in our thinking. Such questions as, "How emotionally stable and pliable is he?" and "To what extent is speech therapy efficiency impaired by his own defenses and insight of deficiencies?" cannot be shunned. We consider these and other issues of such fundamental importance in speech therapy that we have devoted Chapter 2 to a discussion of them.

In addition to considerations of personal problems and questions, conflicts concerning purely professional problems often arise. For example, if a speech clinician accepts the viewpoint that many speech disorders, totally or in part, are symptomatic of underlying personal-social anxieties and must be handled accordingly—if he believes that speech symptoms, such as stuttering, which are to any degree psychologically motivated, are serving an adjustive aim of the individual—he cannot avoid asking himself such questions as, "To what degree is this stutterer's symptom emotionally purposive?" and "what are the implications of this purposiveness in terms of decisions to work directly upon and modify or 'take away' the symptom, as compared to procedures designed to reduce emotional motivants so as to decrease the *need for* the symptom?" Speech clinicians or counselors working with a variety of speech and hearing disorders, and who, let us say, tend to utilize client-centered counseling as their fundamental *modus operandi*, repeatedly entertain this question. This topic has received a fuller treatment in the following observations:

If the disorder is not primarily of emotional origin, must the counselor disregard his basic philosophy and become more directive? If so, how much? There is the possibility of underestimating the intensity of the emotional factors and finding oneself dealing intellectually with the person whose speech problem more and more appears to be psychologically maintained. On the other hand, one easily can be nondirective when perhaps the main approach should be centered on questions and advice.

It appears that the therapist must play the role of a "general" speech counselor who can adapt to the presence of different intensities or to the absence of emotional signs as causal factors in speech problems. However, the term "general counselor" can include so much that it has little common meaning unless defined. If speech counseling is viewed as an omnibus activity which includes the diagnosis and rehabilitation of emotionally stable "organic" clients (for example, cleft palate, hard of hearing, dental and other oral irregularities) in addition to the speech-voice improvement of average speakers, it seems difficult for the speech counselor to be anything but "general" in his approach. From this viewpoint, the student who has been recommended to take a course in "Discussion Procedures in Industry" instead of "Public Speaking" experiences speech counseling just as does the anxiety-ridden Mary, who stutters severely and considers leaving school because of her inability to adjust to class and social situations.

. . . speech counseling is regarded . . . as a process applicable to those individuals having speech or hearing problems which are emotionally motivated, or those clients in which the communicative ability is disrupted primarily or in part by a "non-functional" factor such as organic or intellectual deficits, or a foreign language influence, but which is complicated by a psychological overlay. The aim is to develop insight concerning the nature of the emotional links with the speech dysfunction by the structuring of a communication situation in which the contributing personal and environmental forces are decreased in intensity. In a progressively adjustive process, the individual's realm of consciousness concerning the forces affecting oral communication efficiency and comfort is extended so that the anxiety level may subside, and until he is perceiving self, people, and situations more realistically (Murphy, 1955), p. 261).

The introductory considerations of this chapter will be dealt with at greater length throughout the remainder of the text. They have been mentioned briefly here as an orientation preview of the contents to follow. We shall say this, however: The critical focus or determinant in deciding which therapeutic modality the clinician must choose as a tentative beginning treatment structure is, of course, the stutterer himself. How one decides which "type" or depth of therapeutic approach is appropriate is the supreme and pressing challenge. It is our hope that this book will make some contributions toward meeting that challenge.

REFERENCES

Ainsworth, S. "Integrating Theories of Stuttering," *J. Speech Hearing Disorders,* **10:** 205–10, 1945.

Berry, M. F., and Eisenson, J. *Speech Disorders.* New York: Appleton-Century-Crofts, Inc., 1956.

Boring, E. G. *A History of Experimental Psychology.* New York: Appleton-Century-Crofts, Inc., 1929.

Eisenson, J. (ed.). *A Symposium on Stuttering.* New York: Harper & Bros., 1958.

Hahn, E. (ed.). *Stuttering: Significant Theories and Therapies,* 2d ed. Palo Alto, Calif.: Stanford Univ. Press, 1956.

Hilgard, E. *Theories of Learning.* New York: Appleton-Century-Crofts, Inc., 1956.

JOHNSON, W. *People in Quandries.* New York: Harper & Bros., 1946.

JOHNSON, W., and LEUTENEGGER, R. (eds.). *Stuttering in Children and Adults: Thirty Years of Research at the University of Iowa.* Minneapolis, Minn.: Univ. of Minnesota Press, 1955.

MURPHY, A. "Counseling Students with Speech and Hearing Problems," *Personnel Guid. J.,* 33: 260–64, 1955.

TRAVIS, L. "Laboratory Research of the Speech Pathologist." In *Proceedings of the American Speech Correction Association,* Vol. VIII. Madison, Wis.: College Typing Company, 1938.

———. *Speech Pathology.* New York: Appleton-Century-Crofts, Inc., 1931.

VAN RIPER, C. *Speech Correction,* 3d ed. Englewood Cliffs, N. J.: Prentice-Hall, Inc., 1954.

Chapter **2**

The Self-Image
of the Clinician

I am always envisioned by myself: what I am, all things reflect to me.——Emerson

The most important single variable affecting success in the treatment of stutterers is—*the clinician.* Understanding his own behavior is a prerequisite to understanding the stutterer's behavior. A difficult or facilitating administrative setting, a wealth or dearth of diagnostic and therapy materials, ideal physical plants or mere cloakrooms, a "team" approach or individual responsibility for a mammoth case load, minimal or maximal professional training, limited or extensive experience—all these elements fade in significance when compared to the importance of the clinician himself. It is the clinician who is the key element, most vitally in terms of his emotional stability, pliability, and to a lesser degree, of his level of intelligence.

No two clinicians administer therapy for stutterers in exactly the same way. The clinician's choice of the stutterer's feelings to which he will respond is extensive and varied. Each clinician differs in his understanding of such aspects of the stutterer's behavior as (1) level of ability or disability; (2) state of reality or fantasy; (3) degree of social- and self-perceptual distortion; (4) insight capacity; (5) frustration tolerance; and (6) shifting aspiration level. Thus it is his responsibility as a clinician to continually reappraise his

27

own behavior. This is part of the learning process in becoming a more capable, more understanding worker.

Whether or not a stutterer wants to learn has a great deal to do with the emotional relationship existing between clinician and stutterer. As we look back over the course of our own education, it is probable that most of us can say that we learned most from teachers whom we admired and wanted to be like (although some of these same teachers might have been less liked by some of our classmates). As we recollect personally, we think now that the teachers whom we have considered most successful were those who not only satisfied educational needs but who were also able to form warm, inspirational, and emotional relationships. And where children who stutter are concerned, the necessity for fitting therapy into a functioning framework which is designed to satisfy the child's emotional needs, as well as his speech needs, is even more critical. Psychodynamic speech therapy, especially at deeper levels of treatment, is not taught easily unless the student is especially receptive (if he is not overly defensive, repressed, threatened, or anxious in the learning situation). The successful clinician is the worker who is able to establish the warm, effective relationship on which such new learning is dependent.

WHAT ARE CLINICIANS MADE OF?

When students learn about or observe deviant behavior, they may become troubled because it is similar to their own behavior or to that of their friends. For example, medical students often experience "itches" when studying dermatology, or "palpitations" when studying cardiology, or "swallowing difficulty" in laryngology. In the same way, students of speech therapy sometimes "stutter" during their early academic exposure to the problem.* Usually, these mild, brief,

---

* A common slip of the tongue observed occasionally among student speech clinicians (and experienced workers also) is the use of the word "studying" for "stuttering," and vice versa. The frequent hearing and use of these words in educational and therapy settings plus their acoustic similarity (association value) makes this a most reasonable and understandable, nondeviant behavior.

and transitory speech repetitions occur in such periods as examination or "first case" stress ("this is my first stutterer, and I'm scared stiff"). The student clinician's examination or his first meeting with the stutterer can constitute a test of his own personal worth, conditioned by whatever parent-child relationship may have existed and, thus, by what import the exam or "therapy test" has for the student in relation to the parent substitute (the teacher or supervisor). For a few students, such events are things of horror, manifested by late arrivals for the appointed hour or absences because of "illness." In such instances, of course, a period of individual counseling for the clinician is indicated.

These and similar experiences help to accentuate the facts that all human behavior lies on a continuous range (overlaps) and that individuals are more alike than different. One of the most valuable decisions which clinicians can make is to admit their commonality with the persons whom they are trying to help. Clinicians seldom have an atypical behavior structure, a syndrome which is chronic, repetitive, intense. They are persons different quantitatively from persons with identified problems. But they are not different qualitatively. The principle of being different in degree and not in kind applies to all clinicians, all stutterers, all people. In this sense, stutterers in comparison with nonstutterers are not unique, nor are nonstutterers unique in comparison with stutterers. For instance, just as different clinicians satisfy certain needs of different stutterers, so may stutterers satisfy certain needs of clinicians. Murphy and Ladd have touched on this matter in discussing a similar situation which exists between the classroom teacher and his pupils. In describing various teaching personalities, they tell us of the following:

. . . paternal or maternal persons who derive satisfaction from a temporary relation as parent substitutes . . . ; social, warm, human teachers who enjoy the opportunity for sustained contact with a variety of personalities; protective teachers who, projecting upon students their own . . . (school) frustrations, try to make them happy; detached people who enjoy as spectators the panorama of experience created by each new group of students; intellectuals . . . ; and easy-

going teachers who accept a student . . . with comfortable tolerance
. . . In our sentimental glorification of the teaching profession we do
not always admit that teachers use students just as students use
teachers (Murphy and Ladd, 1944, p. 73).

An immature clinician may be able to establish rapport
with a group of adolescent stutterers, but he may lack enough
insight and vision to make the therapeutic interaction developmental. If he does not have a firm perspective of his
own needs, motivations, goals, and possible conflict areas,
he will be less capable of handling emotionally and socially
disturbed stutterers or others. The more emotionally unstable he is, the greater is the chance of his projecting personal biases and infantile need-satisfying activities into the
therapy structure. He will favor, sympathize, reject, and
misinterpret on the unconscious level. He may emphasize
to adolescent stutterers the importance of attempting a total
emotional split with their parents, rather than working toward
nurturing and increasing insight and acceptance of the
parent-child relationship, thereby revealing his own inadequate, dependent relationship to his own parents. Other
forms of defensive behavior which are seen among speech
clinicians and students would include: (1) feeling misunder-
stood by fellow clinicians, students, or one's cases; (2) a compulsion to adhere to set methodology; (3) aggressive behavior
directed toward less senior persons; (4) extreme passivity
in a therapy situation; (5) chronic disagreement with procedures and ideas of fellow workers; (6) perception of self
as omnipotent therapist; (7) excessive use of abstract, nonaffectual language (intellectualizing).

Capsule recollections of the following sort occur in the
cogitations of a person who has just completed a period of
academic life with student speech clinicians.

ALICE: She was so concerned about asking too many personal
        questions of her cases; always saying she thought it was
        much too aggressive. Very seldom did she ever say anything
        personal about herself. That way nobody could utilize any
        information that might be detrimental to her—or so I used to
        think, and still do. How many private talks did we have

about this? We should have had more time for her to work her way through that little block. It affected her therapy here. How could I have helped more?

BILL: A bright young fellow who should make a contribution to the field. But he never did come to feel relaxed when doing therapy with older persons. Very sensitive about his youthful appearance. Tried to help him throughout the year to see that ability, confidence, and relaxed attitude were more crucial for therapy success than was the factor of age. He agreed to this but emotionally he never grew to believe it. But he did see how his anxiety interfered with the development of a firm therapy relationship. Probably additional experience and maturity will bring him through.

CLAUDIA AND DORIS: Both were quite disturbed after their adolescent stutterers told them in no vague terms that they weren't getting anything from therapy. They thought they had to "change their approach or something." It took several conferences before Claudia came to see that such incidences were to be regarded not as failures but as an actual portion of many therapy relationships. Claudia soon convinced herself that such occurrences were to be handled like any other therapy material—in terms of its significance for the case's adjustment—in terms of how such incidents could best be utilized for adjustment progress. But with Doris, it was different. If she didn't see progress, she felt compelled to alter materials and procedures. Well, maybe it was because of her experience as a regular classroom teacher; there she could see progress, daily progress. It's so utterly different with our speech handicapped. It requires such tremendous patience and tenacity and also faith in one's treatment procedures. And, too, realization and acceptance of the fact that there are no specific prescriptions of therapy possible, but only general, pliable working frameworks based on diagnostic assumptions or inferences—all of which may change. It's a lot to ask of young persons. . . .

ELEANOR: She was so upset when Eddie splashed water onto the floor during the modified play-therapy session, even though we had included this as acceptable therapy activity for him (a five-year-old stutterer). She tried to remain comfortable and within the objective therapeutic structure, but it was so obvious as I watched her from the observation room; she was so concerned with the "dirty messing activity" that she was unable to interact in a therapeutically productive way. Had to change clinicians. . . .

FRANK: His two little stutterers made no observable progress whatever, although our therapeutic approach appeared to be the wisest possible. I think the failure was enough to discourage him from further work with stutterers or the methods used. Did it help Frank to know that clinicians of every philosophy and amount of experience encounter failure? I don't think the fact changed his feeling. The mothers never came to the parent counseling sessions. Who knows what stresses or negative attitudes the children were exposed to? Therapy cannot always give the needed solution. What are two hours of therapy if all the other hours of the week are conflict-ridden? But Frank took it all personally; it was "his" failure; and we couldn't help him to see it otherwise.

Recalling such instances now brings to mind one part of a lecture presented by a child psychiatrist, Thaddeus Krush, at Boston University in the summer of 1955. He was discussing the attitudes of student nurses and various other ward personnel toward in-patients:

. . . the theme of our seminars with these individuals has been centered around, "why are you angry at my patient?" and it usually turns out in the course of the exploration of the ward situation that it is because the patient is doing something which the nurse or attendant has had strongly suppressed by a parental figure during his or her childhood. An attempt was made to get the nurse or attendant to realize that their past attitudes color a good deal how they look at the present problem of the patient.

A similar situation exists in the teaching of children. It would appear that not infrequently the educator is placed in the position of expecting the child to produce or achieve in a definitely predictable pattern. When the child does not conform to this scale, there must necessarily follow a feeling of frustration on the part of the teacher. If the teacher turns the full force of the frustration upon himself, he is apt to become depressed by his feelings of inadequacy. If he turns the force of this frustration upon the child, he is apt to blame the child for the failure of the method. In either of these instances, he gives way to his frustration, and the consequences are deleterious to himself or his student. However, if the teacher turns this frustration to an examination of what is going on in regard to the pupil, studying the problem from several different angles, not the least of which is the pupil's own view of the situation . . . then there is a possibility that a compromise in reality can be reached which is not too frustrating to either pupil or teacher (Krush, 1955).

One implication throughout this book is that, while formal training in speech therapy is important, there are other attributes as fundamental in the worker's professional training and activity. Inquisitiveness, simplicity ("down to earthness"), emotional stability with pliability, accepting attitudes, a knowledge of one's own need-system, creativity, vitality, courage, the ability to empathize with the age levels of the persons in therapy—these are some of the desired basic characteristics. To like the persons with whom one is working is desirable. Occasionally, a clinician will be able to say that he does not like the person with whom he is working. In such cases, it is preferable to try to reassign the case to another clinician. But it is even more important that the clinician try to analyze the elements in the situation which have induced his negative reaction. It is not that every clinician should be able to agree with Will Rogers' statement about not ever having met a man he didn't like. This really is asking too much of most mortals. But if, through introspection or other means, the clinician achieves insight concerning the affect blocks that kept him from best serving the person, then true professional growth has occurred.

Many clinicians have little if any choice to make in case assignments. They simply must work with the persons who are "assigned" to them. In a few instances, then, the situation is likely to be one of the clinician's "going through the motions," and that may be about all there is to it on either side of the therapy table. Perhaps what we really want are clinicians who are not afraid of new ideas; clinicians who can inject a degree of experimentation into their work; clinicians who are sensitive to the forces which comprise the speech therapy *process;* clinicians who consider the attitudes, feelings, and reaction patterns of the stutterer rather than only the words, broken or otherwise, that he utters. Speech therapy is concerned with more than the acquisition of fluent

speech; it is concerned with the individual's complete adjustment, with his whole, human being.

THE NEEDS OF CLINICIANS

This book is concerned with the "need for stuttering" and
the needs of stutterers. Their "rights" are the clinician's responsibility. But at least a momentary glance at a list of the
clinician's own needs is warranted. Oftentimes clinicians are
faced with many difficult workaday problems; low salary,
heavy work load, inadequate equipment and facilities, and
stringent school or clinic policy. But the dominating determinant affecting the general success of a speech therapy and
counseling program, aside from the clinician himself, is *the
administration*. There may be hundreds of stutterers, parents
who are pounding on the door, trained workers, adequate
funds, and available facilities, but with an ineffective administration the program is confused, strained, and significantly
less worthy. The administration needs a sound philosophy,
with the strength and wherewithal to develop and sustain
its philosophy into a working program. Many school administrators, usually through a lack of knowledge concerning
special service fields, avoid their responsibilities to handicapped children. Often they feel that, because they administer a regular school program for all children, those not able
to fit into the pattern are not the school's responsibility. And
if programs should be created, little more than casual administrative lip service is ever forthcoming. Adoption of
principles of sound administration in special education, such
as the few cited below, adapted from Graham and Engel
(1950, pp. 20–21), would do much to increase the efficiency
of such programs.

1. Responsibilities should be definitely fixed. Some person
   should have the authority to make decisions regarding
   policies, budgets, and facilities.
2. Administrators must realize that special educational services will mean greater expenditures—for special space,
   special equipment, and special supplies.

3. The administrator must make arrangements to see that parents of the handicapped child are made aware of the nature and purpose of the program. This would include provision for a portion of the clinician's time to be spent in parent education or counseling.

One of the most difficult tasks is to help the administration to become gradually more and more aware of the clinician's own basic philosophy and preferred operational procedures. Although many school administrators accept without question the principles and practices of the clinician, many feel that childhood problems of any emotional severity do not belong in the school system but rather in a clinic. They may prefer that the clinician confine his activities to formal practices and refer the emotionally disturbed children to the school psychologist (if there is one) or perhaps to a nurse, who will suggest outside aid facilities to the parents. Of course the time when there will be enough clinics to satisfy the needs of America's emotionally handicapped school children is not yet in sight. Waiting lists of six months or of a year's duration are common. It is becoming more and more obvious that, increasingly in the future, the schools will have to add this responsibility to their heavy burdens. Handicapped children, as much as other children, have the right to an educational program adapted to their needs and limitations. Certainly it is the hope of many child psychiatrists and psychologists that the work of the inadequate supply of specialists in emotional disorders can be increasingly augmented by an enlightened army of workers consisting of physicians, teachers, clergymen, nurses, and other specialists, all developing understandings and methods that are appropriate to their own professional framework.

SHOULD STUTTERERS TREAT STUTTERERS?

Some speech clinicians find themselves considering the desirability or wisdom of persons with a stuttering symptom serving as therapists for other individuals who stutter. Some say that those who have experienced the frustrations and conflicts entailed in being stutterers are for that reason better qualified to understand, and therefore to help, others with the same handicap. There is no acceptable evidence supporting such a generalization. One could assert with equal validity that persons with stage fright should provide help to others who experience this problem; that persons who have nervous mannerisms, who are overdependent, or who display other psychoneurotic or psychosomatic symptoms, should practice psychotherapy *ad absurdum*. The basic issue concerns such questions as the following: "If I have emotional blind spots or personality problems, do they distort my perception of the individual who is experiencing problems similar or almost identical to my own? For example, if I experience a feeling of strong jealousy toward my boss's higher position with his greater recognition and reward, will I be able to work objectively with this young man who stutters and who is experiencing the same trouble with *his* boss? If my speech is fairly fluent but breaks down consistently when I use the telephone, does this reduce my efficiency in helping John, who has the same problem? Or is it that, because I have not ever stuttered, I am better able to perceive, analyze more objectively, and work more efficiently with the stutterer's dilemmas? Because I do not have the emotional blind spots stutterers may have, am I able to 'see' the problems more clearly?"

Reaching a conclusion on the basis of the above questions would be too simple, hazardous, and unfair. Human behavior warrants very few universal statements. Rather, we sustain an attitude of inquiry. For do not past studies and our own best observations often reveal that many stutterers have excellent personality attributes, that many seem very well adjusted except for the stuttering? Recalling that a given stutterer is apt to fall at any point along the adjustment axis, our "judgments" as to whether or not he should work with other stutterers rests not on the single, simple behavioristic observation "he stutters" but rather on the carefully considered diagnostic judgment as to *where he lies on the dynamic adjustment continuum*. To judge a person's ability to help another person merely on the basis of a single aspect of his total functioning, such as speech behavior, is indeed naive, dangerous, and unfair. There is no reason why we should not apply as many as possible of the criteria we use in judging adjustment success in our stuttering cases to those *doing* the therapy, be they stutterers *or* nonstutterers. Are there not a few personality problems present in clinicians who are nonstutterers? Though they do not stutter, may they not perhaps be fearful of high places; be extremely insecure; socially withdrawn; chronically verbally hostile; rigidly authoritarian?

Because of personality and speech conflicts, some clinicians who stutter are handicapped mildly or severely in their relationships with and perceptions of their client or in their acceptance or analysis of other stuttering dynamics and findings in books, lectures, and discussions; yet, *exactly* the same statement may be made about *non*stutterers. Stutterers have no monopoly on personal problems. It is just that their particular symptom of an underlying disturbance is more obvious, especially to those attuned to dysrythmia. Thus the real criterion is personal adjustment, not the speech component. Some stutterers should not treat stutterers. Some nonstuttering workers should not treat stutterers. In short, the more that any person is personally nonadjusted, the less he should be encouraged or allowed to treat human beings with personality disorders.

A FINAL WORD

Speech therapy with stutterers is exciting, challenging, and rewarding. The clinician plays many roles on the job: clinician, program director, permissive and accepting listener, scheduler, P.T.A. speaker. Interwoven throughout these roles are the countless distractions which are part of every job. It is quite a trick to keep from scrambling the roles, for it is difficult to make the quick shift from one to another. Every clinician has a special situation, and each must work out his own balance. Every clinician lives, works, and stays vital as long as he responds with spirit and some success to the challenges. If he stops responding, he dies. And he stops responding only if he relinquishes the will and the strength to make his own decisions and abide by his own true conscience. When he has exhausted his intellect on a therapy or diagnostic dilemma, he will not be afraid to use his imagination to lift him still further to more satisfying achievements (Murphy, 1960).

If a day passes in which he has not learned something new from a child, a colleague, or from his own actions, he will know that it is only because he has failed to perceive it and not because the chance was not there. As he listens to the endless chain of broken words from stutterers, he will realize that while he is trying to help them, he is also trying to help himself, and that he should make the teaching process a continual learning experience for himself. He is his own best listener; in this respect he will be selfish. But he will take rightful solace in thinking that, by so doing, he will perhaps be a better listener to the next stuttering person. He will work with what he has and what he believes. He will use doubt as a springboard to more productive reasoning, not letting it become a confusing determinant or a source of anxiety. Finally, after years of work and research in stuttering, he will come to realize that he has added to his knowledge more that is unknown than is known. But this will not be discouraging, for he will come to see that it is the seeking or the trying as much as the finding that matters. New thoughts will not be his enemies. And, at some point in his career, he may say, "Everything is worth knowing; perhaps this is one of the real reasons for living."

REFERENCES

Graham, R., and Engel, A. M. "Administering the Special Services for Exceptional Children," in *The Forty-Ninth Yearbook of the National Society for the Study of Education,* ed. N. B. Henry, Part II: "The Education of Exceptional Children." Chicago: Univ. of Chicago Press, 1950, pp. 18–37.

Murphy, A. T. "Objectivity, Subjectivity and Research," *Exceptional Children,* **26:** 400–405, May, 1960.

Murphy, L. B., and Ladd, H. *Emotional Factors in Learning.* New York: Columbia Univ. Press, 1944.

Part II
The Psychodynamics of Stuttering

Chapter 3

Speech and Language Development

You know also that the beginning is the most important part of any work, especially in the case of a young and tender thing; for that is the time at which the character is being formed and the desired impression is more readily taken.——Plato

All children are susceptible to interpersonal disruptions and self-threats. Most children manage to make their way from one level of speech maturity to the next. Some children do not; among these are those children whom we call stutterers. The difference between becoming and not becoming a stutterer may be slight. Likewise, the difference between being and not being a stutterer may be almost indiscernible. This is in keeping with the view that stutterers are more like than unlike nonstutterers. To cite an old maxim, the difference is one of degree, not kind. A greater "degree" (accentuation) of frustrating, self-debasing, anxiety-provoking interpersonal relationships will increase the possibilities of stuttering within a child. In like manner such conditions heighten the possibilities that the child will acquire other behavioral deviations. The reason that a child "chooses" to stutter rather than to set fires, wet the bed, refuse to eat, lie, steal, speak in an infantile way or not at all, can only be inferred. The point is that basically, for all children who have problems of a psychogenic etiology, the difficulty lies in disturbed interpersonal relations and a distorted self-perception which

41

bring accompanying feelings of confusion and self-inadequacy. Fundamentally the factors that cause stuttering are
like those which are operant in many other types of behavior
distortions. In addition, the treatment methods for children
with psychogenically motivated problems are similar *in
principle*.

FOUNDATIONS OF VERBAL DEVELOPMENT

We are concerned not only with the development of
speech and language in the child but also, more importantly,
with the tasks and influences which can make the acquisition
of normal speech and language a hazardous event for many
children. In the emotively unharmed human, language development is a process of successive differentiations of symbolic behavior. The phrase "stages of speech development"
carries enough logic to warrant its retention as a common
referent. In this respect, speech is little different from all
other aspects of human development; an orderly sequence
of growth unfolds, barring the occurrence of intrusive forces.

Intermeshed with the verbal stages are *physiological* developmental stages involving the gradual acquisition and
refinement of skills connected with basic body structures and
their functions, such as bowel-bladder control and motor
exploratory and sensory discrimination behavior. In addition we may think of *psychosocial* developmental stages as
encompassing differentiation of and adjustment to self and
environment. None of these stages is discreet. Assuming
that the part cannot be understood without relation to the
whole organism, speech development and disruption can best
be understood in relation to what is or is not happening to
the entire human system; i.e., in relation to what conflicts,
comforts, confusions, freedoms, frustrations, or satisfactions
the person may be experiencing and the degree to which the
experiences may be affecting (or be affected by) the verbal
behavior. Chapters 3 and 4 present a clinical chronology of
speech and language development against a background of
psychological development. They attempt to show how

intimately these human systems and functions may be inter-related in both typical and deviant (symptomatic) behavior.

The foundations upon which socially acceptable speech and language development rest may be described as: (1) a sound body; (2) cortical ability within the normal range; and (3) a comparatively stable, pliable, and positively motivated personality (implying a background of an emotionally healthy family or situational climate). Physically a child must have the ability to be active; i.e., to explore and to have varied experiences with the world about him as well as with himself, in order for normal speech to develop. This necessitates a certain degree of neuromotor skill, evidenced as the child learns to sit up, crawl, walk, and so on. Sometimes there is a temporary cessation of vocal or verbal growth during and just following the acquirement of other motor abilities. Following the *stabilization* of allied motor behavior, the vocal output tends to increase, probably partly due to the expanded range of perception and motor experiences which were made possible by the upright positions which the child assumed.

Any child with neuromotor, sensory, and structural soundness has the physical potential to acquire speech and language. But intellectual and socio-emotional conditions will influence the degree to which the physical endowments can be utilized to full capacity. Even in a sampling of normal individuals, there is a broad *continuum* of behavior. Some children, for example, seem to be able to endure much more heat, cold, pressure, noise, and brightness of light than others, seemingly quite independent of environmental motivation. Some have fewer illnesses, greater and faster recuperative powers, stronger and more sustained physical drive, more muscle strength and alacrity, greater sensory acuity, and finer sensory discrimination. Granted that psychological influences alter or set the pattern of these behaviors, the possibility of constitutional motivants cannot be dismissed (Ausubel, 1958; Stone and Church, 1957). Although, to the best of our knowledge, genes cannot directly control a behavioral trait, they do affect bodily structures and functions, although often to unknown degrees (Hall, 1951). Perhaps the least that may be said is that multiple genetic factors tend to influence ultimate behavior (including speech behavior) through the mediation of the bodily structures. Without entering the nature-nurture debate, and without trying to make ascriptions to heredity *per se,* nevertheless there are apparent differences among humans of what may be termed "somatic goodness"—the constitutional soundness of the organism—quite aside from considerations of the person's intellect, psyche, or environment. Physical growth and maturational powers affect the efficiency with which a child will be able to use his physical system in accordance with the demands, realistic or not, that family and society make upon him. In the speech function, the maturation of the speech mechanism determines in part the degree to which a child will be able to speak as the persons around him wish he would or think he should speak.

Our assumption is that "somatic goodness" tends to affect the capacity of the individual to endure and adjust, not only to somatic strains but to psychological tensions as well. The more somatically sound the person is, the better able he is to tolerate and cope with emotional and social frustrations. Although, in relation to stuttering, we do not by any means ascribe primary importance to such an assumed generalized somatic factor—in fact, the imprint by the environment upon the body's functioning is paramount to us—nonetheless, a healthy body is more capable than a weaker one in combating speech and language stresses.* Certainly, many a physically-handicapped person has a far healthier speech facility or personality than many nonphysically-handicapped individuals, but this achievement usually can be traced primarily to a nurturant, positive, emotional upbringing as well as probably to a good intellect, serving as compensation or buffers for the physical disability. In stuttering, if there is a "somatic variant" operating as a partial subsoil or disposition to stuttering,

---

* Of course the reader may react here by thinking that a healthy body derives from a healthy psyche and that it is the healthy psyche which makes the person more capable of coping with stresses.

the assumption becomes one of regarding the stutterer as somatically "weaker" (although still possibly well within the normal range). The clarification or description, much less the identification, of this "weakness" is not possible, of course. We refer to it here as a brief acknowledgement that a constitutional factor in stuttering *may* exist. We do not know whether it does or doesn't. But beyond this verbal tip of the cap to the possibility of a "somatic variant," this book devotes its pages exclusively to the treatment of stuttering phenomena from a clearly psychodynamic point of view.

Just as our interest focuses on the psychological and environmental forces affecting speech behavior, physiologists would be inclined to regard the "forces" as primarily neural, hormonal, and chemical. Psychogeneticists would emphasize the impact of "forces" within chromosomes. As clinical speech pathologists, we consider the life forces in terms of attitudes, interests, motives, needs, and values, though intermittently we look over our shoulder to see if the genetic factor has been clarified; always are we mindful that a somatic differential *may* exist. Certainly, such an attitude is justified if we agree that the current emphasis on environmental factors has not yet been able to provide us with a completely adequate framework for explaining stuttering and other communicative breakdowns.

Sex as a factor in verbal development has meaning beyond the mere interest in incidence or ratios of male to female stutterers. We know that for every stuttering girl, there are about four to seven boys who stutter. We also know that girls acquire language sooner, talk earlier and more often, and with a greater vocabulary. The difference in language development becomes noticeable as early as ten months of age, although as the child grows, the differences decrease in size. However, the female superiority in language growth and fluency is consistent, even when all the usual experimental variables are matched (McCarthy, 1954). Any discussion of stutterers is a discussion of males, for the most part, simply because most stutterers are males, and also because our knowledge of stutterers consists almost exclusively of research based on studies of males. Although we think we know something about male stutterers, we know very little about female stutterers. Discovering what the critical differences are in basic make-up or cultural influences between girls and boys may lead us to our best insights concerning stuttering phenomena.

THE MIRACLE OF LANGUAGE

Language serves (sometimes well, other times poorly) as a mode of communicating with other persons. The greater the similarity of viewpoint between speakers concerning the meaning of the word, the more efficient does communication tend to be. The communicative breach between infant and adult, while initially vast, decreases as the child learns to utilize the signs and symbols with which the elders in his environment feel most comfortable. With time and good fortune, the symbols will come to mean to him what they mean to others, and he will "understand" and "be understood." Unfortunately there are more acts, attitudes, and objects than there are words; i.e., each word is not a "fact," but rather can represent a spectrum of possible meanings. Herein lies the root of much "misunderstanding." In the extreme case, the "word," having no relationship to the deed, thing, or thought (reality), is not understood, and the user's social adjustment is impaired because he is not "communicating." Sullivan has said that ". . . an enormous amount of difficulty all through life arises from the fact that communicative behavior miscarries because words do not carry meaning, but evoke meaning, and if a word evokes in the hearer something quite different from that which it was expected to evoke, communication is not a success" (Sullivan, 1953, p. 184).

People tend to be quite subjective about language. Most of us have had a tremendous amount of experience in talking, and this seems to affect our objectivity toward it. It was Wendell Johnson who observed that people don't very often speak about speaking. Yet our entire culture, our political, economical, educational, and social systems are based upon, and function according to, symbols, a great percentage of them being oral verbalizations. Through language symbols, civilized man has transmitted his knowledge, actions, and beliefs down through successive ages of mankind. Each generation has led its descendants to the threshold of new knowledge, almost completely through symbolic processes. Each parent may lead his offspring to different thresholds. Each child, through symbolic experience, may organize and transmit his thoughts, feelings, and behavior to stimulate himself or others to new or continued action.

It is difficult to say just when language behavior ends and thinking begins. The processes seem inseparable. Just as man's thinking has been conveyed to us via language, so has man used the language of children as the main vehicle by which to understand the thought processes of children. One thing does appear more certain: Thinking and language can be understood only by reference to the total living experience of the individual, as intimate correlates of all human socialization experiences. Speech is social behavior. Observing the variation in verbal values at differing socio-economic levels, for instance, conveys to us this meaning of speech as social action. Middle-class children learn early that verbal functions are important. The father's work involves language, writing, and skill in speaking. Parental attitudes concerning the importance of verbal abilities are likely to be influenced by this situation. With lower-class children, language appears to be not so vital. The father's work is with *things* rather than with words (Davis and Havighurst, 1947).

The gestures and speech sounds of adults, culturally stabilized into a socially useful and acceptable pattern, will be generally consistent as they produce this symbolic behavior recurringly in the presence of the child. The child's gestures and speech patterns, however, will be much more unstable, not having been reinforced through considerable imitation or repetition. Although earliest speech is learned as shared behavior in a concrete social situation, the time comes when the object is *not* present or when the child is not *in* the situation. The differentiation and elaboration of words apart from the concrete object or situation is a mighty step forward in the child's release from the restrictions of purely nonverbal behavior. Of course the degree of variance between the word used and the nonverbal action or concept one is attempting to represent verbally may come to serve as a basis for social maladjustment, especially if the variance between word and event is extreme (language-reality relationship). The overt sharing of one's thoughts and feelings with other persons serves eventually to shape those components of behavior into the prevailing, culturally acceptable mode. Regarding this sharing process as a socially controlling influence, Cameron has stated that "reactions which for any reason are left uncommunicated and unshared with others are likely to play a leading part in behavior pathology, because they lack this controlling influence" (Cameron, 1947, p. 86). Stuttering, for example, may be many things, but one of its persistent characteristics is its uncommunicative nature—the preclusion of thought and attitude and the unknown emotional price the stutterer must pay for his lessened ability to share his feelings with other human beings and to know objectively his own attitudes and drives.

Preverbal Behavior: Crying. "When the human infant comes into this world, he is for all practical purposes a biologically helpless creature. It is safe to say that he is blind, deaf, mute, and paralyzed. It takes him longer to attain any degree of self-dependence than the newborn of any other species" (Kanner, 1957, p. 30). The great bulk of what infants experience must be inferred. In fact, most conclusions concerning infantile behavior are founded on observation, clinical or otherwise, and inference. The earliest mode of vocal behavior, crying, is regarded as the first expression of sensation or feeling. The birth cry, rather than an ejaculation of anger or joy, is simply a reflex act associated with the initial filling of the lungs with air. It is a vocal signal of a physiological event symbolizing the onset of respiratory behavior and blood oxygenation. Later crying is described as a response to some internal or external stimulus.

There is no clear correlation between the types of cry and forms of stimulation, although the cries do appear to reflect an infantile discrimination between comfort and discomfort. We assume that if the cry produces comfort—for example, the mother comes and soothes—it acquires positive value. Concerning variations in the amount of crying, it appears that children who receive the most nursing care do the least amount of crying. Children who have been institutionalized in early infancy tend to smile and babble less than infants raised at home (Bakwin, 1942). Studies are available of children placed in foster homes as compared to suitable control groups. Significant differences are likely to be found, with the foster children revealing overactivity, disorganization, excessive demand for affection and attention, inferior social maturity (Goldfarb, 1945), and quite often severe mental retardation and illness (Spitz, 1946).

Some authorities consider the birth cry to be the infant's initial learning-talking experience. Yet this appears debatable if we regard learning as a relatively permanent change in behavior which results because of previous experiences. It is difficult to conceive of birth-cry behavior in terms of classical conditioning. If we regard it as behavior which accomplishes a result and is not merely reflexive, then it may be considered as instrumental behavior or instrumental learning, but this seems to be pressing the assumption. Perhaps, because the behavior occurs without the infant being motivated or required to respond, because it occurs more or less incidentally, it comes closest to the concept of *incidental learning* (Morgan, 1956), though many learning theorists would argue against this (Hull, 1943) if only from the viewpoint that incidental learning, being a form of *perceptual* learning, implies that some discriminatory response occurs.

Van Riper aptly states: ". . . there are more vowels and consonants used in noncrying vocalization than in whimpering, and more sounds used in whimpering than in ordinary crying" (Van Riper, 1954, p. 95). Research supports his statement (Irwin, 1941). We might deduce that noncrying states are better *learning* states. Studies on the relationship between crying and mothering care indicate that there is a direct ratio between minimal mothering care and maximum infant crying (Aldrich, 1945a, 1945b, 1946). Early crying may be the first sign or association of vocal expression with parental rebuff—witting or unwitting. Parents who steadfastly ignore the crying child in fear that he may be "spoiled" show a form of derogatory reaction to this particular vocal act as well as to the infant himself. At the same time, crying appears to be the infant's most effective means of handling fear, if it brings a comforting mother. In such cases, crying may be true vocal magic—it brings such pleasant results.

One of the major principles of Harry Stack Sullivan is that "the tension of anxiety, when present in the mothering one, induces anxiety in the infant" (Sullivan, 1953, p. 41). The mechanism or process whereby this communication of anxiety happens is not known specifically, but Sullivan refers to it as a "manifestation of an . . . interpersonal process," to which he applied the word *empathy* (Sullivan, 1953, p. 41).

Crying often is self-punishing, too, for it may serve to increase the anxiety of the mother and thus to increase the infant's own anxiety (assuming anxiety to be transferable). If the child has some unmet need (soiled diapers) at the time of the "crying-anxiety" moment, the unmet need (not having diapers removed and affected body parts tended to) may become associated with anxiety through conditioning. Crying, then, early and perhaps easily, can become equated with a helping mother or a hindering mother. In the latter case, the child well may cry in order to get rid of the mother (the anxiety). Thus, crying comes to have *sign* aspects—a signal of comfort or discomfort to the child expressing (and perceiving) the behavior. Later the child may come to use crying as an aggressive stimulus directed toward the offending elders. Johnny, who holds his breath (stops crying) may be getting back at the bad mother (producing anxiety in the mother). This action may produce more anxiety in himself, however, and thus becomes self-punitive.

In such ways, crying may qualify as the first psychogenically motivated vocal symptom or disorder. Older children may utilize crying in these ways, of course. Indeed, the authors have been impressed by the number of children who seem to employ crying as an instrument with which to embarrass the teacher or clinician, especially if mother is present. The sense of the unspoken words, "He doesn't understand me, Mom," couldn't be conveyed more poignantly than by the retaliatory crying. In other cases, crying may be one main mode of emphatic expression for a child not having the words or fluency to do the job verbally.

> Speech, phylogenetically the most recent acquirement, is abandoned quickly if the child is under the influence of affects. Not only in distress does the child cry rather than tell about his situation, but other emotions are also expressed by gesture rather than by word. The child jumps around with joy but does not say, "I am glad," or he hides his face or himself altogether if embarrassed. Children in early years actually communicate by speech only when they are calm and their attention is directed. Under emotional influence, they revert to mimical expression. To this we may add the body language of the urethal and anal functions to conclude that the language of emotions is primarily a body language; the verbal language, on the contrary, brings to the ego a means of communication beyond the purely physiological and emotional patterns of reaction (Benedek, 1952, pp. 75–76).

Babbling and Jargon. The infantile production of indistinct or incoherent random vocal sounds usually begins by the second or third month, and it may continue for many months. (Generalizations here are tentative at best because of individual differences, various manners of investigation, and difficulty in transcription of the vocalizations.) The babbling vocalizations serve as pabulum for primitive auditory differentiation. Gradually the "discomfort" (crying) sounds become mixed with an increasing number of "comfort" (positively conditioned) sounds (gurgling following a meal, for example). Babbling, then, is probably the first play activity of the child, a precursive vocal play of spontaneous, random phonations. It consists of the sounds of no one language but includes the sounds of all languages. Babblers the world over have this common "language."

In time the babblings become differentiated; certain

sounds are repeated more than others. This process is determined primarily by the type of acoustical environment the child is exposed to, by the relative ease of production of sounds, and possibly by the sheer bodily pleasure accompanying the oral movements necessary to the expression of sounds. Eventually the speech circuit grows to a full cycle as, rather than purely reflexive vocalizations, we have a circular process of vocal-motor expression and auditory, kinesthetic, and affective feedback in operation to maintain and develop the speech function. This may be the earliest occurrence of voluntary motor control originating from perceptual processes. As Simon has said, this merging of ". . . sound production and perception, motor performance and concepts of meaning, leads to coded vocal communication: through maturation-paced changes in performance and perception, the child learns the conventionalized code of his language and what means what" (Simon, 1957, p. 32). But ". . . it is not clear just how important babbling is for the development of words. The more frequently used language sounds are not those that babies babble earliest and most often. During the first two months the consonants the child produces (outside of crying) are principally glottal . . . at two months, 87 per cent of the child's consonants are glottal [h] or the glottal stop; whereas in adult speech the more forward consonants are preferred . . ." (Simon, 1957, p. 30). However, by the fifth or sixth month, the child is using vocalization to get attention, to reveal needs, and to control others ("socialized vocalization"). Soon thereafter he begins to use a certain sound or syllable to refer to a particular object or feeling. Many children will now be repeating a few nonsense syllables, while others may concentrate on the repetition of a single syllable. *Echolalia* is the term applied to such repetition; echolalia also refers to the parrot-like repetition of a word or sometimes entire phrases. Most children are echolalic during their speech developmental period, imitating or repeating their own or others' speech, though not usually comprehending the meaning. For most children, echolalia does not persist as a dominant form of speech behavior beyond two or three years of age.

From about ten months to two years of age a large share of the average child's speech consists of *jargon.*

This unintelligible jabber is probably more important for speech development than people realize. It is the lineal descendant of vocal play, but it differs from the earlier babbling in its rich variety and its seeming purposiveness. The child seems to be talking to other people or to his toys, rather than playing with the sounds themselves. He seldom repeats the same syllable . . . jargon is probably the child's practice of fluency. Most young children swim in a river of fast-flowing, meaningless, adult jargon. Why should they not imitate their elders in fluency even as they copy their speech sounds and inflections? . . . A few children never use any jargon. When words fail they gesture or cry or remain silent. Most babies are like adults. They must talk whether what they say makes sense or not (Van Riper, 1954, pp. 104–10).

The Language of Gesture. Eventually jargon will be replaced by the conventional sounds and words of the adult world. But before word comprehension comes gesture comprehension; before word usage comes gesture usage. The child learns that gestures convey information, satisfy wants, and are socially purposive. Turning his head to the side conveys a meaning (he doesn't want any more food). If the language of gesture is especially rewarding, it may not be necessary at all for some children to develop speech as the more socially acceptable substitute. Some children have such an efficient gesture language that no need for speech is felt. "Delayed speech" may be the consequence.

Just as the infant's early symbol comprehensions appear to involve the gestures of others, so the undifferentiated, gross movements of the child, performed sometimes with accompanying vocalizations, become symbolic (gestures) through the selective intervention of adults (gesture conditioning). Through progressive differentiation, most gestures gradually disappear so that vocal behavior becomes dominant. As the child reaches for mother, he says "mama," but gradually the reaching gesture drops out of his repertoire. In certain cases the vocal behavior becomes reduced or doesn't develop at all, and the gross nonverbal motor behavior persists. In very severely involved situations, verbal and general motor performance, through fixation, become nondevelopmental.

The Language of the Body. Perhaps the most primitive mode of communication, even more basic and less symbolically differentiated than gesture, is what might be called the language of the body. The infant's general primitive mode of communication with the mother consists of variations in skin color and temperature, respiratory fluctuations, gross biological oral movements (sucking), and very little differentiated vocal behavior. Gradually, gestural ability will unfold, consisting of hand, foot, and entire body movements along with more specific facial expressiveness ("face lights up"). Lack of responsiveness to this nonverbal, pregestural behavior may, through negative conditioning, serve as a basis for later communicative disruptions. Even in speech-therapy situations, the clinician sometimes has to rely on this body language as the child's major communication mode; this is true not only in severely emotionally disturbed or brain-damaged children but also with stutterers of various emotional involvement.

Nor does the language of the body belong exclusively to children. Many adolescents and adults, to varying degrees, lapse into this primitive manner of "speaking." The stutterer sitting before his clinician with his eyes transfixed and fearful, his face masklike, blushing, perspiring, wiggling, and making sucking movements may not be saying one word, but most certainly he is communicating something. Even in the colloquial language of many nonhandicapped adults there is an evident display of a more sublimated form of body language in which the names of body structures and functions are employed to convey psychological meaning. The reader, for example, may think that the authors should "eat their own words" in some instances because he "can't swallow" certain viewpoints. He might want to "give a tongue lashing" or at least "make a biting comment," but he may merely say that "it gives him a pain in the neck." Most adult sublimated body-language forms appear to concern oral functions, and the majority of phrases are oral-aggressive in nature. Recently one of the authors heard a 24-year-old mild stutterer describe how, throughout adolescence, though he had never stuttered, he had employed filthy language to an obvious extreme in most social situations, though never at home. Upon entering a highly respected eastern university, he had embarked on a campaign to rid himself of this unacceptable language. Within two years he was a social model of propriety, but he had developed a speech block. It seems quite possible that the swearing was serving an aggressive, oral cathartic purpose and that the need to express strong feelings, in conflict with the need to "swallow" the feelings, had resulted in an ambivalence expressed in the form of a speech conflict.

The Language of Inflections. Sullivan used the term *gesture* to include not only facial expressions and body pantomime but also pitch, inflection, rhythm, and emphasis in vocalization and speech (Sullivan, 1953, p. 178). This is a broader conception of gesture than has been developed elsewhere, and it appears to give valuable added dimension to our scope of understanding the verbal behavior of people.

By the seventh month, not only is the baby indulging in much repetitive inflection play, but he is also responding to the inflective aspects of the vocalizations of elders. Not only does he often stop crying when spoken to, but he reacts to *affect* changes in voices, usually much in advance of comprehending or reacting to words. Thus, in accordance with whether these emotional changes or inflections are positively or negatively valenced for him, the baby is stimulated or inhibited in his general behavior, including his vocal behavior.

In particular, restrictions on the tonal scope of the voice probably are the first forbidding gestures that are built into the separate personification of the bad mother in contrast to her physically identical counterpart, the good mother . . . a great deal of what may be called "the way the wind blows" is conveyed tonally; it has nothing in particular to do with verbal content, but is instead a matter of how verbal content is expressed, and the like. So the first forbidding gestures, and among the world's most dependable forbidding gestures that human beings ever differentiate in the interest of avoiding anxiety and pain, are undoubtedly changes in accustomed voice. . . . there are few things more effective at changing the immediate integration of interpersonal situations than certain tonal tricks which come to us very, very naturally . . . (Sullivan, 1953, pp. 90–91).

The Language of Silences. Silence may be as important a part of speech as is sound. Whereas in older children and adults silence may be a sign of social or therapy resistance, in infants it may be, to them, behavior having positive sign value—behavior which the infant hopes will evoke a positive response from the perceiver-interpreter (the mother). Many children of all ages have learned that silence truly may be golden, i.e., that it achieves the sought-for recognition or reward (parental attention or love), the more so if the parents happen to adhere rigidly to this particular gold standard; i.e., if they stress the importance (to them) of silence. With such parents, eating times tend to be popular enforcement periods ("Children should be seen and not heard"). Some very young children learn the destructive effectiveness of silence when it is used by them as a hostile, retaliatory weapon. One form of symptomatic silence, breath-holding, is a not uncommon behavior among emotionally upset children. It is observed as early as the first year of life, but it is seldom seen in children more than five or six years of age. Perhaps the closest thing to infantile breath-holding in older children or adults is seen in the breath-stoppages of stutterers. Kanner (1950, pp. 383–86) has reported that in a study of 188 infants reputed to have breath-holding spells, anger was the precipitating cause in 90 per cent of the cases. Although a definite relationship to physical conditions has often been shown, breath-holding very often is to be thought of as one signal (an oral signal) of a disturbed parent-child relationship.

In older children and adults, in situations where oral communication may be the preferred or acceptable or expected mode of behavior, silence is likely to be a symptom of resistance. The silent one may be fearful of revealing inner thoughts, or he may be apprehensive about the reactions of the audience (parents, fellow students, friends, teachers). He may be fearful of the anxiety welling up within or of the anxiety which may be aroused were he to break his silence and express thoughts and feelings. Silence in any life or therapy situation may serve again as a hostile weapon against the listener (parents, clinicians). This form of aggression will satisfy the immature needs of the silent one to the extent that it serves his purpose (proves upsetting to parents, clinician, or teacher). Estimates of the extent to which such silence is self-punitive are more speculative, but silence probably operates as masochistic behavior in at least some instances. One of the most notable forms of the language of silence is the type of disordered behavior long given great attention in the speech field, namely, "stage fright." Infantile silences can be regarded as oral symptoms and are treated as such; i.e., from the viewpoint of the relationship between the emotions and the oral symptom (silence) rather than only in terms of the curing of the silence itself through such a technique as encouraged or enforced recitations.

The Language of Words. The criteria which adults use to judge whether or not Johnny is "growing up" are well known and rather universally adhered to: age of sitting, creeping, toilet training, walking, and talking. Valuable premiums or "stamps of approval" are given these accomplishments by the adult world which surrounds the child. Certainly the premium placed on speaking ranks high. The difference between "speaking" and "not speaking" may be a mere word or two, but the differences in adult attitudes toward "early" and "late" talkers often are considerable. The moment when the child utters his first word is unconsciously thought of as a milestone in our culture, and children learn the importance of acquiring this kind of behavior, so admired and desired by their important elders. How does Johnny acquire "the word," this magical noise pattern which elicits such reactions from those around him?

Anyone can observe that, from the child's many vocalic productions, certain sounds are more likely to be reacted to than others. "Mama" and "da" usually bring attention and tender responses (rewards) on the sometimes mistaken parental assumption that the utterance is connected with names for mommy and daddy. Incidental babblings are accepted eagerly as words by the anticipating parents. The often accidental sound combinations in the child's babbling and jargon repertoire become reinforced through positive parental reaction more than other sounds which happen not to be as emotionally or culturally meaningful and acceptable to the elders. Through such a selection and differentiation process, the adoption and development of the "mother tongue" occurs. The sounds not receiving rewards, through lack of reinforcement, tend to drop out or to be delayed in developing (Mowrer, 1950).

Nor is listener reaction the sole determinant. We can well assume that the child's reaction to his own productions reinforces or interferes with further production of those sounds. Inability to produce a given sound, especially if the sound is highly valued by adults, may be viewed as a case of negative feedback, inasmuch as the attempt failed (self-defeating). However, the child must be aware of the "failure." He may or may not develop such awareness on his own. But adult reactions condition him to become aware, for better or for worse. Certain socially nonreinforced sounds, however, may persist for varying periods because of "organ-satisfaction," i.e., somatic pleasure in the making of the sound (sucking and lapping sounds, for example).

The process whereby an ineffective sound or word may come to evoke a response which earlier occurred only in relation to another (effective) sound or word is termed *verbal conditioning* or *verbal association learning*. Learning theory maintains, for example, that the number of reinforcements and the additive degree to which such reinforcements have been satisfying to the organism probably have a direct relationship to the number of times a given (vocal) response will happen again in similar situations. When the child comes to use a sound or sound series that has meaning which is generally universal to his setting (i.e., when he uses a word with repeated, consistent, and accurate relationship to an object, idea, or event), we say that he has acquired his "first word." Of course he may understand the word long before he can use it meaningfully and consistently, and he may be able to imitate without comprehending the word as spoken by an adult, but not until he utters the word voluntarily with some socially symbolic accuracy in relation to a thing or act do we say that Johnny has acquired his first word.

Sullivan has discussed this occurrence, saying:

. . . words . . . are consensually validated. A consensus has been reached when the infant or child has learned the precisely right word for a situation, a word which means not only what it is thought to mean by the mothering one, but also means that to the infant (Sullivan, 1953, p. 183).

Mowrer has suggested that:

. . . in both human infants and talking birds, the first stage of word learning is autistic, and by this is meant that a word, having been associated with satisfactions (drive reductions) provided by the parent or "foster parent," becomes satisfying in its own right, i.e., satisfying not only when uttered by another but also when uttered by the . . . baby itself. And from this it is but a short step to the conclusion that the capacity to utter the conventional noises called "words" develops because the organism is automatically or "autistically" rewarded whenever it makes a noise somewhat like a word which has thus become satisfying. The organism is thus prompted to perfect this noise, with or without tutelage (Mowrer, 1950, pp. 707–8).

Continuing this line of thought, a word associated with a *pleasant* object or event is likely to be felt as a "good" word. A word associated with an *unpleasant* object or event is likely to be felt as a "bad" word (Mowrer, 1950). Although such events ordinarily occur initially in the presence of people (usually parents), we infer that the speaking of the good or bad word *later* (in other speaking situations *or* to oneself) may conjure up similar good or bad associations. A child may use a word because he has a good feeling about it (it is a rewarding word)—or he may avoid the word because he has a bad feeling about it (it is a punishing word).

Since the sound of the mother's voice has often been accompanied by comfort-giving measures, it is to be expected that when the child, alone and uncomfortable, hears his own voice, it will likewise have a consoling, comforting effect. In this way it may be supposed that the infant will be rewarded for his own first babbling and jabbering, without any necessary reference to the effects they produce on others (Mowrer, 1950, p. 699).

Berry and Eisenson state that "speech learning, from its very inception, is a process of stimulus and response and strengthening of responses, a process in which associations are formed that are at first unintentional, random, and meaningless, but that later become selective, intentional, and meaningful" (Berry and Eisenson, 1956, p. 22). As has been said, if the sound or word is a "good" one, the child, liking it, will also like to hear himself make it. The infant's own vocalizations may become positive stimuli for him if he "likes" sounds, i.e., if he associates goodness or reward or tenderness or comfort (via the mother) with them. Thus feedbacks of this kind may serve as verbal rewards or punishments. Even in speech therapy, one can see the desirability of getting children (and adults) to *like* to hear and utter speech in general, of giving them positive associations with speech, of giving them "pleasant speaking experiences."

The speech and language developmental and sustaining expressive process, then, consists of stimuli and responses or lack of responses (repression, resistance, or apathy). The responses are strengthened or weakened according to whether they are positive (satisfying) or negative (unsatisfying) to the respondent. The stimuli (sounds, words, silences) likewise acquire positive or negative valence to the degree to which they, also, are associated with satisfying or unsatisfying experiences. Through continued experiences, associations and generalizations occur in relation to these satisfying or unsatisfying stimuli and responses. Sounds or words or silences or gestures similar to other sounds, words, silences, and gestures tend to acquire the connotations of the events to which they are associated. Such speech and language events, formerly unintentional, and with little or no intellectual or affect meaning, acquire "dictionary definition" or emotionally tinged meanings through a continual process of perceptual and motor selection, refinement, and specificity. To put this another way, language events (and again we include "silence" as one form of language behavior) acquire values which vary with each speaker. This is the crucial characteristic of words: they are value carriers. To the child the words "no" or "naughty" or "don't" have negative value, whereas "nice boy" or "honey" tend to have positive value. Words *per se* come to act as punishments and rewards, and parents use them to mold the attitudes of children and thus to affect their behavior in future situations. The values associated with parental words are strengthened intermittently by nonverbal punishments or rewards (lickings or lovings). So, very early in the child's existence, he learns the power of words, someone else's or his own. He learns that words are easy to carry around, and that they can be used wherever he goes—by himself or others. Words are ever-present instruments, available at any time in any situation for use as punishments or rewards. In fact, not only does he learn that the words of *others* may be punishing but he discovers also that his *own* words may indeed be self-punishing, by virtue of using the "wrong" ones (giving the incorrect answer) or giving one "improperly" (at the wrong time or in a faulty manner—stutteringly).

McCarthy (1954) emphasized language's interlaced relationship with the infant's other growth areas: respiratory, nutritional, dental, and motoric. Language emerges as the infant passes through the generic verbal growth stages which are shown in Table 1. But language can never be disengaged from the child's other growth areas, and his internal and external conditions of euphoria or tension. We shall examine these basic internal (psycho-physiological) and external (environmental) forces in more detail in the following chapter, which considers fundamental psychodynamics of infancy and childhood as they relate to healthful or disordered speech-language development.

Table 1 is a plotting of the speech-language stages of development. Of course the chronological indicators can reveal only trends because of the often disparate points of development of a specific common mode or "type" as revealed by different children. From any viewpoint, the chart is to be considered incomplete, inasmuch as it is difficult to consider speech development in isolation from all the psychosocial factors in a child's make-up which serve as basis or subsoil for healthy or deviant speech development.

Throughout the verbal learning process, the extent of positive learning appears to vary significantly in accordance with how much and in what way the child imitates (or doesn't imitate) or identifies (or doesn't identify) with the significant adults in his environment. Mowrer wrote: "When one individual serves as a model for the behavior of the other, with both individuals present, we may speak of imitation; but when one individual acts like, or copies, another individual in the latter's absence, we may speak of identification" (Mowrer, 1950, p. 715). Wyatt (1957) proposed that "partial (temporary) identification with the mother or mother substitute in the form of positive cathexis of the mother's voice and speech is essential in language learning and indispensable for the development of correct patterns of articulation in any given language." She adds that interferences with the desired cathexis of the mother's voice may emanate from the child who may be ill during a learning period; from the mother, who is unable or unwilling to function as a suitable love object, or is nonexistent; or from the situation of separation, in which the mother-child interaction is interrupted.

The toddler's earliest words are likely to be applied categorically by him. "Mama" may refer to any adult female figure and "uncle" to any male adult. There many instances in the early literature (especially European) of children's use of single syllables in contrasting significations (Decroly, 1934; Kaplan, 1957; Stern and Stern, 1907). In

TABLE 1

SPEECH-LANGUAGE EVOLUTION

Communication "Stages"	Approx. Age in Months	Speech-Language Characteristics
I Presymbolic Primitive differen-	0	Crying and undifferentiated, throaty vocalizations
tiations Auto-affectual	1	Crying differentiated for hunger, pain, and discomfort
	1–2	Some vowel sounds
	2–4	Turns to sound of human voice ("tone")
	3–5	Coos and plays vocally: primary auditory self-perception
	4–6	Vocalizations reflect pleasure or displeasure
II Symbol-Differentia- tion	4–7	Babbles, vocalizes when socially stimulated
Autistic (private symbol usage) Affect-exchange		Says several syllables Differentiates friendly and angry talking
dominates mean-	7–9	Syllable-repetitions (mama, dada)
ing-exchange	8–9	Imitates sounds of self ("circular response") and others (echolalia)
		Selective listening to familiar sounds or words, especially if related to need-satisfaction
	9–12	Some gesture comprehension; combining gestures with vocalizations
	9–10	Expressive jargon
	10–14	Word "imitation"
III Symbol-Integration Social-symbolic	10–14	Gesture comprehension, differentiation, social usage
Affective-meaning exchange	11–15	"First word" ("consensual validation") (voluntary accurate usage)
Differentiation and Integration	12–20	Social introjection: adapts and inhibits on simple commands
	12–16	Several or more words Words joined in simple combinations with uncertainty
	21–30	Compulsive repetitions of words or phrases
	22–36	Repetitive speaking of words, phrases. Simple sentences
	48–72	Cultural expectation of verbal fluency and intelligibility

time, words are applied in a more discrete manner; each word having its own history of personal differentiation in meaning. The toddler limits the word to fewer events, or expands its usage to more situations, or shifts the meaning of the word in an application to newer situations. Not only does his dictionary meaning of the word become more specific (more conformant to the cultural norms), but the "affect loading" of the word also becomes increasingly embellished or relinquished. By "affect-loading" we mean the degree of emotional content, as discrete from the denotation or intellectual meaning, a given word has for an auditor or speaker. Ask yourself if there is a difference in your emotional response or association as you read *aloud slowly* the following list of words: "door—ceiling—gun—Negro—fear—kiss—body—money —father—block—Republican—guts—date—truth—nipple—car."

It is impossible to know what you feel and difficult to know what any listener feels when any word is uttered, but experience shows that we differ, from nuance to extreme, in the affect meaning or affect load a given word has for each of us. Measuring the magnitude of the reaction is impossible. But, agreeing that there are individual differences in emotional magnitude of responses to certain words is not so difficult. There is some experimental evidence (McGinnies, 1949) that words which have anxiety-producing components will arouse perceptual defenses in the perceiver; i.e., the perceiver is apt to have a higher recognition or response threshold for words threatening to him. This behavior has been described as defensive on the assumption that the perceiver is trying to avoid (repress) the unpleasant connotations the word elicits. Some critics (Postman, 1954) of this type of experimentation and thinking have replied that, because the person may be fearful of *saying* or even writing a socially tabooed word, even though he recognizes it, he may *suppress* (consciously avoid) his response rather than *repress* (unconsciously avoid) his response. Continued experimentation is necessary to make the issues more precise. Although psychologists have produced and will continue to produce the bulk of the literature on anxiety and word-perceptual defense, it is hoped that an area such as this, with its obvious implications for the psychology of speech-language disorders, will come to hold greater interest for speech pathologists.

Just as the nature of personal experiences with given words tends to "individualize" the speech-learning toddler, the learning of language in a larger sense tends to "generalize" him. The price he pays for his acquisition of speech is an increase in conformity and a decrease in privacy. His adoption of conventional language, which may be thought of as verbal introjection or incorporation, may come to be one of his most powerful instruments in a successful adjustment to his society. On the other hand, the extent to which his words are *un*conventional or "nonconforming" will influence the degree to which his societal adjustment may be difficult (less acceptable to society). This nonconformity may be a "progressive deviation" (a new art form which is beyond its time, the development of a nuclear theory, the writings of G. B. Shaw) or a "regressive deviation" (behavior which society considers negatively atypical and which may lead to belittlement or outright rejection by parents or society). Clinics are filled with persons who are unable to use words acceptably (communicate to others their basic thoughts and feelings). At the same time it probably is symptomatic, too, that the areas around which behavior disorders revolve tend to involve those interest areas about which the average person speaks or thinks most (status, prestige, sex, hostility, power). Perhaps it is this very talking out of basic feelings that keep him adequate ("normally" adjusted) and perhaps it is this lack of talking out or inability to talk it out—the "it" is important—which leads to real trouble for the inadequate (maladjusted) person. It is not difficult to conceptualize stutterers in this framework.

SPEECH AND DEVELOPMENTAL TASKS

Johnny's task, the acquisition of speech, is not a simple one. To some parents it may seem to be an extremely complex and a very slow process. The common question of "when" to "teach" the child cannot be answered categorically. Research is available which shows that practice or training at a later age is, in general, more efficient than at an earlier age, not only for gross or more specific motor tasks—toilet-training (McGraw, 1940), walking (McGraw, 1935), buttoning (Hilgard, 1932)—but for vocabulary learning as well (Strayer, 1930). However, whether the effects of word-learning practice, for example, are relatively permanent or transient, is an important but not a well-defined function. Whether words or fluencies once attained will remain unblemished at a later period of development will depend upon the degree to which the earlier acquisitions are undamaged by later disruptive experiences.

Ausubel (1958) has written an excellent analysis of the principles of readiness with implications for general educational and speech development. Havighurst, discussing child development in general, stated: "When the body is ripe, and society requires, and the self is ready to achieve a certain task, the teachable moment has come" (Havighurst, 1953, p. 5). An interpretation with implications in terms of speech development may run as follows: "When the body is ripe . . . [i.e., when the speech and hearing mechanisms in particular and the entire perceptual-expressive system in general are able to perceive, comprehend, and reproduce with some meaningful accuracy the oral noises we call words] and society requires . . . [this requirement in speech tends to occur in the 9–15 months range under usual conditions] and the self is ready . . . [and this would seem to be the important prerequisite, the extent to which the child wants to mimic, imitate, identify with the elders] the teachable moment has come" [(for speech)—recognizing that the "moment" must be an experiencing through some period in time]. Lack of, or deviation in, speech development may occur if the above "elements" become confused in time or manner; for instance, (1) when the speech mechanism or intellect is insufficiently mature or developed but the parents expect verbal accomplishment, (2) when the communication system is ready for activation but there is no environmental (parental) stimulation, and (3) when the neuromotor branch of the communication system is ready but the child is psychologically unprepared.

The acquisition of speech or the time of "acquisition" of the "first word" may be thought of as one of the tasks of development confronting the child, in fact, as a "speech developmental task."

A developmental task is a task which arises at or about a certain period in the life of the individual, successful achievement of which leads to his happiness and to success with later tasks, while failure leads to unhappiness in the individual, disapproval by the society and difficulty with later tasks.

The prototype of the developmental task is the purely biological formation of organs in the embryo (Havighurst, 1953, p. 2).

Speech-language developmental stages lend themselves to a gross comparison with the notes in the major or minor modes of the diatonic scale. If a full tonal pattern of a scale is to emerge, there can be no omission of any note. If a completely integrated organism is to evolve, there can be no skips in the passages from one physical, psychological, or developmental stage to another. The migratory route over each growth stage is governed by the individual's rate of growth and his capacity for growth. Both of these are related to the successes or failures which he has experienced at previous stages; i.e., to the success he has experienced in being exposed to a beneficial verbal environment, in experiencing positive imitation and identification patterns with mothering figures, in working through the processes comprising the verbal developmental tasks, and in experiencing opportunities for developmental repeating (positive practice) of the learned perceptual-motor verbal behaviors (FitzSimons, 1958). Allen commented that "infancy is not merely a 'flag station' on the road to a more mature period, to be passed by as quickly as possible." He added that "the infant who has been given a real chance to be an infant will be a healthier child emotionally" (Allen, 1942, pp. 28–29).

Speech-language developmental stages occur as fairly orderly related series. We observe progression in the life cycle from cell to embryo to fetus; the motoric sequence of chin up, chest up, and reach up (with a miss); and the speech-language developmental task pattern.

Learning to talk is a developmental task which, if not learned at the "proper" time, renders the individual less capable of learning subsequent speech or language tasks. It is the parents who decide what is the proper time, and their decision is crucial for the youngster. For example, Johnny may be doing as well or even better in speaking than the average child his own age, but if the parents consider this the "proper" time for greater verbal expression or fluency, the consequences for the child (and parents, too) in terms of frustration due to lack of expected achievement are likely to have cumulatively severe consequences. Again, just as parents whose children experience a paucity of vocal stimulation may be missing the "teachable moment," so may other parents miss the "moment" by not allowing the child to experience it, whether he is or is not ready. Parents (and teachers perhaps) who do too much talking to and for the child, who tell the child exactly what to do and say well after he has developed the speech fundamentals, are apt to stunt his vocal growth, independence, and spontaneity. Even in adulthood, similar vocal dependency and suppression are not uncommon.

The child's success in earlier verbal developmental tasks influences the degree to which he will master the task of word learning. The acquisitions of preverbal gesture language, nonlinguistic vocalic utterances (inflective phonations, for instance), echolalic and imitative syllabic utterances constitute a sequence of preverbal or prelinguistic developmental tasks. Forward movement will be measured by successive task achievements. The transition from one task to another may be difficult or impossible according to how disrupted the child-adult relationship or general emotional autonomy of the child may become. In some cases language development interferences of a psychological nature may either fixate language growth or cause the verbal behavior to regress to a more primitive level. Such psychological speech or language comprehension and expression fixations or regressions are due primarily to the disruptive effects of anxiety. The anxiety (or its derivatives) is traceable to a disturbed child-adult relationship.

It is recognized that, for successive integration of new developmental patterns, the child needs opportunities to practice the newly acquired behavior repeatedly in a self-enhancing, interpersonal relationship. In relation to linguistic growth, Wyatt (1958) posited that repetitions of such developmental units should be regarded as developmental repetitions. As such, they are produced without any signs of effort and with apparent pleasure. She added that such repetitions acquire a compulsive character if influenced by anxiety.

In addition to the developmental tasks which, as discussed, are primarily motor or expressive in nature, we postulate the existence of behavioral processes describable as *perceptual* developmental tasks. These include not only the utilization to fullest capacity of acuity and discrimination in the sensory modalities but also the acquisition by the child of an increasing capacity and specificity in the realistic perception of the world about him and of himself. A major portion of the child's successful adjustment to life is the ever-enlarging capacity for, and ever-increasing specificity of, external (social) and internal (self) perception—the challenge of perceiving or apperceiving experiences, situations, or words realistically or "objectively" ("as they are"). The extent to which a child misperceives (misinterprets, misunderstands, projects upon) the real meaning of life events depends to some degree upon whether or not earlier perceptions (gestures, facial expressions, adult voices) have been conflict-ridden or ambiguous. Hypothetically, the earlier the age at which such negative conditioning has occurred, the greater the number of subsequent perceptual developmental tasks will there be affected and, in general, the more primitive the observed verbal behavior will be. The child who has learned to perceive as threatening those vocalizations which are loud and rising in inflection (symbol of rejection or a preface to punishment) is more inclined to experience difficulty in introjecting or accepting (then freely using) language behavior ordinarily learned after the inflection or nonverbal vocalic stage, especially if the later speech-learning tasks happen to include loud, rising-inflection verbalizations.

Disturbed ability in the expression of speech may be traced, then, to *perceptual* fixations or confusions. The process whereby a person unconsciously or consciously perceives an object or situation as anxiety-provoking because of its resemblance to an earlier object or situation which was truly productive of anxiety may be termed *negative perceptual identification*. A child with a particularly rejecting or perfectionistic mother who happens to have a nasal vocal quality may later withdraw or feel uncomfortable in the presence of a teacher or other woman with a similar voice quality. If the nasal-voiced mother is emotionally healthy, the child will be inclined to react positively to the other person. In the first instance, the child makes a negative perceptual identification; in the second, a positive perceptual identification. The degree to which a positive identification develops with elders affects the general quality of the child-parent relationship, which in turn affects subsequent personal relationships as well as language behavior.

Identification usually connotes "being like" some model person. We have assumed that children do not identify as well with persons who are anxiety-provoking to them. The child finds little pleasure in "being like" a person he dislikes, is angry at, is uncomfortable with, or fears. When we refer to poor identification or lack of identification with the mother by the child, or *by* the *mother* with the child, we infer probable deleterious effects on speech and language development and fluency. The degree to which reciprocal identification between mother and child is weakened or confused probably correlates highly with the degree of noncommunication between them. If identification is distorted, the mother (the behavior model) becomes a negative model to the point where the child, now truly the mother's symptom, develops his own anxiety-reducing or protective armor (defense mechanisms or speech-voice symptoms).

SOCIALIZED VERBALIZATION

Many studies concerning childhood speech and language development may be cited (Fisher, 1934; Irwin and Chen, 1946; Lewis, 1951; McCarthy, 1930; Spiker and Irwin, 1949; Stern and Stern, 1907), although the impression left upon reviewing them is that major attention has been placed almost entirely on the child's verbal behavior from the viewpoint of adult grammar analyses systems. Less thought has converged upon the emotional and social motivations and significances of childhood language behavior.

Following the acquisition of the first word, and barring complicating infiltrations, the whole complex process of the verbal developmental structure proceeds. Single words serve as entire phrases or sentences or represent clusters of meanings. The earliest words tend to be nouns or interjections related to the immediate environment; verbs tend to appear next in order, with adjectives, adverbs, and pronouns following (McCarthy, 1954). Personal pronouns appear to be quite difficult for the child to master; we notice that these are more or less "personal words" ("me get ball," "him go out," "me, good boy?" "He bad boy, isn't him?"). Later on we notice an increasing use of "I," and also that it is used more frequently during play with other children than in speaking with adults (Leopold, 1939). By 18 months the typical child may have a vocabulary of 50 or more words which are becoming more firmly attached to objects and actions. His perception, comprehension, and expression of these words produce a more social stabilization of his environment. Usually there is some private vocal play, and jargon may continue in strong evidence. Although there may be much unintelligible jabber, the vocal flow almost always is *fluent*. One of the child's tasks is to acquire words expressive of feelings so that there is less need to show these feelings through frustrated or angry behavior. One of the adult's tasks is to help the child not only to acquire these words but also to help him to be able to *express* these words. The acquisition of words is of far less value if they are not communicable (as in delayed speech, mutism, or stuttering).

We have observed that words are not the same for all children. How a child uses different words, what he does with them, and how he seems to regard them give us some idea as to the significance of words or speech for him. To what degree do words refer to people, things, or self? Are words used socially or autistically? Realistically or fantastically? Aggressively or passively? Intellectually or emotionally? Some children who are constricted verbally may merely be in a "speech absorption" phase. They may simply be operating according to a comfortable schedule of speech development, although their progress falls short of adult-imposed standards. Such children may have a vivid imagination, sensitivity, and a capacity for analytical appreciation which will bloom in language and other ways at a later time. Some bright children appear to relinquish temporarily certain speech behavior until they have acquired a vocabulary which will convey their more abstract or complex thinking processes. This is the period of verbal and vocal uncertainty which most young children reach, remain at temporarily, and relinquish (Ansbacher and Ansbacher, 1956; Johnson, 1955).

By the age of three years, the speaking vocabulary may have skyrocketed to nearly a thousand words, while the comprehension vocabulary exceeds that. The child has been using words to express emotions for a long time now. He has found words useful in testing parental limits, exploring the world about him ("wot dis?"), and manipulating his environment in general. But words are manipulating him also. Mother's "Don't" may be all that is required to make him conform to the adult patterns of behavior and speech. Also, he is learning that he cannot talk whenever he feels the urge and that he may not talk with hesitancy and repetitions. Talk, which was once prized whenever emitted, now is subject to parental and cultural correction, and it is stopped on certain occasions such as mealtime, nap time, company time. At this point, fairly well-defined parental reactions to his speech behavior have developed. The kind of acceptance or rejection of his speech which a child receives at this stage may be decisive in terms of subsequent verbal development and fluency. Often the child will use speech as an obvious form of play. At other times, he will use speech as a security-testing medium: he repeats the same questions no matter how often they have been answered. Repeated derogatory reactions from adults at such times would tend to affect speech-security development.

By the age of four or five years, the child is communicating, for better or for worse, with his entire being. His manner of speech, his loudness level, inflections and quality of voice, his rate of utterance, his loquacity or taciturnity, his attitudes, his verbal spontaneity, inhibition, or stereotypy all combine to give an impression of the child as a "unique" (happy or unhappy) personality. The child's speech, language, gestures, and voice come to reveal his basic needs, motivations, conflicts, and his self-perception. It is these indices which will serve as main indicators of the stability or instability of the individual for the remainder of his existence. For some time now, he has been exploring beyond his immediate motor and perceptual environment, and it has been increasingly a verbal exploration. He experiments with out-of-bounds behavior, and he tests reality limits (Piaget, 1926) through speech ("I don't want to"). By five years, the exploration has become predominantly verbal, although the average preschooler, now learning to restrain his feelings in interpersonal dealings, is also producing speech containing less emotion (Shirley, 1938). The persistence and satisfaction of the inquisitive need via the countless "How's" and "Why's" will be conditioned by the tone of the adult responses which are given to his queries. Six-year olds begin to invite and accept supervision, though some will resist it; others may regress to a two- or three-year old level. In the latter cases, it is as though some inner storm were producing confusions, with an outcropping of somatic complaints ("I have a tummy ache"; "I don't want to go to school today, Mommy") or other symptoms. The seven- and eight-year-olds are apt to become more pensive and less talkative but "good" students (well-controlled behavior).

Egocentric and Sociocentric Components. Throughout the discussion thus far, a question can be raised regarding the legitimacy of accepting the existence of "stages" of development. Certainly there is a great deal of overlapping; many older children show very immature speech, while many younger ones have very mature speech behavior. The vast range of constitutional and environmental differences brought to the thresholds of the various growth phases by different children makes variability inevitable. As Ausubel has stated: "... it is only necessary to show that certain qualitative differences in development in process arose consistently at definite points in a developmental cycle which differentiate the greater mass of children at a given age level from adjacent age groups" (Ausubel, 1958, p. 96).

We have said that the preschooler's amount, type, and fluency of verbalization gives us our major impressions of what "kind" of child he is. Some youngsters are verbally compliant and submissive; their speech may be abortive, inhibited, hesitant, tremulous, and disorganized. There are some who are verbal mirror-images of the parents, giving back perfect imitations of parental verbal and vocal (for example, inflection copying) behavior. Others, more independent, utilize speech more forcefully and freely to express feelings and to manipulate the environment, although the forms of verbal environmental manipulation run a long gamut from the use of a simple cry or "charming" speech to symptomatic speech behavior of a more serious nature (delayed speech and stuttering). Finally, some children may be completely "independent" to the point of being out of verbal contact with their environment (Waal, 1955).

However, not all verbally constricted youngsters should be viewed automatically as behavior problems. Children must be observed in a variety of communication settings, including those which are reassuring, in order to determine to what extent positive verbal behavior is expressed and the degree to which such positive behavior may be more indicative of the child than was the apparently symptomatic behavior of verbal constriction. The younger the child, the better the chance that the seemingly deviant verbal behavior is not an ingrained and dominating speech or language compulsion, and the more should premature induction be delayed. Is Johnny's repeated utterances of "naughty Mommy" while smearing clay on the toy elephant a revelation of a parental attitude? Or is it a projection of Johnny's own guilt feelings and need to be punished? Perhaps he is simply repeating a play activity he observed in his nursery class. It could have been a reaction to temporary anxiety, seldom or never to occur again. Only a consideration of the verbal behavior in relation to many samplings over a reasonable time span will help ensure a more valid analysis of Johnny's verbal dynamics.

The attempt to clarify the often barely accessible regions of children's verbal dynamics is a demanding challenge. The investigator, especially if he is an innovator, will experience both discomfort and pleasure as he searches out the well-springs of the forces impelling and permeating human oral communication. As he seeks the total significance of childhood speech and language, his conflicts or ruminations will arise primarily from three life realms: (1) from *himself,* concerning choice of principles, procedures, materials, and settings for investigation; (2) from the *child,* concerning the often nebulous, often puzzling, often unmeasurable flux and flow of behavior; and (3) from *fellow workers* concerning their support or criticisms, analytical reactions, and terminological frictions regarding his assumptions, hypotheses, methods, or conclusions. Yet, the investigator willing to work his way through these forests of forces is the one who not only may bring new light to bear on old or discarded issues but may also focus thought on theories and practices not hitherto linked productively to the study of speech and language.

The work of Piaget (1932) regarding the egocentric nature of childhood speech serves as an example of an intuitive, systematic worker who developed a newer child-language framework, using a case study approach. His writings have stimulated much additional research, not to mention theoretical controversy, in the past three decades. Piaget's method of studying children consisted basically of (1) *observation,* comprising the recording of the child's questions, reflections, and conversations, and the utilization of these data for the second phase, viz., (2) *the interview,* following which the speech was classified within a fairly elaborate language system. His interest (excessive, some think) in classification probably derived from his early work in biology, a field in which he had published a number of scientific papers by the age of fifteen.

Piaget described egocentric speech as speech in which the child is not concerned with whom he speaks or whether people are listening to him. He speaks for his own pleasure. Three types of egocentric speech were named: (1) echolalia (repetition); (2) monologue, and (3) dual or collective monologue. In sociocentric speech, the child considers the listener's point of view, tries to influence his thinking, exchange ideas, and actually communicate with him. Types of sociocentric speech posited by Piaget included: (1) "adapted information" (thought exchanges); (2) criticisms; (3) commands, threats, and requests; (4) quotations; and (5) answers. Egocentric speech was said to be dominant until the age of five to six years; the ability to understand other people and to speak one's own ideas with efficiency was held not to occur prior to the seventh or eighth year.

Piaget's investigations, based primarily on a functional analysis of about 20 children aged four to seven years, led to numerous studies which revealed contradictory results concerning percentages of egocentric and sociocentric speech. McCarthy's (1930, 1954) analysis of her own data, using Piaget's criteria, showed significantly less egocentricity (40 per cent) as compared with Piaget's (57 per cent), while other investigators found higher agreement; Fisher (1934), for example, concluded that the child is a confirmed "egotist" but extremely sociable, satisfying both needs by incessantly talking to people. McCarthy (1954) reports Buhler as believing that the child's speech is the expression of a need for social contact and that "monologue" speech is primarily an expression of a need to affiliate. There is some evidence that the degree of egocentricity in children's speech may be highly similar to that found in the speech of adults (Henle and Hubbell, 1938). McCarthy (1954) presents an excellent analysis of the difficulties inherent in interstudy comparisons of linguistic variables and of egocentricity and sociocentricity.

To workers today, the distinction between egocentric and sociocentric speech seems overdone. Any bipolar conception is viewed as myopic in relation to a consideration of the child as a fluctuating organism reacting over a period of time to different personal and situational stresses. It is easy in retrospect to find fault with Piaget. Some of his examples do not fit his definitions; there was indifference to individual differences; sampling and reliability procedures were disregarded. But he was a pioneer in a more functional approach to childhood speech. His emphasis on case study and analysis paved the way for more productive research than had been possible with traditional descriptive studies.

Certainly it can be said that, in general, with increasing age, children become more capable of considering the feelings and viewpoints of others and in talking to one another in a social exchange of ideas (Ames, 1952). We observe the gradual addition of such word concepts as "we" to their repertoire (Gesell and Ilg, 1943). Egocentric speech comes to have increasing sociocentric elements; it is used for verbalizing socially; i.e., the child's self-needs are being satisfied through socialized activity. In the clinical setting, when disturbed children talk to people their own size, language tends to be more sociocentric, while with larger people, language becomes more egocentric ("You're bigger than I am—take care of me"). The more threatened the child (or adult) is, the more he is apt to interpret the situation egocentrically.

We have observed that the more egocentric and personalized the language of persons who stutter becomes, the more blocked and impeded their speech becomes. For persons who stutter, the "I am . . . ," the "I feel . . . ," the "I think . . . ," and the "I will . . . ," can be emotionally and communicatively catastrophic. A consequent goal in speech counseling is the self-activation by the stuttering person of the flow of egocentric speech in order to render egocentric, emotionally toned feeling residuals less ominous.

Piaget has been criticized for ignoring the importance of unique interpersonal relationships and the entire constellation of personality dynamics in current personality theory. Whatever the merits of this charge, his descriptions and interpretations of child behavior have an often startling similarity to current psychoanalytical thinking. In some ways, a comparable analogous situation exists today in the area of stuttering theory. Although the assumptions or principles of the several points of view on stuttering etiology appear to be quite disparate, if the student looks beyond the immediate terminology or theoretical models of each "system," he will find they agree on many basic points. Oftentimes the controversies appear to be based on very minor differences, while major similarities are disregarded.

A CONCLUDING STATEMENT

This chapter has attempted to give the reader an understanding of speech development from a psychodynamic frame of reference. It has been suggested that although interpersonal relationships involving speech behavior as such may lead to speech disruptions, interpersonal tensions involving behavior which is not strictly *speech* behavior may be even more important in creating psychogenic speech disorders. We shall turn to a more detailed consideration of these possibilities in the next chapter.

In the subsequent two chapters we shall consider the basic psychosocial needs and motivations which serve as the subsoil out of which mature or disordered behavior develops. We shall attempt to summarize basic psychodynamic concepts so as to reveal their import and implications for verbal learnings and therapeutic procedures. Consequences of the socialization of the child, the experiencing of anxieties and specific fears, and the modes of defense adopted by the child in attempting to cope with exogenously and endogenously derived discomforts will be viewed as related to the development of psychogenic speech symptoms.

REFERENCES

ALDRICH, C. A. "The Crying of Newly Born Babies III: The Early Period at Home," *J. of Pediatrics,* **27**: 428–35, 1945.

ALDRICH, C. A.; SUNG, C.; and KNOP, C. "The Crying of Newly Born Babies II: The Individual Phase," *J. of Pediatrics,* **27**: 89–96, 1945.

ALDRICH, C. A.; NORVAL, M.; KNOP, C.; and VENEGAS, F. "The Crying of Newly Born Babies IV: Follow-up Study After Additional Nursing Care Had Been Provided," *J. of Pediatrics,* **28**: 665–70, 1946.

ALLEN, F. *Psychotherapy with Children.* New York: W. W. Norton & Co., Inc., 1942.

AMES, L. B. "The Sense of Self of Nursery Children as Manifested by Their Verbal Behavior," *J. Genet. Psychol.,* **81**: 193–232, 1952.

ANSBACHER, H., and ANSBACHER, R. *The Individual Psychology of Alfred Adler.* New York: Basic Books, Inc., 1956.

AUSUBEL, D. *Theory and Problems of Child Development.* New York: Grune & Stratton, Inc., 1958.

BAKWIN, H. "Loneliness in Infants," *Amer. J. Dis. Child.,* **63**: 30–40, 1942.

BENEDEK, T. "Personality Development," in *Dynamic Psychiatry,* eds. F. Alexander and H. Ross. Chicago: Univ. of Chicago Press, 1952.

BERRY, M., and EISENSON, J. *Speech Disorders.* New York: Appleton-Century-Crofts, Inc., 1956.

CAMERON, N. *Psychology of Behavior Disorders.* Boston: Houghton Mifflin Co., 1947.

DAVIS, W. A., and HAVIGHURST, R. *Father of the Man.* Boston: Houghton Mifflin Co., 1947.

DECROLY, O. *Comment l'enfant arrive à parler,* Vol. II. Belgium: Cahiers de la Centvale, 1934.

FISHER, M. "Language Patterns of Children." *Child Development Monograph,* No. 15. New York: Teachers College, Columbia Univ., 1934.

FITZSIMONS, R. "Developmental, Psychosocial, and Educational Factors in Children with Nonorganic Articulation Problems," *Child Development,* **29**: 481–89, 1958.

GESELL, A., and ILG, F. *Infant and Child in the Culture of Today.* New York: Harper & Bros., 1943.

GOLDFARB, W. "Psychological Privation in Infancy and Subsequent Adjustment," *Amer. J. Orthopsychiat.*, **15**: 247–55, 1945.

HALL, C. "The Genetics of Behavior," *Handbook of Experimental Psychology,* ed. S. Stevens. New York: John Wiley & Sons, Inc., 1951, pp. 304–29.

HAVIGHURST, R. *Human Development and Education.* New York: Longmans, Green & Co., Inc., 1953.

HENLE, M., and HUBBELL, M. " 'Egocentricity' in Adult Conversation," *J. Soc. Psychol.*, **9**: 227–34, 1938.

HILGARD, J. "Learning and Maturation in Preschool Children," *J. Gen. Psychol.*, **41**: 36–56, 1932.

HULL, C. L. *Principles of Behavior.* New York: Appleton-Century-Crofts, Inc., 1943.

IRWIN, O. "Research on Speech Sounds for the First Six Months of Life," *Psychol. Bull.*, **38**: 277–88, 1941.

IRWIN, O., and CHEN, H. "Development of Speech During Infancy and the Curve of Phonemic Types, *J. Exp. Psychol.*, **36**: 431–36, 1946.

JOHNSON, W. (ed.). *Stuttering in Children and Adults.* Minneapolis, Minn.: Univ. of Minnesota Press, 1955.

KANNER, L. *A Word to Parents About Mental Hygiene.* Madison, Wis.: Univ. of Wisconsin Press, 1957.

———. *Child Psychiatry,* 2d ed. Springfield, Ill.: Charles C. Thomas, Publisher, 1950.

KAPLAN, B. "On the Phenomena of Opposite Speech," *J. Abnorm. Soc. Psychol.*, **55**: 389–93, 1957.

LEOPOLD, W. "Speech Development of a Bilingual Child: A Linguistic Record: I. Vocabulary Growth in the First Two Years," *Northwestern Univ. Stud. Human.* No. 6, 1939.

LEWIS, M. *Infant Speech: A Study of Beginnings of Language,* 2d ed. London: Rutledge & Kegan Paul, Ltd., 1951.

MCCARTHY, D. "Language Development in Children." In *Manual of Child Psychology,* 2d ed., ed. L. Carmichael. New York: John Wiley & Sons, Inc., 1954, pp. 492–630.

———. *The Language Development of the Preschool Child.* Minneapolis, Minn.: Univ. of Minnesota Press, 1930.

MCGINNIES, E. "Emotionality and Perceptual Defense," *Psychol. Rev.*, **56**: 244–51,1949.

MCGRAW, M. *Growth: A Study of Johnny and Jimmy.* New York: Appleton-Century-Crofts, Inc., 1935.

———. "Neural Maturation as Exemplified in Achievement of Bladder Control," *J. Pediat.*, **16**: 580–90, 1940.

MORGAN, CLIFFORD T. *Introduction to Psychology.* New York: Mc-Graw-Hill Book Co., Inc., 1956.

MOWRER, O. *Learning Theory and Personality Dynamics.* New York: The Ronald Press Co., 1950.

MURPHY, L. *Personality in Young Children,* Vol. I. Methods for the Study of Personality in Young Children. New York: Basic Books, Inc., 1956.

PIAGET, J. *The Child's Perception of the World.* London: Rutledge & Kegan Paul, Ltd., 1926.

———. *The Language and Thought of the Child,* 2d ed. New York: Harcourt, Brace & Co., Inc., 1932.

POSTMAN, L. "The Experimental Analysis of Motivational Factors in Perception." In the Nebraska Symposium on Motivation: *Current Theory and Research in Motivation,* I. Lincoln, Nebr.: Univ. of Nebraska Press, 1954, pp. 59–108.

SHIRLEY, M. "Common Content in the Speech of Preschool Children," *Child Develop.,* **9:** 333–45, 1938.

SIMON, C. "The Development of Speech." In *Handbook of Speech Pathology,* ed. L. E. Travis. New York: Appleton-Century-Crofts, Inc., 1957, pp. 3–43.

SPIKER, C., and IRWIN, O. C. "The Relationship Between I.Q. and Indices of Infant Speech Sound Development," *J. Speech Hearing Disorders,* **14:** 335–43, 1949.

SPITZ, R. "Hospitalism: An Inquiry into the Genesis of Psychiatric Conditions in Early Childhood," II. In *The Psychoanalytic Study of the Child,* Vol. II. New York: International Universities Press, Inc., 1946.

STERN, C., and STERN, W. *Die Kindersprache.* Leipzig: Barth, 1907.

STONE, L., and CHURCH, J. *Childhood and Adolescence.* New York: Random House, Inc., 1957.

STRAYER, L. "Language and Growth: The Relative Efficacy of Early and Deferred Vocabulary Training Studied by the Method of Co-twin Control," *Genet. Psychol. Monogr.,* **8:** 209–319, 1930.

SULLIVAN, H. *The Interpersonal Theory of Psychiatry.* New York: W. W. Norton & Co., Inc., 1953.

VAN RIPER, C. *Speech Correction: Principles and Method,* 3d ed. Englewood Cliffs, N. J.: Prentice-Hall, Inc., 1954.

WAAL, N. "A Special Technique of Psychotherapy with an Autistic Child." In *Emotional Problems of Early Childhood,* ed. G. Caplan. New York: Basic Books, Inc., 1955.

WYATT, G. "A Developmental Crisis Theory of Stuttering," *Lang. and Speech,* **1,** No. 4: 250–64, 1958.

———. Personal communication to the authors, April, 1957.

Chapter 4

Personality Dynamics and Speech Development

> *The past will not sleep. It works still. With every new*
> *fact a ray of light shoots up from the long buried years.*
> ——Emerson

DIFFERENTIATION AND INTEGRATION: VERBAL AND NONVERBAL

The maturation of human behavior reveals a trend toward the modification or elimination of generalized and superfluous movements to more specific forms of behavior. Those postural-locomotor activities, for example, which have become irrelevant to the performing of specific tasks are minimized or abandoned. The process is one of increasingly specific inhibitions of alternative responses. We observe the progression of specificity as the child raises his head, sits, crawls, stands, walks, runs, hops, and dances. This process has long been discussed in psychology,* and it has been applied to language development by Jesperson, who theorized that the language evolutionary process was one of progressive differentiation of myriad "mass units." In a conception of personality offered by Kluckhohn and Murray, the authors discussed differentiation and integration in this way:

* Coghill stated it this way: "The behavior pattern from the beginning expands throughout the growing normal animal as a perfectly integrated unit whereas partial patterns arise within the total patterns and, by a process of individuation, acquire secondarily varying degrees of independence" (Coghill, 1929, p. 989).

. . . no conception of personality could be complete without some reference to the developments that occur, most of which can be adequately described in terms of differentiation and integration. "Differentiation" covers all refinements of discrimination in perception, interpretation and conceptualization, as well as detailed specifications in laying out plans and exact directions and timing in action. Mental differentiation is involved in the appreciation of differences, in the intellectual process of analysis, as well as in the isolation and perfection of specialized action symptoms and abilities, verbal and manual. "Integration" includes the ability to perceive similarities, as well as different kinds of relations between objects and events, to develop a coherent conceptual scheme, to resolve conflicts, to maintain loyalties, to rationalize values, to build a philosophy of life, to coordinate different plans, to plan and talk in a logical manner, to organize dynamic systems into a unified whole (Kluckhohn and Murray, 1950, pp. 30–31).

The conception of progressive differentiation and integration is especially important in relation to language dynamics. The movement from one developmental task or "stage" to another is really a process of symbolic individuation and integration, the successful unfolding of which is dependent on a great many factors. The phase of transition from one stage of language development to another may be productive of stress. The biosocial status or conception of self felt by the child serves as a field of reference for the synthesis of his goals and attitudes. It is quite conceivable that disorientation or disequilibrium may occur if the child feels the need to change abruptly his status, his mode of communication, his self-concept. New words, new grammatical structures, and new fluency requirements may be thought of as uncharted regions which require the child to explore, test, repeat, adapt to, and to accept the reality demands of the new verbal domains.

The difficulties of transitional periods in personality development have been described by Ausubel:

. . . the familiar and differentiated roles that [the child] had learned in relation to an earlier pattern of social expectations and the cues that he had employed with confidence in interpreting his interpersonal environment suddenly become useless and confusing. Second, considerable *anxiety* is engendered by the threat to self-esteem inherent in forfeiting current status while the attainment of new status is still uncertain. He is required to discard a painfully acquired portion of his identity, the security of established roles and status prerogatives, and frequently a sheltered and protected position; and in return he is permitted to strive for a potentially more satisfactory type of biosocial status. But in connection with this striving looms the ever-present threat of disappointment and failure, the pull of conflicting loyalties and the awesome responsibilities of freedom and autonomy. And whenever he is forced to choose between two alternatives, each of which offers advantages as well as disadvantages (e.g., parents or peers, dependence or conformity, conformity or individuality), a decision in favor of one inevitably frustrates needs and inclinations referable to the other and gives rise to regret and self-recrimination (Ausubel, 1957, pp. 104–105).

Theoretically, the more the child feels the necessity to progress more rapidly (to move on to another stage), the more a state of verbal disequilibrium is likely to develop. Phases of transition, then, are to be regarded as important way-stations in verbal behavior, deserving of more than fleeting consideration.

Because language behavior develops and exists on the basis of an intricate network of regulatory means, its establishment is not usually impaired easily. The complex requirements involved in learning to use single words socially, for example, ensure a high level of resistance to disruption or dissolution to an earlier stage. Infants, like adults, tend to adjust to new verbal demands or expectations by changing their behavior in the most parsimonious fashion; that is, they alter their actions so as to retain as completely as possible the relative constancy of their existing adjustive dynamics. Changes in speech learnings tend to be gradual and minor. As mentioned above, the more the child feels the necessity to progress more rapidly (to "move on" to another "stage") or to abruptly change a prevailing mode of behavior, the more a state of verbal disequilibrium is likely to develop, and the more crucial the youngster's need to reorganize his verbal structure. But the process of differentiation and integration is hardly begun when the infant encounters the strong influences or pressures of those who comprise his adult world. Interferences with the freedom to explore his own body and external objects, to see and hear everything that surrounds him, to vocalize or verbalize about body parts and functions, as well as constraints on all his interpersonal interactions, can be experienced in a variety of ways. This "variety" is affected by countless determinants, such as the social pressures on the mother to conform to the "code" of relatives or neighbors, which may in turn generate maternal pressure on the child to conform. In time, as we shall see, the child may come to serve as his own most effective suppressor.

Progressive differentiation and integration (the developmental growth pattern) generally is rewarding to the individual. It is only when the process becomes fixated or *less* differentiated and integrated (regresses) that chronically ruptured and nonintegrative behavior occurs. Much of the behavior observed in speech-therapy settings may be described as fixated or infantile. When such behavior becomes *chronic,* we may refer to it as "disordered," "deviant," "defective," or we may call it a psychogenic speech disorder. The roots of such nonintegrative verbal behavior are found in many soils, as we shall attempt to show.

The Principle of Generalization or Association. One of the oldest laws of learning is that things similar tend to be equated. The principle of association, formerly applied to ideas in general, now is used to refer to associations between stimuli and responses. The more an object, event, or behavioral field is *like* one previously experienced, the more likely the possibility that the memory or feeling about the previous experience will be triggered by the present situation. An association may be positive or negative, conscious or unconscious, or a combination of these. An adolescent cruelly punished for years by a father who limped is more likely to have a strongly negative association with men who limp than is the boy whose limping father was a kind man.

Associations may, in the experience of infants, involve bodily structures or functions. There is little need to detail the great similarity in structure among the various bodily orifices. The shape and the muscular and tissue structure of the anus and mouth, for instance, are strikingly similar. The expulsive, retentive, and incorporative characteristics of these structures are easily equated; even anal and oral sounds may be associated, especially by the less discriminating infant. Can experiences in one structural or functional area be associated (positively or negatively) with experiences in another area? More specifically, can repeatedly painful experiences in one bodily area (harsh and early toilet training, for example) condition the infant's attitudes or feelings about his body parts and functions in *general,* especially those body parts and functions which are most similar to the negatively tinged sectors? The concept of generalization as an extension of conditioning principles is applicable here.

A new conditioned stimulus (aunt's voice, for example) that is not previously reinforced may produce a conditioned response (apprehension) at its first presentation. The chances of this occurring are enhanced if the stimulus is similar to the conditioned stimulus which has been reinforced. Thus, if a mother's voice is a conditioned stimulus, a similar voice (the aunt's or the teacher's), though of slightly different character, will also elicit the conditioned-response apprehension (though with less intensity, the more disparate the voices). "This process whereby a novel stimulus produces a response learned to another similar stimulus is known as *generalization*" (Hilgard, 1956, p. 51). Through association and generalization, such reactions fan out and become attached to objects or situations which have features comparable to the characteristics of the original stimuli. The youngster who is severely restrained from speaking during family mealtimes may generalize his response to all situations which involve eating or small group activity. And what happens to the child who, when he moves his arm slightly as though to hit (or to protect himself from) his mother for punishing him, hears her exclaim: "Don't you dare hit your mother! Your arm will fall off!" One may venture the opinion that repeated maternal responses of this kind to the child's attempts or wishes to express his feelings physically could culminate in a general inhibition of any expressive behavior, including speech-expressive behavior. Another instance of generalization is observed when the child calls all women "Mommy" or all men "Daddy." Again, the more similar the women and men (conditioned stimuli) to the mother and father, the higher is the probability that the men and women elicit reactions similar to those which are produced by the original stimuli, the father and mother. The child who stutters principally in the presence of male authority figures may be doing so as a consequence of having unwittingly generalized from his early experiences with elders who elicited anxiety.

THE PRIMARY SOMATIC ZONES OF INTERACTION

Just as the stages of language development discussed in the preceding chapter have been thought of in terms of verbal differentiation and integration processes, so the allied psychosocial stages of development constitute additional developmental tasks. Eventual harmonious functioning of the organism depends on the degree of success in psychosocial differentiation and integration. All task processes are interdependent in varying degrees; not only are verbal task disruptions likely to produce psychosocial disequilibrium, but psychosocial task disruptions may produce verbal disequilibrium, such as stuttering. For a greater understanding as to how psychosocial experiences may be related to psychogenic verbal dysfunctions, we shall consider some of the dynamics of the psychosocial differentiation and integration processes. The following discussion of psychosocial development is not to be thought of as anything but arbitrary. The "stages" represent convenient conceptual divisions which are used to convey some important features of behavior. This kind of verbal economy allows us to achieve a general glimpse of what is, in reality, a fascinating but very complicated panorama of the young human in action.

Oral Differentiation and Integration. In addition to the auditory and visual modalities, the infant's main communication pathways to the world about him occur through the three basic bodily orifices, viz., the anus, urethra, and oral cavities. Two of these constitute the end stations of the gastro-intestinal tract. These sensorally rich mucocutaneous openings serve as the chief arteries linking the infant's inner processes with outer reality, and although they are fundamentally biological in function, they are peculiarly susceptible to functional disturbances stemming from emotional conflicts (Alexander, 1950; Dunbar, 1943; Wolfe and Wolff, 1947). Each of the bodily orifices may be thought of as a "zone of interaction" (Sullivan, 1953). The oral zone of interaction embraces all the neuro-glandular-muscular complexes which are connected with breathing, crying, eating, and speaking. Other bodily parts or functions may be critically involved in the given behavior (for example, the *formulation* of speech occurs beyond the mouth), but the oral zone serves as the hub in the network complex.* Sullivan stated:

> The zone of interaction may then be considered to be the end station in the necessary varieties of communal existence with the physiochemical world, the world of the infrahuman being, and the personal world.
> Processes in and pertaining to these zones of interaction must have a great deal to do with the occurrence of experience . . . of living. So far as experience is, or effects, useful durable change in the functional activities of the living organism, it must relate backward and forward—that is, in phenomena of recall and foresight—to the zone of interaction to which it is primarily related. . . ."
> From the data of later life, I hold that experience takes special color from, or is especially marked with reference to, the zone of interaction which is primarily concerned in its occurrence (Sullivan, 1953, pp. 64–65).

Much of the child's first 18 months is taken up with oral activities. His early life is pretty much an oral-intake process, with the mouth the main contact with the universe around him. Due to biological development, the oral zone is a structurally sensitized pathway which is more important,

* To Sullivan, the oral zone also included the auditory function which later becomes a zone of interaction in its own right (Sullivan, 1953, p. 123).

stimulating, and pleasurable than any other bodily area, and though serving initially as a nutritional carrier, the oral zone soon is experienced erogenously, quite aside from the ingestive function. That is, sucking, lapping, and blowing are done for the pleasurable feeling afforded, independent of the need for nourishment. Watching an infant as he plays with an object, we see how he manipulates it, withdraws it, looks at it, puts it back into his mouth, drops it, picks it up, mouths it, and so forth.

In the original Freudian formulations, three primary developmental phases were said to occur: the "oral phase," the "anal phase," and the "phallic phase" (Freud, 1933, pp. 136–137). The oral phase was divided into two periods: the oral receptive (also termed the oral incorporative, oral passive, or oral sucking stage), and the oral sadistic (also termed the oral biting stage). In the first phase, which occurs roughly in the first six months of life, the oral zone of interaction may be described as primarily passive-dependent in character. The infant's very life depends on how well he masters this passive sucking activity. In addition to its nutritional importance, sucking serves as the infant's first motor pleasure. Also, we note that sucking involves not only the tongue and lips but the palate and cheeks as well, and that the basic biological movements of sucking, swallowing, belching, and smiling are the events out of which speech movements and sounds emerge. The infant's major adjustments are through oral zone interaction. He lives with and because of his mouth. He loves with his mouth, the love-object usually being the mother. To the infant, the mouth is the zone not only for the intake of food and liquids but for the intake of his entire outside world, a world consisting almost entirely of the mother upon whom he is completely dependent. As the child takes in with his mouth, he incorporates with his eyes, his hands, his whole body. As will be discussed later in this chapter, he may also take in some of the attributes of the tending elder (Fries, 1946). Oral gratifications will occur through the sucking of his own fingers, toes, and other available objects. The major portion of his

orientation is very much an oral "in-out," "in-hold," and
"out-in" process.

As oral zone experiences increase in number and complexity, the child begins not only to associate them but to
discriminate among them. He individualizes his attitudes
and reactions to them. He differentiates the various experiential modes and meanings. He tends to favor some forms
of experience and to avoid others. He increasingly differentiates and integrates his perceptualizations, conceptualiza-
tions, and behavioral styles, all the while consolidating oral
zone processes with auxiliary zones and processes. During
approximately the seventh to the eighteenth month, newer
kinds of oral functions emerge. Oral expressiveness, often
in the form of biting, spitting, and mastication, mixes with
the older passive sucking behavior. The child becomes more
active orally. He learns that he can bite (hurt) things, even
bite them off sometimes, and that he can take things and
hold them involuntarily. "With all of this a number of
interpersonal patterns are established which center in the
social modality of *taking* and *holding on to* things—things
which are more or less freely offered and given, and things
which have more or less a tendency to slip away" (Erikson,
1950, p. 72). This incorporative-retention-expulsive development may be considered the foundation of the total verbal
and social differentiation and integration processes.

In the active oral phase the child may experience concurrently *both* the passive oral needs and the active, incorporative needs; i.e., the condition of ambivalence, wherein opposing, conflicting feelings (want/not want; love/hate) are felt
toward the same person. This infantile experience appears
to be the prototype of future ambivalence development. The
child is frustrated in satisfying some need (while nursing at
the breast or during crying). He becomes aggressive (bites
or yells). His aggression brings a negative reaction, perhaps
punishment, from the parents. The negative reaction makes
the child angry at the parents, and he wants to retaliate (bite
back or reply angrily), but he is fearful of what will happen
if he does. If he displeases the parent, he may be deprived

(of her nurture, comfort, love) and "left" (hungry, rejected, or deserted). Also, if he displeases (bites or speaks out), additional punishment may result; he may even be laughed at, ridiculed, or sent away (to the crib or to his room). Overtly "giving in" to the adult may offer the least apparent discomfort, although the covert feelings may actually produce great internal stress.

If, for various psychosocial reasons, the child finds it impossible to move on to the next developmental task, we may say that a general or an oral fixation has developed; i.e., that the child is "fixated" at the oral phase of development. This may occur if the child has not been satisfied adequately in his earlier experiences.* Also, if the earlier period is made so pleasant that it is too difficult to change, or if the child is compelled to remain at the earlier phase (not allowed to bite or be orally expressive), fixation may occur. To the degree that a person is fixated at a certain phase of development, to that degree will he tend to have personality attributes emanating from that period, even though they are now inappropriate (infantile) (Hutt and Gibby, 1957, p. 89). Clinical experience indicates that during periods of stress, the person will tend to regress to the dominant infantile modes of adjustment: passivity (to be taken care of) or aggression (to get back at). This will occur if he has not completely worked his way through (differentiated or integrated) the oral or allied developmental tasks.

Anal-Urethral Differentiation and Integration. The anal-urethral zone of interaction is centered in those mucocutaneous junctions which serve as end stations pertinent to the expulsion of food and water residues. The primitively felt needs in this zone are related to bowel and urinary evacuation tensions. As in the oral zone, there is a rich supply of

---

* In comparing "nursing indulgence" and "age of weaning" of 22 societies, Whiting and Child (1953) have demonstrated that, at least in the middle class, our tendency is to "indulge" the child little and to wean him early (a little over six months); in fact, the American middle-class ratings were second lowest in the groups compared, the least indulgent society being that of the Marquesans, who feel that prolonged nursing makes the child hard to raise.

receptors which makes it possible for the child to experience strong sensory satisfaction. From approximately the fourth to the twentieth months of life, the anal zone components of experience assume an increasing primacy for the child. In the early months, the child evacuates loose stools, a situation which in our culture calls for fairly rapid cleaning of the soiled parts by the mother. He is washed, wiped, patted, and powdered in the general region of the buttocks and anus. Urine soiling, on the other hand, tends not to be reacted to with quite the dispatch given the anal products.

The anal zone of interaction thus necessarily comes to involve factors of an interpersonal character from very early in life. The functional activity centering in the anal zone often becomes involved in the manifestations of infantile anxiety, especially when the mothering one is made anxious by these details of her mothering function. By this I refer to those who find it extremely difficult to deal with the infant's soiled diapers, and so on (Sullivan, 1953, p. 133).

In addition, manipulation by the child of his own anal parts may be repugnant to the mother, for the hands that reach the anus may soon reach the mouth, and most cultures have rather strong, deeply ingrained attitudes concerning fecal matter, its acceptability, and its harmful aspects, real or imagined. Even if the mother is not anxious about these events, she is very likely to be in touch with other adults who are sensitive about such processes and structures.

In the infant's early days, every urination or defecation is a coronation. Parents smile, praise, and if there are relatives or neighbors in the house, their praise may be solicited by parents who wish to convey to the infant the idea that it is wonderful to give. Indeed, toilet time may be the only occasion when the family gets together regularly, as they collect to shower words of encouragement and praise upon Johnny. But Johnny's day of reckoning arrives, sooner or later. He learns that his body treasures are no longer thought of as joy-giving "gifts." Perhaps he presents his gifts at the wrong place (in the yard or the living room), or at the wrong time (grandmother is visiting), or else the next-door neighbor mentions that her own son, who is no older than Johnny, is already "trained." Johnny's mother now has an important decision to make: Will she let him develop, at a reasonable pace, the ability to control his anal functions? Or will she start to pressure him verbally—mildly, warmly, sternly—or imply nonverbally, through facial expressions and gestures, that she wants more toilet efficiency? The child's developmental task here becomes one of learning to defecate or urinate at the proper time.

And what is the proper time for the acquisition of voluntary control? The answer must be made in consideration of the anatomical, physiological, and psychological components involved. Usually, anal control occurs prior to urethral control, possibly because of the stronger societal reactions to anal processes and the greater frequency of urethral functioning. Usually a conscious, cortical control of the external eliminative sphincters does not occur until walking ability is fairly well established. The child should be aware of eliminative tensions; be able to comprehend and respond to some language; and be capable of imitating his elders. (Of course it is possible that anal-urethral integrity may be delayed because of slow maturation of the pyramidal pathways which affect this zone or by structural anomalies of the tracts, but in the present discussion we are assuming dysfunctions which are psychogenically determined.) Available research and clinical observations indicate that attempts to establish voluntary control of anal functions prior to 18 months should be considered coercive (Leighton and Kluckhohn, 1947; McGraw, 1940; Whiting and Child, 1953).

In one study (Huschka, 1942) of 163 problem children, about one-half had been toilet-trained prior to 18 months. In another study (McGraw, 1940), using the co-twin control method, children receiving systematic, daily bladder training instituted within a few weeks of birth did not differ significantly regarding age when trained as compared to those children whose training had been delayed from one to two years. There is evidence, too, that the more a child is punished for "accidents," the earlier he tends to be "trained" (Whiting and Child, 1953).

The mother's attitude toward the eliminative processes and products conditions the child's feelings in relation to them as well as to her. (Of course the mother's own childhood experiences and conditionings are important.) If she experiences excessive anxiety *or* excessive pleasure in her role, the negative or positive loading associated by the child to the structures and functions increases. In addition, the elimination process itself may have both positive and negative associations, for expulsion can be not only pleasurable but painful too. Here ambivalence is felt in the anal mode, as it was in the oral mode. Later anal differentiation, sometimes referred to as the anal retentive stage of development, which begins around the end of the first year usually, is characterized by stool retention as compared to the earlier stool expulsion. The child may find pleasure in the holding of the feces, a pleasure which can become overvalued if the holding serves other needs for him—irritating the parents ("anal sadism").

Compared to some other societies, the American culture is premature and harsh in toilet-training practices. Here, also, most evidence pertains to our middle-class families, who tend to start training very early and punish rather severely (Davis and Havighurst, 1946, 1947) in comparison to other socio-economic groups and culture. Whiting and Child, using ratings made of the anal training practices of 22 societies, have stated:

The median estimate for the beginning age of serious toilet training [for the 22 societies] falls at the age of two. Slightly over half of the primitive societies (fourteen out of twenty-five) begin toilet training somewhere between the ages of one and a half and two and a half. At the upper extreme there is one society (the Bena of Africa) where toilet training is not begun until the child is almost five years old. At the lower extreme there are two societies which begin toilet training during the child's first year. Our American middle class group falls near this extreme, as they . . . start toilet training when the child is only a little over six months old; this is earlier than is reported for all but one of the societies reviewed (Whiting and Child, 1953, p. 74).

In relation to *severity* of toilet training, the same authors rated 20 societies and found a numerical range of 18 (most severe) to 6 (least severe) with a median rating of 11. The American middle-class group was given a rating of 18, based on data from Davis and Havighurst (1947). This was the same rating given to the Tanala, the most severe of all the primitive societies studied, and reflects the extreme severity in toilet-training practices of the American group (Whiting and Child, 1953, pp. 76–77).

Some cultures have older siblings take the responsibility of bringing the child to toilet, but Western civilization has considered the "battle of cleanliness" so important that adult hands are delegated to avoid the social stigma of a "dirty" child. The higher the premium placed by the parents on rigid orderliness, punctuality, and neatness, the earlier and the more rigorous the toilet training will be, and the better the chances that the child will tend to incorporate or introject these attitudes, make them "his." Harsh parental control of elimination activities may produce conformity, but the unsatisfied wishes for anal indulgence will manifest themselves later, if not directly then through such substitute materials as mud, sand, water, and other substances more acceptable to elders. If these sublimated messing activities are denied also, more dissociated displacements will occur, as in the form of "dirty" or "filthy" talk, or by way of reaction-formations such as excessive neatness or overly pure, moralistic speech.

Western culture, then, more often places the mother in a conflictful position of having to choose between satisfying her neighbors or relatives and satisfying the child in terms of what appear to be his desires and abilities in anal activities; of course the resolution, though it may be only temporary, occurs primarily as a result of what is most satisfying to the mother. The emotionally mature mother will be more sensitive to the child's signals, more acceptant of his need for longer maturational periods, and more tenderly secure in her actions; and she will impart this tenderness and security to the child. On the other hand, the mother who is overanxious about toilet training imparts her anxiety to the child.

Such a mother is also apt to be the early diagnostician, to "diagnose," perhaps, that the child must be constipated. As an auxiliary to toilet-training procedures, laxatives or suppositories may be used. The more extensively they are used, the better the probability that this mother is fulfilling her own needs instead of the child's. Impatient with the child's "not learning," she absolves herself of failure by attributing the difficulty to a need for "medicine." Of course medicine may also be punishing, from the child's viewpoint, as his reactions may reveal upon having an enema administered to him. And, in fact, the anal insertion may be quite painful if the sphincters are not relaxed. On the other hand, if the child does care to relax, the procedure can become desirable if it has components of pleasure. Bowel evacuation produces equilibrium of a sort, and the consequent relief may serve as a forerunner to later passive-receptive attitudes to others in general. Overindulgence in such passive receptivity by the child can lead to a persistent parasitical relationship to the mother.

The nuclear issue concerns the rapidity and severity with which the child must relinquish his self-esteem in the face of possible derogation, conflict, and doubt. Will he give, or will he hold back? Will he use his holding back as a retaliatory weapon against those frustrating him? Will he become independent or give in to their wishes, do their bidding, make no decisions but those they want? Will he accept the responsibility which accompanies the accepting of these social demands? Will he retain a *status quo* (fixate, neither *give* nor *take* but *hold*). Or will he regress in behavior? At one moment he is pliable; the next, intractable. Now he lovingly cuddles; now he resists physical contact. The process of anal differentiation is a series of alternating or ambivalent feelings through which the child struggles to maintain an equilibrium and achieve a more mature integration of behavior. Toilet training, with all its implications of societal obligation, is really the first moral training to which the child is exposed—with its approval and disapproval, reward and punishment.

To offset or avoid disquieting impulses, the child may surrender to the toilet-training demands in order to "keep the peace." If severely cowed by elders who are unable to countenance any resistance to their authority, he may eventually stifle (inhibit) all overt anger behavior, including angry speech behavior. Deep concern about disapproval or withdrawal by the important adults may produce a speedy and complete conformity to the desired pattern. If conformity behavior is rigidly, sternly, and persistently reinforced, the end result may be a child with an extremely docile spirit. Chronic adult reactions of head-shaking, reprimand, disgust, tongue-clicking, harsh handling, and even slapping in anger are bound to bear bitter fruit.

In a healthy training environment, the mothering person rewards the child by cooperating tenderly in helping him to learn the social requirements of anal functions. The more the mothering one truly enjoys the activities (satisfaction in a job well done), the more effective, positive, and developmental will the learning be. Here the child is not forced to make a choice suddenly, prematurely, or under threat of pain. It is true he is going to be mildly frustrated, no matter how well-timed or unexacting the procedure may be, for after all, he has to relinquish some of his freedom by confining his expulsions to certain times and places. But even though the adult may be reacted to with some resistance, the secure child feels free to rebel somewhat and, in fact, is given some freedom in this behavior. Casual, firm, but tender handling helps to strengthen the child's own sense of inner goodness, from which will grow a deeper sense of autonomy, assurance, confidence. Rigid, stern management probably contributes to what we may call a sense of inner badness, from which will grow shame, doubt, and general self-derogation.

In the healthy anal-training setting, the child is not given too many developmental tasks to be accomplished at one time. For example, initiating sphincter training during the weaning period or the early word-learning period tends to be too demanding in terms of task load and differentiation necessities for many children. Developmental processes which are conflict- or anxiety-laden increase the possibilities for confusion among the various zones of interaction. Anxiety-motivated hyperconsciousness of cleanliness related to either the oral or anal functions may result in the apprehensions and taboos originally linked with one zone being equated, generalized, or displaced to another zone and function. Anal anxieties, confusions, or conflicts may "infect" oral processes, and vice versa. Everything that comes out of the body may be equated. The child's conception of cleanliness is tied up with bodily products. Feelings associated with anal cleanliness may be further generalized or associated to other body products such as urine, saliva, foodstuffs in regurgitation, oral sounds, or *words*. Both the oral and anal cavity produce sounds, and sounds, being highly similar, may be equated. Resentment due to toilet-training restraints often take the form of problems in eating. Previously untroublesome, the child, in rebellion against the overdemanding mother, refuses to eat, spits out his food, smears, throws, spills, and screams (Sterba, 1941). Just as he closes off, holds in, or ejects via the anal orifice, he may close off, hold in, or eject via the oral opening (and the urethral, also). The structural and functional similarities or equations of oral and anal pathways are revealed in our common language: holding back or pinching off = shutting up, not talking (delayed speech?); expelling, exploding = verbal explosion or blasting, popping-off; pleasurable elimination = babbling; diarrhea = logorrhea ("running off at the mouth"); and ambivalence = hesitant speech (stuttering) (approach-avoidance). Verbal displacements carrying strong emotions and occurring as profane language representing bodily products, parts, and functions are not uncommon; more diminutive forms are spoken by three- and four-years-olds (pee-pee, poo-poo, ka-ka, etc.). Belching or "giving the bird" have anal likenesses. Such behavior may be regarded as upward affective and motoric displacements from the anal to the oral level.

With time, even if toilet training is not administered *per se*, the child comes to assume self-control. In time, through voluntary repetition of the appropriate behavior, he comes to accept and use the behavior as his own, even though originally it was an introjection of parental wishes. To the degree, however, that the child has been unsuccessful in the differentiating and integrating requirements of the developmental task, he will be less capable of proceeding on to and adequately coping with successive tasks. Individuals who never really achieve full integration in this orificial function, especially those "fixated" at the oral level, are inclined, according to Freudian theory, to possess certain rather distinguishing traits. To illustrate, persons fixated at the anal-expulsive period of development are said to be suspicious, conceited, ambitious, and extremely interested in money (equated with valued objects, such as body products). They are apt to bear grudges, indulge in odd hobbies, and feel unappreciated. Anal-retentive fixations may be revealed by rituals or extreme meticulosity and pedantry. In addition, such persons may be duty-bound, regardless of the effect on loved ones or self; they may anger easily, be rigid in discipline of self and others, and be regarded by those around them as being basically unhappy. In therapy, their verbalizations are likely to reveal messing proclivities and hostile eliminative wishes, especially about important figures in their environment. This may be followed by guilt feelings, attempts at atonement, or thoughts of self-punishment, which in turn may lead to the development of docility as a form of self-defense in the therapeutic process (Erikson, 1950, p. 55).

Many people find it difficult to believe that inhibitions of zonal pleasures can have such more or less typical characterological results. We would agree that it is too extreme to think that specific character traits originate solely from frustrations connected invariably to the orificial functions and structures. It seems to us more logical and acceptable to believe that the child-rearing practices just discussed are primary components of a much larger configuration of environmental or parental attitudes. The parent who initiates toilet training prematurely and follows through harshly is the one more inclined to initiate and pursue other child-training procedures similarly, including the speech-training practices. In short, the individual's eventual speech or general behavioral integrity or disequilibrium is determined by the *totality* of cultural and family demands and by the *unique pattern* of the attitude systems which permeate the total behavior of the elders. Ausubel has made a strong point of this view, asserting among other things, the following:

> . . . the characterological consequences of a specific toilet training practice may be expected to *vary* depending on the particular generalized attitude it typifies in a given parent. For example, *one possible* general orientation toward child rearing that *may* be expressed in coercive toilet training is undue emphasis upon conformity, orderliness, self-control, and punctiliousness. But even if this is the case, the parent undoubtedly inculcates these same values in countless other direct and indirect ways throughout the entire period of childhood. Under these circumstances, it seems more credible to believe that if a school child treats his money, clothes, and notebooks with exaggerated care it is because of the cumulative impact of such indoctrination rather than solely because of the rigid toilet training he experienced as an infant (Ausubel, 1957, p. 251).

The mistake of linking a discrete behavioral deviation with a highly specific training method or function is very much like the situation which existed for many years in speech pathology in which some workers and many laymen assumed that a change in handedness caused stuttering. Although some significant differences were found in the incidence of handedness changes between stuttering and non-stuttering persons, it seems evident to us today that the changing of handedness is merely one reflection of a general system of attitudes found among parents who are inclined to be coercive in many other training procedures involving the "changing over" of unacceptable behavior.

LATER CHILDHOOD DIFFERENTIATION AND INTEGRATION

From about the third to the seventh year, a great many challenges and changes occur in the life of the developing child. We recognize this as the period during which children are usually judged as being "non-fluent," "deviant," "delayed," or "normal" speakers. Freudian theorists maintain that this span of life can be best viewed as revolving primarily around two behavioral cores: (1) the ascendance to primacy of genital eroticism, and (2) the presence of the oedipal situation.

The genital zone serves as the important erogenous foundation-structure in psychosocial development, with the focal surmountings being the penis in the boy and the clitoris in the girl. The genital zone has already been prepared for its role as an excitation focus by the earlier contacts by the mother in the activities of cleaning, diaper-changing, and powdering, and by the child's own manual manipulation of the genitalia. The following account by Hutt and Gibby is a clear and representative explanation of the psychoanalytic conception of the "oedipal conflict":

The boy has already developed a strong emotional attachment to his mother. . . . He has come to be emotionally dependent upon her, he has been fondled and played with by her, and his physical and most of his social needs have been met by her. . . . This relationship takes on a sexual quality, since erotogenic satisfactions become greatly heightened. She now becomes . . . his love object. During this same period, the boy also has learned to like his father. But the intensity of this relationship seems pale by contrast with the other. . . . The boy's relationship with both parents is complicated and contains contradictory elements. While he normally loves his mother, he also is irritated and frustrated by her and at times feels he hates her. . . . His relationship with the father also contains some hostile elements, since the father is not as available as the boy would like, he may be "rougher" and more punitive. . . . The little boy is quite content during the day to be with his mother . . . , to receive her attention and affection. . . . But when father comes home, . . . the mother devotes her attention to him and thus the father . . . becomes an object of special hostility . . . depriving the boy of his intense emotional satisfactions from the mother. Moreover, the father . . . appears to be a rival for the mother, because he is much bigger and stronger and because he becomes the external representation of the little boy's own guilt and fears produced by his own ambivalences.

This is the crux of the oedipal situation. Many factors complicate it.

In normal emotional development, the boy learns gradually to identify with his father . . . to repress successfully his oedipal wishes

for his mother and to assume a more masculine role. During this period he will more often "act up" in opposition to his mother. . . .

[If the parents are not mature, healthy adults] the resolution of the
oedipal conflict is vastly complicated, an *oedipal complex* develops,
and becomes the "nuclear core" of subsequent neurotic patterns. Even
when favorable conditions do obtain . . . there is some period of
turmoil. . . . Boys become (more) aware of their penises . . . are
afraid that they are not big enough; they may be concerned lest they
should lose them . . . as surely must have been the case with girls.
. . . In short, they may have experienced some *castration fears*. . . .
They will not, however, develop *castration anxiety* if good conditions
for effective growth . . . are present.

. . . If the parents are neurotic, effective identification and changes
in identification are virtually impossible. If the mother is a phallic
person and the father is a passive . . . person, the appropriate role
development will not take place.

. . . in the girl, we find the situation more complicated. Like the
boy, she also identified first with her mother and obtained . . . gratification from her. Also like the boy, her area of sexual primacy has
now become the . . . clitoris (phallus) . . . but the girl has to give
up her phallic organization and . . . accept a feminine organization.
She has to go through one additional step . . . she will learn to
identify with her father, as the boy did, but then she will have to
renounce this in favor of a *reidentification* with the mother and the
role of a woman.

The girl's problems are also complicated by . . . other factors
[such as] . . . *penis envy*, for little girls become aware that they do
not have a penis like a boy, nor do they yet have the compensating
feature of breast development (Hutt and Gibby, 1957, pp. 95–99).

Freud's early hypothesis regarding neurosis was that the
traumatic experience of sexual seduction by an older person
was the origin of the disorder. He later observed, however,
that the frequent production of such materials by patients
in therapy often were merely recollections of *fantasies* of
childhood. From this he concluded rather unequivocally
that, since all neurotics seemed to have such fantasies, children who became neurotic adults must have experienced
such wish-fulfilling fantasies. Ultimately, Freud contended
that all children experience such fantasies. Such were the
origins of Freud's theory of the Oedipus complex.

The issues of whether or not boys experience sexual feelings toward their mothers, become their father's rivals, and develop neurotically if unable to handle the anxiety and resolve the situation are fertile areas for argument among childhood specialists. For instance, Freud's basic postulations included the concept of a biologically predetermined instinctual system in the organism. Some think this overlooked the importance of a *cultural* inheritance. The attitudes of the child's parents are molded by cultural influences, and the fact that such experiences as castration anxiety, masturbation repressions, and the like are not culturally universal but are found only in certain societies (Kardiner, 1947) cast a shadow on the assumption that psychological processes are biologically determined. Also, it is very difficult to specify accurately the degree to which infantile pleasure-seeking is "orally" or "genitally" focused, or whether the pleasures are related to the entire gamut of tender experiences which are associated with the mothering one.

In our society, the boy's friendliness with his mother is a logical effect of the close emotional relationship and support which the child has experienced since birth. The father has been a part-time visitor who remains rather vaguely defined until the child reaches school age. Whereas affection between mother and son is quite acceptable in our culture, such exchanges between father and son may elicit feelings of discomfort or embarrassment on the part of father, son, or onlookers. In addition, studies show that the mother is the preferred parent, not only by boys but of girls also (Mott, 1937; Simpson, 1935). That preschool children have sexual interests is undeniable, although it is part of a broad pattern of interest in and exploration of the world around them and of themselves. There is ample evidence (Ford and Beach, 1951) that young children indulge in sexual activity: frequent masturbatory practices, inquisitiveness about sexual parts and functions and procreation, and "doctor" and leg-riding games. But such behavior is qualitatively different from the sexual behavior of adults. "It lacks the social significance of adult eroticism, its significance in the total economy of personality organization, its rich feeling tones, its urgency and regularity, and its status as an absorbing interest in its own right separate from other play" (Ausubel, 1957, p. 254).

The genital and oedipal differentiation phase can, for our purposes, be more parsimoniously dealt with as a period during which the child's main problem is one of coping with the cultural and parental demands upon him to conform or to submit to their authority. The pattern of parental attitudes to which he was exposed in completing earlier developmental tasks is more than likely highly similar to the pattern he will experience in genital/oedipal differentiation tasks. When he has experienced a supportive, permissive, realistic relationship with his caretakers, differentiation and integration will occur. When he has experienced a rejecting and punitive relationship with his caretakers, fixation or regression (disintegration) will occur. The emphasis in our thinking is not on the "sexual" interplay between parent and child but on the broader configuration of parental attitudes and reaction-patterns, past and present, as they appear to be affecting current behavior, *including* "genital" or "oedipal" behavior. The child who is made to feel guilty about genital parts and processes is in most cases the child who is made to feel guilty about *other* parts and processes (feeding, evacuating, vocalizing). The guilty child is the one who is fearful of irritating the feared ones, and in severely holding back his impulses, he humiliates, derogates, punishes, and frustrates himself. In general he represses the drive to release his fullest potential because of this stultifying self-control.

During approximately the fourth year, the child, if he has successfully developed and integrated his skills in language, locomotion, and exploration, moves on to newer and more complex situations, meeting other people and interacting with them. He broadens and enriches his spheres of action beyond the immediate family. He experiences greater variations in handling and attitudes by the new elders (neighbors, teachers) who supervise his activities. His is a learning ground of animal land, fantasy land, nursery school, social mixing, and speech interaction. In his play, he verbalizes many things, including perhaps the wish that father will go away or not come home from work today. He may reveal his competitiveness with his rival through comparisons of the father's bodily parts to his own. Physical aggression toward the father is observed commonly, often without evident reason ("Let's fight" or "I beat you, all right?" or "You be the bad guy, O.K.?"). Whether or not such attitudes or behavior become anxiety-laden depends on the nature of the father's reaction to them, as well as on the child's previous history. Yet even when the father's response is merely a mildly negative one, the child may, out of proportion to reality, assume that he himself would certainly be angry were he to be treated (or thought of) in this hostile way. In this case might not his father become angry? In some children's thinking, the more effective the victory over the father concerning the winning of mother's time and affections, the angrier the rival must become. The authors have encountered a number of stuttering individuals whose behavior in therapy reflected this kind of dynamic: the feeling of complete attachment with and dependence on the mother; the feeling of rivalry and hostility toward the father; the presence of maternal overprotection; and the heightened fear of the father, owing to the person's successful "ensnarement" of the mother.

From approximately age six or seven to puberty, in most cultures there is a decline in the amount of observable or expressed curiosity concerning "private" parts and functions. Children tend to become more well-behaved or "moral," generally inhibited. Not that the forbidden impulses are denied entirely, for many children will continue such activity but more covertly. Healthy children will tend to rechannel their energies into more socially acceptable pursuits. Anxious ones will tend to "overlearn" their defensive behavior, and in so doing, repress and encapsulate the tabooed desires. In such instances, curiosity in general is likely to become inhibited. The child may become overly pensive or withdrawn, his language more restricted. The experience of formal education occurs, and schooling may not only educate and cultivate, but it may also frustrate. For, unlike the relative freedom associated with the preschool period, there are now desks at which to remain seated; groups to which one must conform; adult-chosen work materials which are to be used at certain times and in specified ways; new authority figures who are likely to have rather definite expectations of what children should do and who tend to reward in accordance with degree of compliance shown. At about age 8 or 9 the child's need to identify more closely with groups grows stronger. Even at this age "in-groups" and "out-groups" are readily observable. The child who is different may wear the invisible stripes of rejection and become, in the case of a stutterer for example, multiply handicapped.

The onset of puberty may further intensify the conflicts which are unresolved in earlier life. Sometimes this "return of the repressed" may manifest itself in the recurrence of verbal symptoms which have perhaps disappeared or become more quiescent during the latency period. The adolescent's new biosocial urges threaten to overwhelm his capacity for self-control. His drive for a sense of individuality and independence requires not only that he rebel against his elders but that he also rebel against himself, against his own *conscience*.

THE ACQUISITION OF CONSCIENCE

The neonate has little awareness of the world beyond his own body. His experience is permeated with unlearned ("instinctual") drives which demand immediate satisfaction. He is, in short, dominated by the "pleasure principle," completely *self*-centered. When he is hungry, he wants to eat without delay; when he feels the need to suck, he mouths whatever is available. By doing so he achieves sensory gratification, a sense of comfort, a feeling of closeness. When he is soiled, he makes his wants known clearly and immediately. Soon, however, his own wants encounter those of other people whose wishes may not agree with his. Perhaps he is put on a feeding schedule which is most convenient for mother but which may not be suitable to his individual hunger cycle. Maybe his hands are covered or confined so as to keep him from sucking his fingers. Perhaps he is allowed to cry a little longer before being changed. He experiences increasing amounts of pain and frustration as the elders strive to mold him to prevailing customs. He has little tolerance for delay, but delay he must. He does not understand why he must wait for satisfactions; still, immediate denial of gratifications continues. But he is helpless and completely dependent on those around him. Denied the help he seeks, he needs it all the more and increases his demands. As he grows older, he strives more vigorously for what he wants; yet, he continues to be blocked and impeded in his attempts. As he tries to explore pots, pans, ash trays and wastebaskets, he is countered with "do, don't, must, must not, nice boy, and naughty." The pleasurable handling of body parts or products is interfered with and the "right" ways of eating at the table are enforced. Certain things he cannot do; others he can, but even then only at certain times, in certain places. When? Where? It is difficult for him to know. He fears that he may do the wrong thing—perhaps, out of fear, he does nothing, *says* nothing.

In such ways are the concepts and attitudes of "right" and "wrong" derived from the process of parental checking. The child learns that parental love is forthcoming when he acts as his parents wish him to act. To retain them as love objects and sources, he adopts their behavior, demanding of himself what they demand of him. Rather than resistance or evasion, there is more docility and self-criticism. He learns that by making parental-societal standards his own, he can not only quiet parental reactions but he can also quiet certain of his immediate inner disturbances. Basic urges become throttled or expressed in more socially acceptable ways. The "parentalization of the instincts" will occur, harshly or tenderly, throughout childhood. This process of introjection or internalization of the parental wishes ensures that the child never again will be a completely independent unit. The parents literally have gotten "under his skin." Never again will he be alone. He will reflect, in some way, his parents' attitudes toward money, play, sex, religion, politics, and people for the remainder of his life.

The conscience may be thought of as a set of inhibitory reaction patterns whose genesis lies in the introjections by the child of early parental prohibitions and dicta. These inhibitory reaction patterns are triggered by acts or wishes which transgress the parental moral code. The child, once punished by the parents for overstepping the moral boundaries, now not only punishes himself at so doing but also, for the most part, is unaware of the sources of his attitudes and reactions. They are deeply a part of him, though largely an unconscious part of him. If his conscience is not a harsh one, he is apt to be an adjusted person—independent, aware of self, pliable, confident. In fact, as we shall note later, the strongest conscience probably is a strongly differentiated and integrated ego or self.

The person with a healthy conscience is one whose childhood training or "checking" process was administered by parents who were creative and democratic; who made the restrictions fit the occasion and the child's needs; who always associated fundamentally positive feelings with the training; who conveyed that they loved the child even though they were frustrating him at the moment; who were realistic in their wishes; parents who themselves were sufficiently acceptant of self not to be threatened by the everyday minor transgressions of their child. In such a case, the hand of the potter would not go awry. Certainly, the ideal is difficult to reach in today's mode of living—close friends, neighbors, in-laws, many offering advice, reacting negatively to one's ideas of raising children; the conflicts between having a spotless house or happy children in a confusion of toys; eighteenth-century furniture or something less expensive that will cause little concern if the children mar it; a child meticulously clean or one often muddy; toilet training to begin at six months or two years. The choice is not an easy one. The child in jeopardy of acquiring a harsh conscience and thus of experiencing adjustment discomforts is the one who probably had parents having, more or less chronically, several or more of the following characteristics: rigidity or automaticity of attitudes and opinions; an overly strict code of conduct; punitive manner; righteousness or overambition; extreme self-sacrifice (demanding payment for their relinquishments).

Perhaps it is helpful to distinguish between a self-debasing conscience,* which inhibits and stereotypes behavior, and a self-enhancing conscience, which aids the individual in remaining within the accepted behavior boundaries of his group while developing purposive ideas and ambitions. The former is closer to the Freudian concept of *superego*, which refers primarily to inhibitory reaction patterns, restraints, and the stern and steretyped behavior which we associate with righteous, puritanical persons. The self-enhancing conscience is more similar to the Freudian *ego-ideal*, wherein, through positive identification with loving, supportive parents or parent-substitutes, a person pursues standards of goodness and accomplishment which relate not only to what he thinks *ought* to be but also to what he genuinely *wishes* to be. The self-enhancing conscience functions so as to retain, shape, or release basic and more complex impulses in a manner geared to the attainment of ideals. The self-debasing conscience functions as a control or suppressor of impulses, as a forbidding censor.

The parental frustrations or punishments arouse in the child feelings of hostility which, if expressed, produce parental retaliation which further increases the child's aggression. Fearful that open rebellion may produce not only punishment but desertion by or loss of the parents, and thus loss of need-satisfaction sources, the child accedes to parental wishes. He takes into and makes as part of his own system their attitudes, ideals, and prohibitions. This is the process of *introjection*, which will be discussed in the next chapter.

* To speak of superego, conscience, ego, self, id, or basic impulses structuralizes any conceptualization out of proportion to the true dynamic nature of the processes involved. It is recognized that these descriptions are arbitrary constructs employed as referential verbal landmarks for the sake of discussion.

For now, let us say that a person may introject not only negative or restraining tendencies but also positive tendencies,
such as kindness and tolerance. The child with consistent,
moderate, firm but kind parents recognizes societal obliga-
tions, and he wishes to do what is reasonably expected of
him. He is pliable and susceptible to change when he is
given suggestions or advice. He assumes patterns of attitudes from both parents. He perceives his parents in a way
which is in close agreement with what they actually are.

In general, harsher threats increase the severity of the
conscience. Parents who are unreasonable or sternly derogatory in their treatment of a child's abortive speech attempts
generate anxiety within the child. And the child, striving
to be what they wish, introjects these parental attitudes and
demands. The code which he adopts is so demanding, however, that he is constantly fearful of breaking it, i.e., not
behaving as the parents wish and as he himself thinks he
should. He finds himself in a conflict. He may project the
internalized restrictions onto those about him and behave
toward those persons in a rebellious or aggressive fashion
(including hostile speech behavior). Or he may repress or
suppress the introjected parental feelings in addition to
thwarting his urge to release such anxiety-provoking feelings
(through projection or outright rejection); i.e., he may keep
his feelings (and his speech) to himself, thereby intensifying
his own state of inner conflict. Finally, he may waver between these two basic alternatives, releasing (speaking) at
one time, holding in (not speaking) at another. Stuttering,
in this light, would be regarded as a symptom of the conscience in a quandary. Stuttering individuals would be
thought of as persons with overwhelming, harsh consciences,
whose struggles to quell their anxiety were being revealed
by "speech in a quandary"; speech alternatingly expressed
and repressed (or suppressed).

It is important to note, however, that the severity of
parental demands may be either minimized or exaggerated
by the introjecting child. Moderate parental restrictions may
be perceived as severe suppression by the child, for introjec-

tion is not only a function of external reality but of internal experience as well. The child perceives and introjects according to his needs and not merely according to "what is there." If he projects negative feelings into the parental figures (i.e., attributes feelings to them which they actually do not possess), he introjects *these* attributes also in addition to whatever elements the parents bring to the situation. In such cases the child may come to censure himself much more severely than his parents ever intended. The higher the correlation between what is *perceived* and what is externally *actual,* the more differentiated and integrated is the child. The greater the *discrepancy* between what the child perceives and what is external reality, the less differentiated and integrated (more anxious or neurotically inclined) is the child. The more harsh the demands of conscience within the child, the greater will be the internal conflict with its feelings of inferiority, guilt, and tendencies toward self-effacement or self-derogation.

The infusion of conscience, then, starts as soon as parental restrictions begin. The process embraces the parental restricting behavior of early infancy, as in the regulation of eating times. It grows in intensity and frequency during the toilet-training days. It continues to develop and becomes consolidated as the youngster is cautioned about touching certain objects; seeing certain forbidden acts or situations; using certain words, speaking in certain ways, or speaking at all in various settings. If feelings of jealousy or hostility toward the parents are felt, the child learns to "join forces" (take the parents' point of view) in order to keep the peace and the parental love. The socialization process is contributed to by older siblings, teachers, and others who assume responsibility for managing or educating the child. In all these interactions the conscience of the child is being strengthened and consolidated, for better or for worse.

In later life (during and after adolescence), the harsh conscience may manifest itself most strongly as a feeling of *obligation* toward the earlier generation (the "founding fathers"). Is it not because of the sacrifices and struggles of the parents that he is here at all—and does this not demand "payment"? In such ways do the elders exist, even after they have passed on, as persistently powerful "spirits" requiring homage, respect, and, sometimes above all, obedience. Through such transmissions do humans submit or become compelled, adjusting themselves to the rules of the elders.

The conflict-ridden or undifferentiated conscience is revealed in infantile ways of perceiving the attitudes, reaction patterns, and feelings of others. It is revealed by distorted perceptions of reality and by attributions of traits which are extremely inconsistent with truth. The nonintegrated conscience is actually in conflict with the basic self-system of the individual, for its infantile and harsh nature clashes with the person's ideal concept of self and with his basic self-wishes. The person is torn between the need to satisfy the demands of conscience (for example, to keep high moral and speech standards; in fact, his speech *is* his morality) and the need to satisfy his own basic urges. Often a compromise solution is effected, with the person attempting to satisfy both masters. Behavior becomes oriented to the attainment of basic gratification while simultaneously appeasing the demands of conscience. Such behavior may partially satisfy the need to be aggressive as well as partially gratify the desire to be nonaggressive (conform to conscience demands).

In therapy settings, one of the most common goals in working with stuttering individuals is the modification or reduction of the demands of an overwhelming conscience. The person must be helped (1) to release and to gain more understanding of the repressing forces of conscience which are plaguing him (by seeing the unreality and the nonproductivity of its demands); (2) to re-experience and reassess his introjected objects—to perceive his parents, siblings, and teachers as they are, to perceive himself as he really is; (3) to accept others and himself as they actually are with all their strengths and weaknesses; (4) to learn socially acceptable and development modes of satisfying the demands of the conscience; (5) to increase his awareness or consciousness of his world in every way; (6) to chart and to activate his own behavior rather than be driven by the twisted and archaic introjections of childhood.

REFERENCES

ALEXANDER, F. *Psychosomatic Medicine.* New York: W. W. Norton & Co., Inc., 1950.

AUSUBEL, D. *Theory and Problems of Child Development.* New York: Grune & Stratton, Inc., 1957.

COGHILL, G. E. "The Early Development of Behavior in Amblystoma and Man," *Arch. Neurol. Psychiat.,* **21**: 989–1009, 1929.

DAVIS, W. A., and HAVIGHURST, R. J. *Father of the Man.* Boston: Houghton Mifflin Co., 1947.

———. "Social Class and Color Differences in Child-rearing," *Amer. Sociol. Rev.,* **11**: 698–710, 1946.

DUNBAR, F. *Psychosomatic Diagnosis.* New York: Paul B. Hoeber, Inc., 1943.

ERIKSON, E. H. *Childhood and Society.* New York: W. W. Norton & Co., Inc., 1950.

FORD, C. S., and BEACH, F. A. *Patterns of Sexual Behavior.* New York: Harper & Bros., 1951.

FREUD, S. *New Introductory Lectures in Psychoanalysis.* New York: W. W. Norton & Co., Inc., 1933.

FRIES, M. E. "The Child's Ego Development and the Training of Adults in His Environment." In *The Psychoanalytic Study of the Child,* Vol. II. New York: International Universities Press, Inc., 1946.

HILGARD, E. R. *Theories of Learning,* 2d ed. New York: Appleton-Century-Crofts, Inc., 1956.

HUSCHKA, M. "The Child's Response to Coercive Bowel Training," *Psychosom. Med.,* **4**: 301–8, 1942.

HUTT, M. L., and GIBBY, R. G. *Patterns of Abnormal Behavior.* Englewood Cliffs, N. J.: Allyn & Bacon, Inc., 1957.

KARDINER, A. *The Individual and His Society.* New York: Columbia Univ. Press, 1947.

KLUCKHOHN, C., and MURRAY, H. A. *Personality in Nature, Society, and Culture.* New York: Alfred A. Knopf, Inc., 1950.

LEIGHTON, D., and KLUCKHOHN, C. *Children of the People.* Cambridge: Harvard Univ. Press, 1947.

McGRAW, M. "Neural Maturation as Exemplified in Achievement of Bladder Control," *J. Pediat.,* **16**: 580, 1940.

MOTT, S. M. "Mother-Father Preference," *Charact. and Person.,* **5**: 302–4, 1937.

SIMPSON, M. *Parent Preference of Young Children.* New York: Teachers College, Columbia Univ., 1935.

STERBA, E. "An Important Factor in Eating Disturbances of Childhood," *Psychoanal. Quart.*, **10**: 365–72, 1941.

SULLIVAN, H. S. *The Interpersonal Theory of Psychiatry.* New York: W. W. Norton & Co., Inc., 1953.

WHITING, J. W. M., and CHILD, I. L. *Child Training and Personality: A Cross-cultural Study.* New Haven: Yale Univ. Press, 1953.

WOLFE, S., and WOLFF, H. G. *Human Gastric Function: An Experimental Study of Man and His Stomach.* New York: Oxford Univ. Press, 1947.

Chapter 5

The Self-Process, Anxiety, and Speech Dysfunctions

Which can say more than the rich praise—that you alone are you.——Shakespeare

DIFFERENTIATION AND INTEGRATION IN THE SELF-PROCESSES

In a very deep sense, the fundamental process around which the speaking, socializing, and total behavior of a person revolves is the *self-process.** To a very considerable extent a person's stuttering is determined by what he thinks of himself or of his "speech self," consciously or otherwise. His (1) attitudes toward, his perceptions of, and his feelings about himself and his speech, (2) his value concepts of himself and his speech-self, (3) his mode of enhancing or protecting himself and his speech-self, all will determine not only what and how he speaks but also when and where he speaks.

The self-process consists of consciously or unconsciously experienced feelings, thoughts, evaluations, and wishes which relate to the individual's present, past, or future concept of "me or mine." The self-process operates, in conjunction with external stimuli (the environment), as the most important

---

* The *self* is regarded in this book not as a *thing*, which would connote a topological entity similar to the psychoanalytic concepts of id and superego, but as an organismic process, a "self-process." In like manner was *conscience* regarded as process, rather than a thing.

determinant of the individual's speech behavior and inter-personal adjustment. It has as its purpose the maximum life- and speech-integration of the individual. Although on the one hand the self-process is an interaction of the different "parts" or dynamic focuses of the total organism, it is also a *resultant* and *affector* of the organism's interaction with his surroundings. The self-process is, in short, *subjectivity*, the feeling and apprehension of a person about himself and the world around him as experienced in terms of the needs of his self-structure.

The self-process, then, is the quintessence of human be-havior. A person may have not only conscious evaluations of self or speech but also evaluations of which he is only subliminally aware, plus evaluations which may be uncon-scious. He may have a conscious perception of self which is self-enhancing, but he may also have an unconscious self-percept which is derogatory, as has been revealed experi-mentally (Huntley, 1940). Stated differently, a person's total self-image or speech self-picture may differ from the objective or actual self. The greater the difference, the more nonintegrated or maladjusted the person will become. The stuttering adolescent who "honestly believes" that he does not stutter, but who has been judged to be a stuttering person by four qualified clinicians, is an individual unable to perceive his own behavior without distortion and to assess and interpret his deviant speech realistically. His self-image does not correlate well with objective fact (see the case of Steven, Chapter 11).

The kind of self-structure a person develops in the course of his acculturation derives mainly from his cultural group (which provides the frame upon which his role behavior is built), from the personalities of the people with whom he lives; more specifically, from the way in which his early socialization is worked out by his elders. For it is in infancy that self-differentiation begins. Increasingly, the infant dif-ferentiates his own body from the environment as he becomes more aware that his body has an intimate connection to his experiences. Tactual, kinesthetic, and somasthetic sensations accompany all his experiences, and it is not long before he recognizes that hitting a toy car with a hammer is not quite the same as hitting a finger. The successful completion of successive developmental tasks increases self-integrity by giving the child a feeling of satisfaction with himself (satisfying his need for self-esteem or approval), increasing his self-confidence, and nurturing continuing self-differentiation and self-integration. As the child grows, he needs to believe that certain decisions are his own, that regardless of whether he is, for example, speaking more or less, or not speaking at all, the choice is very much his own. Otherwise, he will reject himself as unworthy or inferior. Increasing and prolonged self-rejection may lead to overt or covert expressions of self-criticism or self-abasement, feelings of guilt and anxiety, and oftentimes extreme submission and depression.

A child who has just completed a developmental task, for example, one who has learned to name objects, repeats the achievement again and again. As he does so, he is aware of himself as "a person who can name things," with whatever connotation this behavior may carry in his particular life space. Erikson believes that the incorporation of this new status into the self-system, particularly if associated with environmental mastery and social recognition, strengthens the child's self-esteem. "The growing child must, at every step, derive a vitalizing sense of reality from the awareness that his individual way of mastering experience (his ego synthesis) is a successful variant of a group identity and is in accord with its space-time and life plan" (Erikson, 1950, p. 208).

The nature of the child's experiences governs largely what his self-concept will be. This speech or general behavior, whether acceptable or not acceptable, elicits reactions. These reactions, especially from the important elders, may be essentially positive (developmental, self-enhancing) or negative (disintegrating, fixating, self-derogatory). Such reactions—physical, expressionistic, "labelistic" ("naming")—when consistently used, will come to be accepted by the child as a part of himself. The reacting elders can be thought of as psychological mirrors which give back to the child a reflection of himself which is realistic or distorted, which is gratifying (self-integrating) or belitting (self-disintegrating). Likewise, his self-concept will determine considerably the kind of role he will portray in his life situations. His attitudes, reactions, and manner of speaking will affect greatly how others will react. These reactions are fed back into his own system, further contributing to his positive, negative, or confused self-concept. If a person's stuttering speech often provokes painful reactions from the environment, self-underestimation is strengthened, producing nondifferentiating and nonintegrative behavior which is even more intractable. In one way, a stuttering person's self-concept may be thought of as his *expectancy* of what may happen to him in various situations. These *expectancies* are major determinants of behavior. They are especially disintegrative or disruptive if they are imbued with fear or anxiety.

In child rearing or in therapy with stuttering persons, the major goal is to help the person to strengthen his self-process; to regard himself as a person of worth, a person of abilities, acceptant of his limitations but aware of his capabilities and without excessive egocentricity or excessive humility. We wish to extend the person's realm of consciousness, to make him aware of and acceptant of basic life urges. We wish to help him to perceive himself and the world around him in a realistic, undistorted fashion; to be able better to assess or evaluate himself as he actually is; to develop self-initiative, self-direction, self-consistency, autonomy. In short, the goal of child rearing and therapy alike is to establish the self-process as a differentiated, integrating life force geared to the attainment of fullest self-realization. Perhaps, most basically, the goal is to help the person to *like* himself, deeply, acceptingly, and realistically. Although the individual's struggle is to attain the fullest actualization of self, the ultimate goal is reached when the person becomes a *social self*, one who not only is self-acceptant but also one who identifies and lives fully, happily, and productively with his fellow man.

ANXIETY, FEAR, AND SPEECH DYSFUNCTIONS

The root experience which interferes with maximal self-integration or speech integration is *anxiety*. Concepts of anxiety have been very troublesome because of the great number and range of meanings which have been developed by workers who have differing theoretical starting points. A review of the anxiety literature will reveal that generalities, contradictory descriptions, and multiple definitions abound even within the same work. Even the most fruitful literature is phrased tentatively, and general agreement occurs on only one point—that much remains to be learned. Clarification problems occur because of the close relationship of this experience with almost all other personality dynamics. In fact, all nonintegrative personality dynamics involve anxiety as causal or effectual concomitants in some degree. In addition, the very attempt to be specific in analyzing or describing the nature of anxiety or in relating it to particular objects or situations is artificial because we remove one of the primary conditions necessary for anxiety arousal; namely, the presence of threatening stimuli of which we are only dimly aware or which we cannot identify.

Anxiety may be thought of as being either *generalized* or *specific*. In the speech pathology literature, Wischner (1952), for example, has suggested the terms "general situational anxiety" and "specific word anxiety." Van Riper speaks of the stuttering person's fear as being an "expectation of unpleasantness," and he, too, speaks of generalized fear and specific, or word, fear in the following manner:

. . . the first feared words or sounds to develop are either (1) those that by frequency of occurrence under communicative stress have had more association with past stuttering, or (2) those that have been severely and vividly penalized by other people when a block appeared on them. The first situation fears develop in the same way.

Gradually these fears spread to other words and situations. As the fears increase, they become attached to certain sounds. Words themselves become invested with various other cues which set off a specific expectancy of stuttering. . . . Words become things. Letters become either hard or easy. In a similar manner, other cues develop which precipitate fear of stuttering in a general situation. . . .

When a stutterer has developed such decided fears of unpleasantness . . . he immediately begins to devise tricks to prevent or reduce that unpleasantness (avoidance, postponing, use of starters, anti-expectancy devices). These . . . at first offer temporary relief, but finally they become only a habitual reaction to the fear of block and thus a part of the handicap (Van Riper, 1947, p. 283).

In the psychological literature, anxiety is differentiated from fear. *Fear* generally refers to apprehensive states which are related to *known* objects or situations that are, to a great extent, consciously understood and susceptible to appraisal. Such a concept of fear would have been termed "objective anxiety" by Freud. The critical feature of *anxiety* is its element of the *unknown*. Anxiety is a diffuse apprehension which at the moment of experiencing cannot be linked in awareness with its objective referents. Usually it is accompanied by a feeling of helplessness. To illustrate, the stuttering individual who is consciously aware that he dreads speaking to a hostile audience is experiencing fear. He is able to point to, or name, the objective fear-stimulus, the hostile audience. The same person, in conversation with a friend with whom he usually feels at ease and is verbally fluent, may experience vague feelings of apprehension, tension, or general discomfort, but he may be unable to connect this feeling state to specific objects or situations. He is unable to "point to" or "name" the instigator. This is anxiety, and it may be a brief or chronic state. The term "free-floating anxiety" has been used to describe such an experience. The person is upset, but he doesn't know what upsets him. Even in the apparent fear situations in which the individual is aware of the object of his fear, for example, fear of a hostile audience, there may also be anxiety; i.e., there may be factors in that particular setting which create inner tension but which are not recognized or identified by him. He may attempt to give meaning to the situation when objective meaning is really not there; i.e., he will strive for closure, perhaps by rationalizing. He may relate the uneasy feeling to one object, then to another, without realistic differentiation.

We observe that anxiety and fear can be differentiated on the basis of degree of perceptual discrimination, the source of anxiety being less discriminable, if at all. Fear and anxiety states may also be distinguished on the basis of response specificity. The stuttering adolescent may react to fear by (1) removing the fear (deciding not to elect a course in public speaking); (2) fleeing from the fear (failing to arrive for a job interview); (3) neutralizing the fear (getting the listener to like him—or to fear him); or (4) ignoring or denying the fear by apathetic behavior (rationalizing not speaking to strangers: "Why speak to them anyway? It's not important, and I'm really not interested.") But response to anxiety, due to the diffuse, unidentifiable nature of the threatening feelings, is much more randomized, generalized, and even haphazard. It is difficult or impossible to (1) remove, (2) flee from, (3) neutralize, or (4) deny a threat which cannot be identified or actualized.

For our discussion, *anxiety* is defined as a state of apprehension or dread due to some threat to the integrity or developmental progression of the self-process caused by frustrating forces of which the individual is only vaguely aware and with which he feels incapable of coping. The threat may be stimulated exogenously (situational fear with loss of objective environmental referents) or endogenously (internal promptings in the form of intolerable feelings, thoughts, and desires which threaten to expose themselves). In most instances, there is probably accompanying somatic tension, and in all cases the root danger is a threat to the goodness of interpersonal relationships.

As has been stated earlier, the original experience of anxiety probably occurs in relation to the early infant-mother relationships. Sullivan has said that "The tension of anxiety . . . in the mothering one induces anxiety in the infant" (Sullivan, 1953, p. 41). The dynamics of this process are not completely clear. It seems certain, however, that the young child is not very capable of identifying and differentiating sources of discomfort. He cannot easily discriminate or relate his tensions to specific sources in his environment or to specific body structures and functions. This non-specificity is the core of anxiety. It is the ingredient which makes it difficult for the child to differentiate (be aware of, perceive realistically, discriminate, adjust to). He learns no consistently effective response to the disturbance. Nor is there differentiation in the infant's still generalized and vague mental state between fear and anxiety, for his cognitive differentiation is still very much in evolution. The ability to make such fine discriminations as between internal and external threats, real and fantasied dangers, and angry and happy voice is an advanced phase of the evolving intra-personal and interpersonal differentiation and integration process.

The increase in specificity of *cognition* proceeds in conjunction with *perceptual* and *motor* differentiations and specificity. Throughout, the child is faced with the challenge of acquiring new and more difficult discriminatory and self-monitoring behavior. In an infinite number of ways the responsible elders communicate to him that they "expect" him to do this task; for example, sucking the nipple instead of biting it, speaking or crying only at certain times, saying a new word, or speaking more clearly or fluently. The very point at which he is to move on or not move on to the next level of development is the decisive moment. Will his efforts to prove adequate to the task be met with adult acceptance and affection, leading to feelings of personal worth *regardless* of success or failure? Will he be reacted to with retaliatory behavior, apathy, or general dissatisfaction, culminating in feelings of frustration, self-debasement, and possible anxiety? In addition, feelings of inadequacy or helplessness regarding developmental tasks may arise out of sheer physiological incapacity or immaturity—the more so, if the tasks "expected" are presented prematurely. On such grounds the plain fact that the child simply does not know what to do to relieve his discomfort may be fear- or anxiety-provoking. The dread that he may lose parental affection and protection because of not fulfilling the elders' desires; the consternation wrought by implied or stated dissatisfaction by the superiors; even the expression (following introjective processes) of self-dissatisfactions due to task "failures"—all these may create anxiety. Incrementally the child, feeling hostile toward the frustrating, task-setting elders but fearful of emitting aggression, represses (ejects from awareness) the unacceptable impulses. This intensifies the state of anxiety.

Finally, the child recognizes that he must relinquish familiar behavior, behavior which was learned to the point of comfort and security. He must thrust himself into strange behavioral settings and tasks which may serve as a threat to self-esteem inasmuch as the child is forced to relinquish the old while constructing new types and levels of competency. In essence he is compelled to give up hard-won competencies and to strive for the accomplishment of new tasks. Such is the price he pays for the promised increase in social status. Part of this admission fee may be in the form of anxiety which may be engendered by the challenges. The accomplishment of any developmental task and the successful integration and maintenance of that competency within the self-system will be made more strenuous if the process is permeated with anxiety.

Childhoods that are imbued with anxiety, especially in nuclear developmental task areas, are those in which (1) the child has been severely suppressed or dominated to such a degree that self-autonomy is threatened (the child has no opportunity to exercise his own initiative or to make some of his own decisions); (2) adult handling has been extremely and chronically inconsistent, so that confusion, doubt, dread, and a feeling of incompetence grow; (3) the child has been derogated, belittled excessively, or generally rejected, so that feelings of self-rejection, guilt, and perception of self as unworthy and inadequate are present; (4) there is a complete lack of external controls, in which case the child may become anxious or fearful lest he express too much hostility (or he may become anxious or guilt-ridden because of aggression that he *has* released, since there is no one to set reality limits or provide the supportive acceptance necessary to offset the guilt reaction); and finally, (5) because of the build-up of the child's hostility feelings, the child comes to fear or feel guilty about these suggestive urges, thereby adding to his own anxiety ("If I am hostile toward those who care for me, they may care less or not care at all, so I must not express my anger"); this latter may be viewed as conscience-derived anxiety.*

The Effects of Anxiety. Anxiety's immediate felt effect is a sense of *helplessness* and *dreadful expectancy*. The very anxious person experiences feelings described by such words as awe, dread, consternation, guilt, and terror. Anxiety, being an apprehensive response to *anticipated* danger, functions as a threat to the integrity and progression of the self-processes. It is an experience which is mildly or profoundly incompatible with the basic needs of self-equilibrium, comfort, and self-acceptance. Anxiety, being an apprehensive experience related to earlier frustrating experiences or to anticipated threat experiences, diffuses and fractionates the organism's energies and capacity to cope with (differentiate and integrate) successive developmental tasks, including speech and language tasks. Extreme anxiety may inhibit or fixate behavior or cause behavior to regress to more immature levels of development which were found to be more acceptable, tolerable, or self-enhancing.

Anxiety, in accordance with principles of conditioning and association, tends to become generalized. Original anxiety experiences are accompanied by peripheral cues which originally do not evoke anxiety. Through temporally contiguous equating with the anxiety-eliciting elements in the situation, these peripheral stimuli may prompt anxiety. Continuing anxiety experiences may mask the original anxiety motivants, making more difficult the differentiation and identification of anxiety sources, thus rendering the path to self-integration increasingly arduous.

---

* Although the common Freudian view of anxiety is that it derives principally from socially unacceptable wishes which the individual dares not to put into action, Mowrer has theorized that anxiety comes from acts the individual has already committed but wishes he had not. Mowrer calls this a "guilt theory" of anxiety (Mowrer, 1950a, p. 537).

Anxiety disrupts learning. The greatest interference will occur in relation to novel tasks, rather than to problems which are more familiar (Ausubel, *et al.*, 1953). A history of unsuccessful attempts at task accomplishment, with its consequent diminution in self-esteem, renders the individual more threatened upon subsequent presentation of these or other more socially involved tasks. Often the stuttering individual will seek opportunities to prepare in advance for such tasks (such as giving oral recitations in the classroom). He considers such a practice to be anxiety-reducing. However, this mode of adjustment can build more anxiety, for extemporaneous speech enlists a different pattern of dynamics. As Ausubel has stated: "Neurotic anxiety impairs problem solving because feelings of inadequacy about ability to improvise in unfamiliar situations leads to (a) an habitual and rigid learning set to adhere to stereotyped response patterns, (b) reliance upon such patterns as a learning 'crutch' and means of anxiety reduction; and (c) a face-saving attempt to produce any 'visible' response where panic associated with initial or cumulative frustration would otherwise result in blocking or utter confusion" (Ausubel, 1957, p. 332).

Anxiety tends to distort perception (Abt and Bellak, 1950). Any perceptual task which is ill-defined or ambiguous may elicit some degree of anxiety in the perceiver. As the anxiety increases, the stimulus is perceived increasingly in a way which is more a function of the perceiver's affectual investment in trying to relate to the object than a function of the actual stimulus. This is what appears to be happening when we say that an individual is using the defense mechanism of projection. The severely anxious individual not only is unable to perceive his environment realistically but he is also unable to perceive himself realistically. He is inclined to "read into" a situation his own meaning. There is some evidence which shows that increasing suppression of affect tends to facilitate perceptual distortion (Feshbach and Singer, 1957).

Anxiety imbues the person with a self-defeating interpretive mental set. The anxiety-provoking stimulus, perceived on the periphery of conscious awareness, or unconsciously, indeed does not have to be present at all. The person has but to *anticipate* or expect its occurrence to feel uncomfortable. As Freud stated, ". . . one feels anxiety *lest* something occur" (Freud, 1936, pp. 146–47). Also, "Anxiety is the expectation of the trauma on the one hand, and, on the other, an attenuated repetition of it" (Freud, 1936, p. 150). Although realistic adjustment measures against possible threats can be triggered by states of discomfort in well-adjusted persons, the anxious person, reacting excessively and undifferentiatingly to the actual or imagined threat, perseverates in his ineffectual adjustment attempts.

Bloodstein wrote an intriguing article (1950) in which he related reductions in stuttering to a single hypothetical condition—*reduced anxiety about stuttering.* Under important conditions in which anxiety about stuttering is reduced, he included the following: (1) distraction; (2) reduced punishment; (3) insufficient time to anticipate stuttering; (4) reduced bodily tension; and (5) the absence of cues which might elicit anxiety. He summarily stated that ". . . the less the anxiety about speech difficulties, the less the effort to avoid it, and consequently . . . the less the stuttering. Accordingly, the most general hypothesis which we can make about reductions in stuttering is that they represent reductions in the stutterer's effort to avoid non-fluency, under conditions of reduced anxiety about non-fluency." Bloodstein held that reduced anxieties *about stuttering* reduced stuttering severity. The present authors would maintain that reduced anxiety *about anything*—making a pleasant appearance, wearing the right clothes, using correct table manners, feeling hostile toward the teacher, or achieving insight as to why one dislikes older girls—reduces stuttering severity. The anxiety *need not be* and probably is *not* in the majority of cases involved most intimately with the speech per se. The nonfluencies are an outer expression of inner discomforts and apprehensions which involve threats to deeper and more universal dynamics of interpersonal relationships, threats to basic needs of love, acceptance, autonomy or self-integrity, acceptable self-image, esteem, safety. The threat of danger to any of these, the confusions, doubts, and conflicts regarding any or all of these basic self-process needs may, because of the anxiety elevation, produce or intensify stuttering behavior. Anxiety about stuttering as such does exist, insofar as the stuttering behavior represents a threat to self-esteem, since it may elicit societal disapproval; but such origins are regarded in most cases as secondary sources of tension. The process wherein personality disruptions produce deviant observable behavior (symptoms) such as stuttering, and wherein the symptom (stuttering) in time comes to serve as a stimulus to anxiety, has been referred to as a "circular process" (anxiety, stuttering symptom, anxiety). The most self-shattering fear of stuttering persons is the fear of the *unknown*, of being helpless, *the fear of anxiety*.

Can anxiety be a developmental, integrating force? Rollo May, for example, has spoken of "normal anxiety," maintaining that "when the person reacts in a manner which (1) is not out of all proportion to the threatening experience, (2) does not involve mechanisms of defense, especially repression, and (3) allows him to perceive realistically and consciously the obstruction, or which allows the regaining of a feeling of comfort if the threat is removed or modified, normal anxiety may be said to exist" (May, 1950, p. 194). This conception is more closely allied to what we have termed *fear,* and it is possibly even more related to what can be better regarded as "developmental tension." Culturally induced, constructive tensions serve as necessary and important motivations in the socialization processes. Tensions that concern the necessity to "do one's best," to please the loved ones, and to be "true to myself" serve to heighten effort, maintain vigilance, and elevate achievement goals. In such a manner we may say that there are normal tension states; however, the use of the term "normal anxiety" is not compatible with anxiety as we have defined it.

From another point of view, Mowrer has discussed anxiety as a constructive force in stating that ". . . if we are right in assuming that anxiety is repressed guilt which is struggling for recognition, then we may look upon anxiety as likewise leading to hope, to change, and to a new way of life" (Mowrer, 1950b, p. 40).

Also, if we regard anxiety as the motivating force which propels the stuttering person to seek help, to keep seeking it, and to persist in the struggle that is therapy, then anxiety is indeed developmental and a contributor to the growth of the self-process.

Self-Defenses Against Anxiety. Because of the vague nature of anxiety, it cannot be easily dealt with in a forthright manner by either the patient or the clinician. An anxious individual will more or less randomly attempt different ways to reduce the tension. Often, quite "accidentally," he will "come up with" techniques which are anxiety-reducing for his particular need system. In this way, anxiety serves as a vitally motivating force. These particular kinds of self-preserving responses are sometimes referred to as defense mechanisms, the overt manifestations of which, if of sufficient severity and endurance, may be called symptoms. A psychological symptom may be defined as any chronic or repetitive behavior which arises and persists as a defense against anxiety, serves to decrease anxiety, but which does not lead to insight as to the anxiety source or to the means of resolving the anxiety.

The prime purpose of self-defensive behavior is to reduce anxiety or fear. Research has revealed how animals that have experienced frustration or discomfort in the presence of certain cues eventually make *avoidance* efforts in the presence of these cues; i.e., when the discomfort is merely *threatened* (Mowrer, 1940). Anxiety can be reduced by appropriate avoidance reactions. The reinforcement in these avoidance responses involves the principle of tension reduction (Freud, 1936, p. 299, the "law of effect"). It is conceivable that self-defensive or symptomatic behavior such as stuttering may arise in this way inasmuch as tension reduction is a rewarding experience, and hence it serves as a reinforcing agent in learning to avoid anxiety, even though that behavior which is learned may be deemed deviant by society. A stuttering symptom may produce social rejection, derogation, or ostracism, but it is still the most efficient behavior possible for the individual at any given moment. It serves the vital function of reducing anxiety—although, as we have stated, the stuttering may in time come to serve as an anxiety-elictor in its own right.

Travis and Baruch (1941) have provided a perspective of functional symptom behavior which we shall categorize under two main classifications: (1) symptoms of deficit, and (2) symptoms of release. In symptoms of deficit, the individual uses great energy to keep his feelings under control, making continuous attempts to hide unacceptable feelings. He becomes "emotionally impoverished." He creates a *deficit* for himself in the quantity and quality of feeling he expresses. He develops symptoms of withheld emotions such as indifference, loss of sensation and movement, inability to initiate and carry out activities, even loss of consciousness and inability to speak (hysterical aphonia or mutism), or perhaps just a general absence of spontaneity (lack of variation in pitch, loudness, and rate patterns in speaking). With symptoms of *release* ("symptoms of disguised emotions"), the individual finds it impossible to contain the unacceptable urges completely; to some degree the affect leaks out. But he cannot express this unacceptable feeling directly (in its "pure" form). He cannot, for example, *directly* express his hostility because of fear or guilt. He evolves an indirect means of expression for it, a disguised form of expression of which he is mainly unaware. Repressed emotions break through in a distorted form. Symptoms of deficit may include such behavior as tics, skin eruptions, eating disturbances, enuresis, perfectionism, timidity, nail biting, intolerance, exhibitionism, and phobias. We would also include "functional" delayed speech and articulation disorders, verbal aggressiveness, and stuttering.

Symptoms of deficit tend to elicit societal sympathy; symptoms of release tend to elicit societal disapproval. Yet, release symptoms are probably, in terms of self-integrity, somatically healthier inasmuch as partial release of pent-up emotions and thus diminution of anxiety is occurring. This concept will be explored more completely in the next chapter. For now, may we emphasize simply that a symptom *is* purposive: It is one form of adjustment, the best possible for the individual at the time. But a symptom is basically nonintegrative; it is a danger signal, but it is not the danger itself. Much difficulty and confusion have stemmed from the fact that the stuttering symptom has been regarded as *the* disorder. It has been interpreted and treated literally and descriptively, whereas in fact it is sometimes no more "the problem" than a fever is the problem in cases of pneumonia.

Our discussion will be aided by a brief consideration of some of the modes of defense which take place as means of dealing with the self-disintegrative threats of anxiety. These forms of adjustment may be used by anyone; by well-adjusted as well as maladjusted persons, except that with the latter, these adjustive attempts tend to be more perseverative and deep-rooted or more automatic, rigid, and unconscious (therefore less susceptible to self-integrative learning).

The socialization of the individual originates in a process in which he absorbs and considers as his own the feelings, attitudes, reaction patterns, restrictions, and ideals of important elders and the group. This incorporative process, called *introjection,* is the child's first attempt to collate the outside world with inner life (the environment with self-concept). It is the first phase of the process of self-differentiation and integration.

We may distinguish between two kinds of introjection—developmental and disintegrative. In *developmental introjection,* the person takes into his self-system the ideals, attitudes, and modes of behaving which are compatible with the self-ideal; i.e., the introjections are enhancing and acceptable to a differentiating and integrating (maturing) self. Such introjections serve as bases for a realistic and fair conscience, the construction of a healthy moral structure, the growth of positive values, desirable ideals, and the nurture of compatible yet progressively advanced aspirations. Although such incorporations occur under varying states of tension, they are distinguished by the fact that the tension states are not so severe as to be regarded as anxiety derivatives. They are absorbed into the self-system, not as a consequence of threat but as a consequence of being presented as adult behavior standards which, though challenging to the individual in terms of the necessity of his acquiring new and more difficult behavior, are not so harsh, unattainable, or incompatible with his basic needs that he becomes anxious concerning his eventual choice in adopting or rejecting them, or becomes anxious as a consequence of having introjected them.

In *disintegrative introjection*, on the other hand, the internalizations occur because of threat or extreme conflict, and in turn they become themselves anxiety elicitors. The individual will introject the behavior of important elders in order to avoid discomfort, belittlement, punishment, and the denial of love, as well as to avoid feelings of *self*-disapproval, such as guilt. The child learns that if he cannot "beat them," he should ("ought to") join them. He learns that being like the parents means being liked by the parents. Instead of expressing his actual feelings ("to mine own self not being true"), he adopts those of the elders. Instead of fighting them, he accepts their dicta.

Introjection, then, is the first defense against anxiety. At the same time, as was discussed earlier in this chapter, it is the source of self-control or conscience. In some instances, the standards a person comes to hold for himself may be far more severe than those to which he was exposed. In cases where the significant elders themselves become less threatening or more permissive, the person's introjections, now an established part of his self-system, may continue to operate. Finally, disintegrative introjection should not be confused with *imitation*. The latter term should be reserved for *conscious* efforts to adopt the behavior patterns of another, and it lies closer in meaning to what we have termed developmental introjection. Throughout this book, whenever the word *introjection* is employed, it signifies disintegrative introjection unless otherwise stated.

The intimate companion-dynamic of introjection is *repression*.* The person, more or less vaguely aware of unacceptable impulses which are threatening to reveal themselves, becomes anxious concerning the fearful consequences which may engulf him if the impulses were allowed expression. One way of avoiding this anxiety is to repel the impulse, if possible. The more fearful the threat that the self-ideal will be damaged, the greater the discomfort. As a defense against this hazard to self-integrity, the self-process may function unconsciously so as to "divorce" the impulse, to "forget" it, to keep it out of conscious awareness; in short, to *repress* it. An additional condition must be mentioned here; namely, that the repressed wishes or impulses continue to function even though the person is not conscious of their existence. Repressed materials consist, therefore, of the thoughts we dare not think, the feelings we do not feel free to express, the wishes we cannot reveal. Any impulse that can create anxiety is subject to repression. Most repressions are in deference to the demands of the conscience. Others occur because of the fear of environmental frustration (fear of punishment).

Although repression is a response to anxiety, it also functions as an anxiety elicitor. Such is the case when repression "breaks down" and unacceptable feelings filter through into consciousness, not necessarily in a way which provokes overwhelming anxiety but in sufficient degree to create discomfort in the person. This is what seems to be happening when persons commit "slips of the tongue," laugh suddenly at the plight of another, "forget" to come to the therapy session on time or at all, forget an acquaintance's name, and so forth—the unconscious is betrayed. It is not the repression per se which produces these behaviors; it is rather that the repression weakens and the restrained forces break through (the "return of the repressed"). Such behavior, if chronic, is to

* The term *repression* is usually distinguished from *suppression*, which is thought of as a conscious and voluntary removal or denial of thoughts and feelings from awareness.

be regarded as symptomatic. Freud clarified the nature of such behavior in the following words:

> I give the name of symptomatic acts to those acts which people perform, as we say, automatically, unconsciously, without attending to them, or as if in a moment of distraction. They are actions to which people would like to deny any significance, and which, if questioned about them, they would explain as being indifferent and accidental. Closer observation, however, will show that these actions, about which consciousness knows nothing or wishes to know nothing, in fact give impression to unconscious thoughts and impulses, and are therefore most valuable and instructive as being manifestations of the unconscious which have been able to come to the surface (Freud, 1953, pp. 92–93).

It may be concluded that repression is related in some important way to any self-process geared to alleviate or ward off the threat of anxiety and therefore is involved to some extent in all self-defensive processes discussed in this section.

It sometimes happens, when unacceptable wishes and ideas threaten to break through, that a person will ascribe these painful feelings to some other person or group. The anxious person becomes hypersensitive to the presence in other persons of these characteristics. Such a self-defensive operation is termed *projection*. A stutterer may feel that a teacher does not like him, whereas in actuality she may be fond of him, but he has repressed feelings of hostility toward her. As another example, in a study of anti-Semitism (Ackerman and Johada, 1950), it was found that persons with persistent anti-Semitic attitudes rather strikingly attributed to Jews those self-attributes which were intolerable within themselves.

It probably is very difficult for anyone, especially anxious persons, to make any evaluation or judgment without revealing something about his deeper self. It is, in fact, this very assumption on which, in the realm of psychodiagnostics, the practice of projective techniques is based. The general procedure underlying projective methods of personality appraisal is to present to the subject a comparatively ambiguous stimulus, such as an ink blot or an incomplete story or picture, and simply ask him to interpret it. The assumption is that the subject will respond according to his perception of the stimulus situation and how he feels when so responding; i.e., he will reveal unconsciously how he organizes experience, interprets stimuli affecting him, and how he feels in general. The individual who is projecting, owing to anxiety, is unaware that the given motive is a function of his own self-system. Unconsciously denying its existence, he is able to realize (accept) it in consciousness only as a function of others. Thus the exhibitionist is able to conclude that others will enjoy viewing him (as he would enjoy viewing others); the sexually repressed coed is content to believe that all the boys "try to get fresh." In the same way, the person who stutters may come to believe that his listeners are "just waiting for me" to stutter. No doubt much of the difficulty of interpersonal relationships stems from such one-way or mutual attribution of unworthy traits from one human being to another. Projection has the unfortunate effect of permitting the person to become suspicious, prejudiced, or vindictive toward the one "at fault." By placing himself in a position of righteousness, the projector wards off encroachment by self-doubts. The most glaring example of projections in action are to be found in the delusions of paranoids.

As with the other defensive reactions to the threat of self-disintegrations, projection, through an anxiety derivative, becomes in its own right the instigator of more anxiety than it serves to relieve. Inasmuch as projection is a *misperception,* or a false perception, the projected characteristic being in the person's unconscious and not in the object to which the projection is directed, the individual is bound to experience additional discomfort. Not only does he misunderstand the motives of people, he also reacts to these ascribed motives as though they had objective reality.

Just as all anxiety-motivated, self-defensive dynamics are linked with repression, so too they may be linked with *regression,* another primary reaction to intolerable situations. In regression, there is a reversal in the self-integration process to a more primitive, less differentiated form of behavior that is typical of more immature developmental stages or younger persons. Thus regression is a common feature in the break-down of self-integrity associated with developmental tasks which become unbearable: from eating solids to taking only liquids; from self-controlled behavior to uncontrolled temper tantrums. The 18-year-old stuttering person who has come to dread the prospect of telephoning may decide to ask his mother to make all his calls for him; the six-year-old, upon the birth of a sibling, may revert to "baby talk," bed-wetting, or thumb-sucking. Regression denotes not only a return to behavior patterns which have been used and relinquished but also to less individuated or more primitive behavior not necessarily used previously. However, it should be noted that anxiety is not a major determinant, if present at all, in temporary regression, as during certain recreational activities or the period just prior to sleep; or during transitional stages of development, wherein the person, focusing on the acquisition of a new developmental task, temporarily allows previously integrated abilities to relapse. Such regressions are to be considered normal. When behavior reversals endure obstinately, the assumption is that anxiety was the stimulus to the condition. It is in this sense that the word *regression* is used here.

The consequence of regression, the culmination in behavior which is *persistently* more primitive, is called *fixation,* a term applicable also to situations in which the individual, owing to anxiety, fails to progress to more advanced levels of self-integration and differentiation; i.e., fails developmental tasks. In cases of development cessation due to reasons other than anxiety, such as illness, physical injuries, or a paucity of environmental stimulation, a term such as *agenesis* may be better indicated. However, *fixation* is commonly used in such instances. In our own usage of *fixation,* the condition's origin in anxiety is implied.

A stuttering person may become a debater, an actor, or a speech teacher as ways of satisfying in a socially acceptable manner the need to be verbally competent and commanding.

Such processes have been called *sublimations* by some, *substitutions* by others, and in certain cases, *compensation,* and *displacement* by still others. The process with which we are concerned involves the replacement of more or less non-developmental satisfactions by those which propel more effectively the on-going progress of the self-growth processes. This sounds like the behavior of well-adjusted persons, and in truth it is difficult and perhaps not really necessary to distinguish between healthy channelization of motives and sublimation. Perhaps we need only add that if the replacement behavior is *elicited* and *accompanied* by some degree of anxiety, we may label this self-defensive process "sublimation." In situations entailing nonpersistive anxiety or no anxiety at all but rather involving tension without enduring apprehension, the term *substitution* or *substitute activity* may be acceptable.

Compensation also involves substitute activity but connotes that the replacement behavior is a more socially acceptable, and thus more self-enhancing, *direct* reaction (or compensation) to real or imaginary threats to self-esteem. This is one explanation of how a lisping child becomes a great orator, and also perhaps why a stuttering individual, unable to give vent to his hostile feelings, becomes a boxer, or failing in speech fluency, becomes extremely proficient in abstract language usage in writing, or perhaps becomes a "language expert." *

Finally we may consider the situation of the third-grader, berated by his teacher but unable to speak in his own defense owing to the fear of stuttering and other reasons, arriving home and releasing his suppressed hostility upon his younger brother. When the mother intervenes, however, the frustrated child thereupon goes into his room and tears the arms from the brother's teddy bear. In both alternative expressions used by the boy, one object is replaced by another.

---

* This brings to mind an observation made by Zipf, the psycholinguist, of the linguist studying the mother tongue who was asked by a discerning psychologist if he had discovered anything new concerning the laws of his mother's tongue.

Such behavior may be termed *displacement,* and although the behavior finally expressed is socially unacceptable, it is still *more* acceptable socially than would be the direct release of hostility onto the original objects of anger, the teacher and the brother.

Other forms of defense against threats to self-integrity may be represented by the following examples. *Rationalization* denotes the offering of a "nice" or more socially acceptable justification for behavior which is basically self-devaluating. The parents of stuttering persons may be heard to say such things as the following: "He must have inherited the stuttering from his uncle. This stuttering is a thing you can't beat, so it's silly even to try." The stutterer himself may say: "Oh, I didn't want the part in the play, anyway. I'll never get anywhere with girls or with jobs because of my speech—that's the only thing holding me back. They don't want to hear what I have to say. It's a waste of time to talk to girls; they're so silly." When such statements are defensive productions of plausible reasons for behavior which is confused or nonintegrative, we may agree that rationalization is occurring. The greater the threat of self-debasement, the more repressed or disguised the self-defensive behavior becomes. Feeling incapable of adjusting to the demands of reality, the person may flee, utilizing the coping mechanism of *withdrawal.* He may, for example, abandon the developmental task at hand. He may "give up" the goal of trying to please those around him. He may become chronically "preoccupied." He may resort to fantasy solutions. He may become physically rigid or stilted. He may even stop talking altogether.

It is clear that some of these arbitrarily distinguished defensive modes may fall within the realm of normal adjustment, depending on the intensity and frequency with which the anxiety, tension, or defensive mode occurs. If the mode is basically self-incapacitating or self-devaluating, it is a self-disintegrative defense. If the mode is, without undue delay, self-enhancing, it is an integrative defense.

Psychogenic Speech-Disruption as a Self-Defense Against Anxiety Threats. In many speaking situations, the speaker's delivery breaks down in fluency because of the threats of anxiety or of fear of a consciously perceived danger. This disruption is seen, not only in stuttering behavior but in what has been called "stage fright." The dynamics of stage fright are extremely similar to those operant in stuttering. The word *fright* may be considered as a synonym for *fear* and has so been considered in the appropriate literature. Thus "the fear of speaking" or "speech fear" would be appropriate equivalent terms for the condition as it has been dealt with in the great majority of the speech literature. But, as the reader will recall, we have used the word *fear* in a particular way, to refer to apprehensive states connected with *known* objects or situations which are for the most part *consciously* understood and susceptible of appraisal. We have stated also that the person in such a circumstance may adjust to the threat by removing, fleeing, neutralizing, or denying the feared situation. All this seems compatible *if* we assume that the threat lies in the situation in which the speaker perceives it to be, namely (1) the fear of the listener or audience and (2) the fear of his own speech performance. We have said, however, that *awareness* of impulses or threats is the prime requirement in the resolution of threatening or conflict circumstances and that fairly complete awareness of "what it is that disturbs me" should enable the person to make an appropriate adjustment and, therefore, to diminish or extinguish the fear response. If, after a period of "practice," of learning to prepare for speeches, of learning to choose speaking topics which are of interest to himself and in which he is knowledgeable, the person *persists* in showing the disorganized speech behavior, our conclusion must be that other factors are operating and that these "other factors" are, in essence, *anxiety* feelings. It seems appropriate here to repeat our definition of anxiety:

. . . a state of apprehension or dread . . . due to some threat to the integrity or developmental progression of the self-process caused by frustrating forces of which the individual is only vaguely aware and with which he feels incapable of coping; the threat may be stimulated exogenously (situational fear with loss of objective environmental referents) or endogenously (internal promptings in the form of intolerable feelings, thoughts, and desires which threaten to expose themselves). In most instances there is probably accompanying somatic tension, and in all cases the root danger is a threat to the goodness of interpersonal relationships.

In both stuttering and stage fright, the speaker is indeed apprehensive of threats to his self-esteem; he is the personification of conflict or frustration, yet he is not altogether conscious of what the frustrating forces are; he feels utterly incapable of handling the situation; somatic tension is painfully obvious; and most certainly the interpersonal relationship and communication are damaged.

From this vantage point, therefore, both stuttering and stage fright are more closely identified as overwhelming anxiety in situations which happen to involve speaking and in which the most obvious behavior disruptions are observable as failures in the speech functions. If we were to chart the course of such anxiety-speech disorders, it might reveal the following pattern: The speaker, just before or while speaking, experiences a state of tension and mild discomfort. He becomes somewhat more vigilant (controlled), concentrating on the speaking task before him. Tension increases to apprehension, doubt, and fear. As he exercises more control (suppression), his speech becomes more restrained, meticulous, and mechanical. He perceives himself to be in a situation of loathsome dread; he wonders if he will "pull himself together" (remain self-integrated); countless impulses surge within him. He can no longer identify or cope with his anxiety state. He struggles to "remain calm at all costs," but he is paying a price. He shifts about, pulls at his jacket button, picks at his lip, blushes, or blanches. His voice becomes harder to handle. The loudness level falls, then rises. Perhaps the mean pitch level rises while the pitch pattern becomes monotonous. His heart pounds; his hands clench. Perspiration breaks out. His breathing becomes spasmodic. Eye contact is lost. Disjointed thoughts increase. Speech becomes stilted with odd pauses. Words are mispronounced, stumbled on, repeated, or blocked; there follows an uncanny confusion, panic, total speech disruption, stark rigidity or escape through fleeing or fainting. Such can be the horror, in extreme cases, of overwhelming disorders of stuttering and stage fright.

In stuttering, and in stage fright, too, the speaker's behavior tells us what he thinks of himself. He is usually acting out of proportion to external reality. He reveals many of a great array of traits, consciously or unconsciously—feelings of self-debasement, self-rejection; conflict between expressing and withholding hostility or love; guilt reactions; a dread of "facing up" to his own basic desires and motives; a fear of expressing his deeper feelings. The fear of speaking turns out to be a *fear of anxiety* in which the person, as a function of the unavoidably noticeable manifestations of the anxiety fear, *consciously* perceives the disorganized *speech* to be the "thing" to be feared. In every case of stuttering or stage fright in the present authors' experience, the current, fractured interpersonal relationships have been related to earlier interpersonal disruptions. The professor is "seen" as the father or earlier punitive teacher and the audience as parent or other early elder substitutes, so that the present speaking situation, through conditioning, generalization, and projection, operates as a stimulus which taps old, repressed conflicts and fears. Inner and outer realities clash. The person may be fearful of exhibiting himself, of "putting himself on trial," because he fears retaliation; he may be fearful of exposing himself to the verdict of the authority figures and of losing approval; he may be fearful of a loss in self-esteem. Just as the important elders in his childhood perhaps did not like his performance, so, too, these important listeners may be displeased.

With the abatement or resolution of the anxieties through psychotherapy or counseling, and with the diminution of fears through the use of speech correction or public speaking experiences, such conditions can be resolved. The important point is that in severe anxiety-speech disorders, a counseling or dynamically oriented therapeutic process is necessary as a first step. Dealing from the outset directly and solely with the speech behavior itself will not solve the basic problems. Such suggestions as "Anticipate a pleasing audience," and "Realize that everybody makes mistakes," have been found to be extremely helpful with the great majority of persons who, for example, have enrolled in college public-speaking courses and who have experienced speech fears. The use and acceptance of such proposals by the average person is, for the most part, reasonable and helpful; their validity with or applications to persons with pronounced anxieties breaking through in the form of speech disruptions is open to very serious question. Clearly, with anxious individuals, such appeals to the intellect will be far less self-integrating. Rather, the person will need to become aware of internal conflicts and basic impulses, to extend his realm of consciousness —to expand, differentiate, and integrate the self-enhancement processes. Speech drills will not accomplish such purposes, although later, when the anxieties have been diminished through counseling or psychotherapy, speech techniques can be extremely effective. The development of specific speech skills that will better equip the person to manage fear situations appears to be helpful in many instances, just as a gradual exposure by degrees to similar situations and, eventually, to the actual feared situations may achieve the goal of making the original fear stimulus a more pleasurable, developmental one. This speech-conditioning process is most helpful in cases of fear related to *specific* objects or situations. If the speech disorganization is symptomatic of a diffuse, underlying anxiety, this approach will be more difficult.

REFERENCES

ABT, L., and BELLAK, L. *Projective Psychology*. New York: Alfred A. Knopf, Inc., 1950.

ACKERMAN, N., and JOHADA, M. *Anti-Semitism and Emotional Disorder*. New York: Harper & Bros., 1950.

AUSUBEL, D. *Theory and Problems of Child Development*. New York: Grune & Stratton, Inc., 1957.

AUSUBEL, D.; SCHIFF, H.; and GOLDMAN, M. "Qualitative Characteristics in the Learning Process Associated with Anxiety," *J. Abn. Soc.
Psychol.*, **48**: 537–47, 1953.

BLOODSTEIN, O. "Hypothetical Conditions under which Stuttering Is
Reduced or Absent," *J. Speech Hearing Disorders*, **15**: 142–53,
1950.

ERIKSON, E. H. *Childhood and Society.* New York: W. W. Norton
& Co., Inc., 1950.

FESHBACH, S., and SINGER, R. D. "The Effects of Fear Arousal and
Suppression of Fear upon Social Perception," *J. Abnorm. Soc.
Psychol.*, **55**: 283–88, 1957.

FREUD, S. "Fragment of an Analysis of a Case of Hysteria," in *Collected Papers*, vol. III. London: Hogarth Press, Ltd., 1953, pp.
7–295.

———. *The Problem of Anxiety.* New York: W. W. Norton & Co.,
Inc., 1936.

HUNTLEY, C. W. "Judgments of Self—Based upon Records of Expressive Behavior," *J. Abnorm. Soc. Psychol.*, **35**: 398–427, 1940.

MAY, R. *The Meaning of Anxiety.* New York: The Ronald Press Co.,
1950.

MOWRER, O. H. "Anxiety Reduction and Learning," *J. Exp. Psychol.*,
27: 497–516, 1940.

———. *Learning Theory and Personality Dynamics.* New York:
The Ronald Press Co., 1950.

———. "Pain, Punishment, Guilt and Anxiety," in *Anxiety*, eds. P. H.
Hoch and J. Zubin. New York: Grune & Stratton, Inc., 1950.
Chap. iii, pp. 27–40.

SULLIVAN, H. S. *The Interpersonal Theory of Psychiatry.* New York:
W. W. Norton & Co., Inc., 1953.

TRAVIS, L. E., and BARUCH, D. W. *Personal Problems of Everyday
Life.* New York: Appleton-Century-Crofts, Inc., 1941.

VAN RIPER, C. *Speech Correction Principles and Methods.* 2d ed.
Englewood Cliffs, N. J.: Prentice-Hall, Inc., 1947.

WISCHNER, G. J. An Experimental Approach to Expectancy and Anxiety in Stuttering Behavior," *J. Speech. Hear. Disorders*, **17**: 139–54,
1952.

Chapter 6

A Self-Process Concept of Stuttering

Resolve to be thyself: and know, that he who finds himself,
loses his misery.——Matthew Arnold

In considering theoretical frameworks for stuttering, certain questions are properly in order. What is a theory? Is it something that isn't a fact? Something less firmly established than a law? Something having more evidence than a hypothesis? An impracticable principle? Something that's "good" but "doesn't work"? To fully appreciate the thinking of the logicians of science, one would need to become well acquainted with methodology by studying leading sources which provide extensive treatment of the subject (Cohen and Nagel, 1934; Conant, 1947; Northrup, 1931). Hall and Lindzey define a theory as "an unsubstantiated hypothesis or a speculation concerning reality which is not yet definitely known to be so; . . . a *set of conventions* created by the theorist . . . theories are not 'given' or predetermined by nature, the data, or any other determinant process" (Hall and Lindzey, 1957, p. 10). Theorists are like artists, several of whom, let us say, are interested in painting the same objects but who depict them in a variety of ways. Like the artist, the theorist selectively perceives the object (or "data"), interprets it in accordance with his own experience (frame of reference), and depicts it in countlessly different ways (through color shadings, form, texture, and the like). He perceives empirical events selectively in accordance with his own needs and wishes. He evaluates them in the light of his own frame of reference (learning theory, semantics, psychoanalysis, etc.), as he depicts them in different ways (nomenclatural deviations). A theory, in short, is a way of looking at things. It is not a vehicle carrying full clarification of the empirical facts with which the theory is concerned.

The theorist, as he builds his "system," uses existing empirical information. A good deal of this information may derive from observations made by workers in the field of clinicians and stutterers in therapy settings. Information will also be obtained from written and oral reports on promising processes and procedures. On such bases, the theorist constructs systematically interconnected assumptions which are relevant to his particular subject of study; in this case, stuttering behavior. Ideally, on the basis of such assumptions, whether specific or general, it should be possible to make valid predictions. A theory also should include operational definitions whenever possible in order to provide means for empirical translation, i.e., to reveal the degree to which chosen concepts correlate with empirical data. If, however, definitions are formulated too precisely, the amount of inquiry that occurs may be curtailed. Briefly, then, what does a theory do? Hall and Lindzey answer:

First, and most important, it leads to the collection or *observation of relevant empirical relations not yet observed.* The theory should lead to a systematic expansion of knowledge concerning the phenomena of interest, and this expansion ideally should be mediated or stimulated by the derivation from the theory of specific empirical propositions (statements, hypotheses, predictions) that are subject to empirical test. . . . It is only the derivations or propositions or ideas derived from the theory which are open to empirical test. The theory itself is assumed and acceptance or rejection of it is determined by its *utility,* not by its truth or falsity . . . [the] capacity of a theory to generate research by suggesting ideas or even by arousing disbelief and resistance may be referred to as the *heuristic influence of the theory* (Hall and Lindzey, 1957, p. 13).

WHAT IS STUTTERING?

The word *stuttering* has so many meanings that it becomes almost meaningless. Stuttering may be thought of as speech which is characterized by any of or all the following: repetitions, hesitations, prolongations, or blocks; in addition there may be breathing irregularities and sometimes accompanying articulation and voice deviations. Such a definition is a purely descriptive one, inclusive of only the speech act, and with no consideration of etiology. Thus it is inadequate. A fuller definition, embracing both etiology and motivation, is therefore needed, and the authors would propose the following:

> *Stuttering is a learned, nonintegrative, self-defensive reaction to anxiety or fear of threatening circumstances with which the person feels incapable of coping.*

The remainder of this chapter will be devoted to interpreting the various concepts contained or implied in this definition. First, stuttering is *learned behavior.* Learning refers to any relatively constant alteration in behavior that is due to past experience. Second, the *roots* of stuttering originate in interpersonal relationships, most specifically around *verbal or nonverbal* developmental tasks during early socialization experiences with important elders. The stuttering behavior *persists* primarily as a consequence of old and contemporary interpersonal discomforts. Third, the stuttering disorder may range in severity from very mild to very severe, not merely in terms of the speech symptom but in terms of total behavior. The reader will note, also, that our viewpoint consistently maintains that stuttering behavior may be due not only to *speech* experiences but to any or all other *non*speech experiences, too. We may enlarge again upon this point by drawing a comparison with a few statements by Johnson.

(a) The person who stutters has been influenced by his experiences with speech to be uneasy and concerned about whether he can say the words he wants or needs to say. . . .

(b) He fears stuttering. . . .

(c) So it is that he does not want to stutter—again. And he tries not to whenever he feels that he might. Now—what he does trying not to stutter is his stuttering . . . a definition might be, then: stuttering is what a speaker does trying not to stutter again (Johnson, 1956, p. 216).

Johnson amplifies his definition, stating:

(d) Stuttering is an anticipatory, apprehensive, hypertonic avoidance reaction. In other words, stuttering is what a speaker does when (1) he expects stuttering to occur, (2) dreads it, and (3) becomes tense in anticipation of it and in (4) trying to avoid doing it (Johnson, 1956, p. 217).

Johnson's statements may be compared with those following, which attempt to reach a more inclusive level of understanding:

(a) The person who stutters has been influenced by his experiences with speech and other behavior to be anxious and apprehensive lest he fail in adequately accomplishing *any* act, including speaking, that he wants or needs to do.

(b) He fears *anxiety*—which means that he does not know specifically what he is fearful of—only that he feels inept, confused; or he experiences *fear* [as defined in Chapter 5]—of specific noxious stimuli which he does "know" (become aware of).

(c) So it is that he does not want to experience the anxiety—or the fear—again. And he tries not to (i.e., he represses, escapes, etc.) whenever he feels that he might be overwhelmed by unacceptable or dangerous events. Now, what he does trying not to allow these impulses to escape is his stuttering. A definition might be, then: stuttering is what a speaker does in trying to cope with (e.g., repress, deny, or avoid) threatening circumstances from without or within.

(d) Stuttering is what a speaker does when (1) he consciously or unconsciously expects a threatening circumstance (2) is anxious or fearful because of it, and (3) becomes disintegrated in behavior and (4) utilizes self-defensive processes as coping, or anxiety-reducing, mechanisms.

Johnson's statements accurately describe, however, what often happens with stuttering persons who have gone beyond the original stuttering phase; their stuttering is no longer largely a result of nonverbal (and mainly unconscious) anxiety-linked functions but rather is characterized by reactions to the speech behavior per se (even in such cases, however, the accompanying effects of nonspeech-focused anxieties or fears tend to remain lethal). In general, the older a stuttering person is, and we are thinking here of adolescence and beyond as a detectable difference line, the more a stuttering problem is likely to revolve around a specific fear of stuttering. But with many stutterers the fear is not simply a fear of speech, of stuttering; it is something much more pervasive and deeply ingrained within the stuttering individual's self-structure, and it is usually unconscious (thus, it is basic *anxiety*).

The following portion of a therapy protocol, in which a 21-year-old male stutterer is speaking with a speech clinician, will show the meaning that such anxiety can hold for a stutterer. Roy has been talking in a very general way of feeling inadequate in all situations:

ROY: I've tried different ways of handling it. One way is to get angry with it for no logical reason—and then by just submitting and saying that the whole thing is hopeless—and sometimes by just trying to pretend it wasn't there.

CL.: It?

ROY: Whatever it was that bothered me—some idea or something I had to do or something like that.

CL.: This "it." I'm wondering if this is an undefinable thing.

ROY: I'd say I don't know how to handle a situation and it would be the method of handling the situation.

CL.: And it's really hard to pin it down, isn't it. This "it" and the "situation."

ROY: The parts of it that bother me are the parts that show a promise of being able to *hurt* me or to sort of *hold* me—so as I am not able to do anything.

CL.: They're unpleasant.

ROY: Not because they *are* unpleasant but because they show *promise* of *being* unpleasant. . . .

CL.: Anything else come to your mind about this?
(*Pause*)

ROY: Yes, I think so. It's a fear—a panicky fear of things that I don't know.

(*Pause*)

CL.: Things you don't know?

ROY: Yeh.

(*Pause*)

CL.: Anything else come to mind on this?

ROY: Sometimes I think that I *use* this in some way.

CL.: Would you like to tell me more about that?

ROY: This fear of what I don't know can work two ways. One way is that I can just *run* and the other way is that I can *find out*. There are some things that lend themselves more easily to being investigated—things that can be laid out with a mathematical pattern, and there are other things that I can-*not* put down in any mathematical pattern. Maybe because I just don't know how. Things like this would revolve around people—things that have to do with the emotions, like art, music, literature, and things like that. In arts, for example, I seem to lean toward traditional aspects, possibly because they can more easily be fitted into a pattern, and the traditional forms seem to visibly interlock with other things like history and that makes them a little more under-standable to me. Yes, I seem to lean toward things that other people have already dissected and laid out and cata-logued for the reason that they *are* more easily understood.

We present this as an example of a person who is anxious, who is unable to identify the objective referents in reality, and who is trying to become aware of the anxiety-eliciting cues in his environment. He is struggling to achieve "closure" by becoming more aware of the elements which trigger his anxieties. He wants to know how his life process during and because of these experiences is being affected in a way which is contributing to stuttering.

"THE STUTTERING PERSONALITY"

A review of the literature will produce evidence which supports the general thesis that stuttering persons, as a group, tend to have more personality and social problems than "average" persons. For example, Despert (1946, 1943a, 1943b), using a variety of projective techniques, has worked fairly extensively with young stutterers. In an excellent study of 50 stuttering children between the ages of 6 and 15 years (and their parents), she used recorded observations of projective tendencies displayed by the subjects during interviews and various play activities. In addition, she collected verbal responses to a set of fables devised to test emotionally sensitive areas such as parental fixations, sibling rivalry, hostility, anxiety, self-punishment, and so on. A large majority of the mothers were found to be too domineering, with the fathers playing more passive roles. Seventy-two per cent of the mothers were overanxious, especially concerning feeding and physical health. They were oversolicitous, overprotective, and tended to be compulsively perfectionistic. Sixty-two per cent of the mothers and forty per cent of the fathers were considered "definitely neurotic." The majority of the children showed poor social adjustment even prior to the onset of the stuttering. Seventy-four per cent of the children reported a variety of intense fears and anxiety dreams. Fifty per cent of the children revealed early indications of compulsive behavior. Despert concluded that the most common finding is primary anxiety (not secondary to the stuttering), and she stated that "pressure on the part of neurotic, often compulsive, mothers at critical periods of the speech development in somatically sensitized individuals is viewed as a catalyzing agent for speech and associated pathology" (Despert, 1946, p. 108).

In a long-range psychiatric study of more than 75 family units of stutterers, Glauber (1952) observed that the mothers as a group were narcissistic, with strong feelings of guilt and aggression, poor self-image, and competitive attitudes toward males. In regard to mother-child relationships, there were almost always feeding difficulties during the first year, and the mother found it difficult to let the child grow up. Often the mothers were speech-conscious; and, in general, great anxiety was experienced concerning speech, general behavior, masturbation, school, and social life, with repressed envy, hostility, and often disappointment. Although there was often much maternal affection and patient care, for the most part social anxiety diffused and distorted the mother-child relationship. One final observation reported was the tendency for the mothers as a group to prod their children toward active, perfectionistic goals, this striving for achievement occurring within a framework in which an overdependence upon the mother was being nurtured.

Glasner (1949), in a study of 70 stuttering preschool children, found that all had some degree of emotional disturbance in addition to the stuttering; for example, 54 per cent had had eating problems, 27 per cent had been enuretic problems, 20 per cent experienced fears or nightmares; over 50 per cent had two or three other behavioral deviations. Glasner arbitrarily grouped the children into three classes: (1) relatively healthy children who, upon removal of disturbing factors, regain fluency; (2) children with a galaxy of neurotic symptoms; and (3) children somewhere between (1) and (2) who were described as not highly neurotic but generally dependent, confused, fearful, restless, sensitive, often asocial children. The majority of the youngsters were rated in this latter category. It was observed that the parents tended to be overprotective, overanxious, perfectionistic persons who set high standards for their children.

Such findings lend powerful support to the dynamic theories of stuttering, although additional review of personality studies in stuttering produces findings that are something less than in full agreement with those cited. In fact, a selective review of the literature allows one to construct a healthy case for the thesis that stuttering persons differ slightly or not at all from normal nonstutterers (Johnson, 1956).

The confusion in personality findings concerning stuttering persons has been highlighted in an article by Sheehan (1958) in which 20 research studies of stutterers were analyzed and compared in order to ascertain if stuttering persons differed from nonstuttering ones in several dimensions of personality, and also if there was a common personality pattern among stutterers. Six Rorschach studies, five Thematic Apperception Test studies, four Rosenzweig Picture-Frustration Test research projects, two self-concept studies, and three level-of-aspiration investigations were critically compared and analyzed.

Prior to a tabular analysis of the studies, Sheehan notes that, "The separation of statistically significant findings from the interpretations offered by the authors [of the studies considered] is necessitated by the frequency with which various authors have arbitrarily interpreted their data in accordance with their various philosophical predilictions" (Sheehan, 1958, p. 18). Sheehan concludes that the findings "are not particularly consistent with each other," that stutterers "do *not* show a definite personality pattern" on the basis of the studies selected, and that very meager evidence is available "to show that stutterers are different from anyone else." The analysis did reveal agreement that lower aspiration levels existed in the groups of stutterers evaluated. Sheehan interprets the lower levels of aspiration of stutterers as "probably a manifestation of their defensiveness" apparently stemming from "the ego-protective level of conflict." He particularly emphasizes the low degree of correlation among most of the projective studies, a finding which he judges "should be discouraging to those who are fond of claiming that stutterers show a definite personality pattern" (Sheehan, 1958, p. 23). In this respect, he refers specifically to the viewpoints of Travis (1940, 1957) and Wolpe (1957), which are essentially psychoanalytically based.*

* Probably it would be a difficult task to show that the writings of Travis and Wolpe, among others, reveal anything like a strict adherence to the doctrine that "stutterers show a definite personality pattern." The assumptions and operational conditions upon which the approach to stuttering persons is made by these and other clinicians is perhaps more properly regarded as a point of view in stuttering, a theoretical system within which these workers function. The reader will recall our earlier citation which stated that a theoretical system is *assumed* and that acceptance or rejection of it is governed by its ultimate *usefulness*, not by its truth or falsity. A theory, to repeat, is simply a way of looking at things. If Travis, Wolpe, and others of similar orientation have predilections about the personality of any stutterer, it is probably only that he is *unique* and is not most productively perceived in the light of principles derived from *group analyses*.

Pursuing this issue, Sheehan (1958) cites a study by Krugman (1946) in which that author had concluded that stutterers manifested personality traits of the obsessive-compulsive type, as Sheehan says, "in line with [Krugman's] prior leaning toward Fenichel's psychoanalytical theory." Sheehan observes that analyses of the statistically significant findings "exactly contradict" Krugman's conclusions; thus they "undermine rather than support the notion that stutterers are obsessive-compulsive."

It is possible that different conclusions might be reached were workers with different orientations to evaluate data of such investigations, or were they to reformulate conclusions on the basis of internal inconsistencies in the study's design. For example, let us take one of the studies analyzed by Sheehan. We shall choose, for the sake of continuity, one which dealt with the behavior just discussed, viz., obsessive-compulsiveness in stutterers. Sheehan concluded that the study by Bloodstein and Schreiber (1957) (using the Thematic Apperception Test) revealed that as far as obsessive-compulsive tendencies are concerned, there were no significant differences between stutterers and nonstutterers. However, analysis of the Bloodstein and Schreiber article reveals the following facts. As stated in the article, the three judges used in the study "could not be considered skilled in the interpretation of the Thematic Apperception Test . . ., although some emphasis must be given to the fact that the judges were not required to make psychological diagnoses." Prior to the scoring, "the judges familiarized themselves with Rapaport's criteria and studied his illustrations. . . . It was assumed only that they had roughly the same understanding of these terms that Rapaport had." The judges were scoring such variables as concern with unessential detail, peculiar circumstantiality, psychological pseudo-insight into the feelings or behavior of the characters, free-association-like ideas, and the like—not a simple task. The coefficients of correlation obtained among the judges were .72, .74, and .93. The two judges represented by the .93 coefficient were a married couple, which the authors felt "apparently reflects the greater opportunity these judges had for preliminary discussion . . . as well as the frequently observed similarity of husbands and wives in matters of attitude and opinion. The smaller co-efficients probably must be regarded as more representative. . . . While the amount of agreement . . . was not high, it appeared to warrant at least a guarded interest in the findings." Now, if we regard the conclusions in the light of these conditions, our reaction tends to become more tempered. The authors themselves stress that careful verification of their findings is needed; also, that their findings do not imply that some stutterers are not abnormally obsessive-compulsive in personality structure. Thus the Bloodstein-Schreiber article does not completely support the view that stutterers are not different. The reader will realize that almost any investigation could have been chosen for a similar analysis with the probability that similar qualifying conditions would be found, regardless of the comparative excellence of the design.

One wonders if the best approach to the problem may not be in the form of a concentrated emphasis on the stuttering *individual,* in terms of identifying pertinent personality determinants, rather than on the stuttering *group.* This does not necessarily imply that such an individual evaluation would be processed around a battery of clinical diagnostic instruments, although we must assume that many such tools would be helpful. Perhaps the hub around which the evaluation should or perhaps even *must* revolve is the clinical *relationship* between the stuttering person and the clinician. The "goodness" in appraisal of "what the stutterer's personality *is*" will depend on the "goodness" of perception, discrimination, inference, and intuition of the clinician as the most sensitive diagnosing instrument (Murphy, 1959).

A reasonably broad interpretation of the great number of research findings on the stuttering personality may be that the personalities of stuttering persons can be distributed along a very broad adjustment *continuum* extending from psychotic (Freund, 1955) to normal adjustment (Johnson, 1956). Perhaps this is the one inherent message in past research—that a given stutterer may be functioning at any "point" in the range of adjustment. Clinical experience points to the fact that the majority of stuttering persons appear to cluster toward a below-average range, which some workers may label "neurotic"; and, in general, the younger the stuttering person, the better the chance that he has emotional problems of somewhat more than average frequency and intensity. Likewise there appears to be no *specific* etiology of stuttering other than the fact that it arises out of fractured interpersonal relationships. It seems necessary to think of *causes* of stuttering as lying in a diffuse constellation of dynamic forces which revolve around basic life processes and the degree of success with which a given child meets the challenges of the speech and related developmental tasks. Although the initial stages of the stuttering disorder function as anxiety derivatives, later stages of stuttering (adolescence and beyond, most observably) may function as fear derivatives—a consideration about which we shall have more to say later in this chapter.

The point is that we cannot generalize—we cannot think of stutterers as "obsessive-compulsive personalities" or "speech defectives" or even "normal persons who happen to stutter" and proceed from that generalization. The very fact that the research and clinical findings are often so different suggests that stuttering persons are definitely varied, somewhat in kind but mostly in degree. The needs and motives of the individual stutterer are so numerous, complicated, and different from those of many other stutterers that it is virtually impossible to categorize dynamics in patterns descriptive of these persons as a group. There must remain, however, the deep hope that there will be found some principles of sufficient general applicability to operate fruitfully in consideration of a nosological group such as stutterers. The point being stressed here is that stuttering persons are unique. Indeed, the disparate findings in stuttering personality research may stand as a monument to the uniqueness of the individuals studied.

In any case, the mere attainment of facts is not enough. In order to help those who stutter, we should strive for (1) the development of a point of view; (2) the ascertainment of some fundamental *principles* of behavior; (3) the utilization of the principles as evaluative guides and as direction markers for the choice of therapeutic approach; (4) an increased sensitivity to rock-bottom emotional forces; (5) an acceptance and fearless use of inference, intuition, and imagination; and (6) greater understanding and emphasis on the intimate interpersonal dynamics between the stutterer and clinician.

In Chapters 3, 4, and 5 an attempt was made to orient the reader, and they were directed primarily to the student reader or the clinician with little background in psychodynamics, to develop a way of thinking about the stuttering persons they would be serving. The dynamics discussed are the critical determinant processes in personality development. These personality dynamics were not, however, thought of as applying to all stuttering individuals. A given stutterer can experience stress in any or all the areas mentioned. More specifically, certain developmental task experiences were regarded as particularly crucial in the etiology of psychogenic speech disorders such as stuttering. Looking at stuttering persons in such a perspective is a more sensitive, even "just," way than regarding them merely as "stutterers" and thinking very little beyond whatever the label conjures up in one's mind.

Let us consider again the principle of generalization, and specifically the generalization process in relation to orificial equating (see Chapter 4, pp. 85–87, 98). This principle, used as part of a point of view in trying to understand stuttering persons, is helpful in many ways. For instance, behavior learned in one situation will tend to be transferred to other situations, according to how similar the new conditions are to the original situation. A child who has learned to avoid bowel movements until rigidly scheduled times may eventually, if the training is severe enough, become generally apprehensive about "letting himself go" in any way, including speech. As he grows older, he speaks only when spoken to (only at the "proper time"). He is fearful that he will speak at the wrong time or that he will not speak at the right time and in the right way. He has generalized the restriction to situations and behavior which were not the original ones but which were similar enough to be equated (in this case, confused) with the original. Part of his problem becomes one of learning to differentiate among situations and behaviors that are similar—and of course this includes speech and speaking situations. In therapy, oftentimes the question arises: Why am I so fearful in this particular situation? Or, why do I stutter in talking with *him* and not with *her?* Discovering what the often unconscious cues are that elicit the discomfort is a frequent goal of therapy; it is a process of particularization of what has become diffusely generalized.

Descriptions of such processes are available in the literature (Lewin, 1933), including discussions of similar processes in stutterers (Spring, 1935). In an intriguing study by Haney (1950), each of six young adult male stutterers was given 90 hours (4 hours a week) of experimental "projective" therapy in which each subject was asked to use his imagination and visualize a white rectangular card in space. As he perceived the card, he was to report anything or everything that he saw and also to attend to any feelings that accompanied whatever he saw. He was asked to assume a passive role and to allow his visualization to have free and random fluctuation. The clinician observed and recorded the verbal productions of the subjects, offering no suggestions, giving no advice or indication as to any possible meaning of the materials produced by the stutterer. If questioned, the clinician either repeated the question or restated it, placing the responsibility for answering on the subject. The Thematic Apperception Test and Rorschach Ink Blots were administered to each subject before therapy began and at the end of the fiftieth experimental hour.

The pertinent findings in Haney's research may be summarized as follows: The statements of the stuttering subjects revealed that the speech mechanism was perceived as confused in structure and space with other bodily orifices, anal, genital, and urethral. A great deal of the verbalizations revealed that the mouth was perceived as behaving biologically; activities such as ingesting, retaining, molding, and expelling were visualized. These were concerned usually with the manipulation of body objects, both parts and products. The subjects repeatedly perceived specific orifices functioning in the manner of other orifices. Much of the oral activity was confused with the functions of other orifical pathways. All subjects seemed to have difficulty in differentiating and assigning gender to their own body parts and activities, and they showed a marked tendency to interpret sexual behavior and vegetative functions in terms of their own oral activity, although in a confused way. Haney's main thesis was that these perceptual distortions are motives implied by the subject's speech maladjustment of stuttering. He posited that the act of stuttering was a symbolic representation of the perceptual distortions. In other words, distortions in perception were regarded as motivations producing the symptom of stuttering.

STUTTERING AND ANXIETY: ADDITIONAL CONSIDERATIONS

Not only do stutterers tend to be more anxious than nonstutterers, but their strength of anxiety, if measured by galvanic skin response and reaction-time methods, also correlates significantly with the frequency and intensity of stuttering (Kline, 1958). We have said previously that stuttering behavior is likely to occur when the person becomes anxious *lest* something threatening occurs; the occurrence may not come about, but if the person *anticipates* that it will (the "it" being difficult to identify), then the effect may be the same. The more apprehensive the anticipation, the more distintegrated the behavior will be; i.e., the more frequent and intense the stuttering will be. From one point of view, then, stuttering can be considered an *expectancy disorder;* Freund (1955), in fact, referred to it as "one of the classical expectation neurotic symptoms." More than two decades ago, Johnson and Ainsworth (1938) were writing that the "expectation of stuttering" should be considered a part of the stuttering disorder.

The present authors have indicated that what the stuttering person "expects" is not necessarily only "to stutter." In many cases the stutterer does not know what he is expecting. This would be the case in instances in which he experienced a feeling of apprehension having unidentifiable sources (anxiety). That is, the expectation experience is an apprehension concerning threatening or self-effacing circumstances which could occur, and these circumstances may be any of many noxious events (internal or external, verbal or nonverbal). Expectation phenomena of a less disintegrative kind include *fear* experiences (thus, consciously perceived threats, according to our definition) connected ordinarily with specific objective referents. Here, one of the most common and most important fear experiences would be the actual fear of the stuttering speech, with its self-debasing aftereffects. However, anxiety expectations, we repeat, are not simply expectations that stuttering will occur but expectations that any threatening circumstances may occur (overwhelming external forces or self-inadequacies concerning abilities to handle threats). Wischner (1950) has stated that "the stutterer is avoiding, not nonfluency as such, but the original nonfluent behavior" (the adult reactions). Wischner's "original behavior" is regarded as the nonfluent speech. We have said that the original behavior could be any critical developmental task experience in addition to the speech developmental tasks. Wischner goes on to make the following amplifying statement:

Historically, the sequence of the development of anxiety in the child might be described as follows: The child's normal nonfluent speech serves as a stimulus to adults in his environment to which they respond with disapproval or censure. The reactions of adults, in turn, have stimulus value for the child and elicit painful reactions in him. These painful reactions become, in turn, response-produced stimulation which evokes a state of anxiety. This anxiety (anticipation of pain) possesses drive properties and motivates the child to activity designed to avoid the noxious stimulation . . . the stimulus cues which are present at this time include persons and words, cues which serve so adequately as instigators to anxiety in the adult stutterer" (Wischner, 1950, p. 329).

In continuing his skillful probe of stuttering dynamics, Wischner asks, "How does anxiety lead to stuttering behavior?" Although it seems reasonable that the anxiety may become focalized about the act of speaking, Wischner offers two alternative responses: (1) although the anxiety is learned, the stuttering speech is not; rather it represents a breakdown of speech behavior consequent upon the anxiety which is specific to the speech behavior, or (2) both anxiety and stuttering are learned; acquired anxiety is a drive state which motivates the person to behave so as to escape pain; successful escape behavior is reinforced (as a result of the anxiety reduction); the stutterer may even stop talking, but the urge to speak is so strong that a conflict occurs; the stutterer will try different ways of speaking; the least painful one (the most anxiety-reducing one) will tend to endure. The bases of this type of analysis may be found in the writings of Mowrer (1939) and other learning theorists.

Sheehan has been another pioneer in the application of learning theory to stuttering behavior, regarding stuttering as an approach-avoidance conflict at various levels between opposed urges: the urge to speak, and the urge to avoid speaking owing to fear of stuttering (1951). Sheehan is in substantial agreement with Wischner (1950, 1952) in concluding essentially that the approach-avoidance conflict is resolved by actually stuttering, thus reducing the intensity of the fear of anticipation of stuttering. "Stuttering persists even though it is more punishing than rewarding in the long run because . . . the stuttering response is continually reinforced . . . the point at which the stutterer is able to go

on to the next word is the point of reinforcement . . ."
(Sheehan, 1951, p. 62).

Sheehan later made his theoretical viewpoint more inclusive, stating that the approach-avoidance conflict which causes stuttering may occur at different levels: "word, situation, emotional content, relationship or ego protective." According to Sheehan, "the blocking in speech may reflect a conflict between speaking or not speaking a feared word, meeting or avoiding a threatening situation, expressing or inhibiting unacceptable feelings, accepting or rejecting certain social roles or interpersonal relationships, and entering into or retreating from certain lifelong endeavors, aspired roles, and other competitive callings" (1954; also, 1953). The statement is certainly an all-inclusive one and appears to cover any conceptual eventuality. It describes in a cogent fashion most of the processes that could be functioning when stuttering behavior is going on, and the present authors concur most completely with it; the only difference is that Sheehan has placed the conditions within the framework of an approach-avoidance theory.

Now, at this point, if we ask ourselves the questions, "What is the stutterer *approaching?*" and "what is he trying to *avoid?*"—what can be said? Here are several possible responses: (1) He is approaching "the word"; (2) he is appoaching the speech act per se; (3) he is trying to avoid nonfluent speech. These are indeed possible answers, correct in some instances. But from our viewpoint the basic conflict may be in *non*speech experiences. Perhaps as the stutterer walks to the front of his class to give his oral report, his "approach" determinant is the desire to achieve status by showing the class how much he knows about stamps, his hobby, but his "avoidance" determinant is the discomfort at the thought of standing before the group, especially the girls, because he is obese, or he has acne, or he feels intellectually inferior. He may stop or vacillate whenever these opposing forces reach an equilibrium. This may be his basic approach-avoidance conflict, and it may be far more serious than the *speech* approach-avoidance conflict. The reader will note that our example is not in disagreement with Sheehan as long as we realize that conflicts may occur, as Sheehan says, at different "levels." That is, they may occur at the situational-conflict level, the emotional content-conflict level, and the self-protective conflict level, in addition to the word-conflict level.

The approach-avoidance conflict represents a conflict in *motives* within the stutterer. He needs or is driven to do one thing while at the same time he needs or is driven to do just the opposite. But it should be remembered that not all conflict behavior can be so dichotomized. The stutterer may experience an *avoidance-avoidance conflict,* which would consist of two negative goals. Jim doesn't want to speak in the public speaking class, yet he doesn't want to flunk the course. Henry doesn't want to work after school at the soda-fountain where he has to speak to the customers, but he doesn't want to lose the income. This is the classical Scylla and Charybdis conflict. Vacillation is a common response to this discord, as is flight from the field of disturbance.

Double approach-avoidance is another type of conflict in which two or more behaviors or goals have both positive and negative significance. Consider the stutterer who wants to join the debating team or dramatic club but also wishes to make the school baseball team; each would satisfy basic needs, and up to this point the situation appears to be an approach-approach conflict. However, home pressure may be on choosing the debating team while peer-group pressure dictates going out for the ball team. Failing to satisfy one of the parties brings loss of prestige; thus each goal has negative value. In an *approach-approach* conflict the conflict is between two equally desirable goals. Socially this may include wanting to go to a basketball game and a school dance when both are scheduled for the same night. Referring to life adjustments in terms of these several "conflicts" is one way of achieving some commonality in thinking about reactions to stress or frustrating circumstances. But an infinite number and complexity of conflicts are possible, and at any moment in time the perceptual-motor processes of the human must encompass a countless and intricate array of such conflicts of different types and intensities, including the stuttering "moment."

STUTTERING AS REWARDING

We have seen that stuttering can be considered as "beneficial" inasmuch as, once the stuttering occurs, anxiety and tension reduction follow as a consequence. It was stated earlier (Chapter 5, p. 128) that a psychological symptom is any chronic or repetitive behavior which arises and persists as a self-defensive process against anxiety. Such a symptom serves to decrease anxiety, but it is not accompanied by insight as to the anxiety source or to the means of resolving the anxiety. Also, we termed stuttering a psychogenically motivated symptom. We said that the *primary* purpose of self-defensive behavior is to reduce anxiety or fear. Therefore the stuttering symptom is a self-defensive behavior which functions primarily as an anxiety- or fear-reduction process; and, in this sense, it is most rewarding. In general learning theory, the *law of effect* says simply that responses (such as stuttering) are learned as a function of their consequences; "liked" states are enforced, "unliked" states are not. Stuttering, being tension reducing, is "satisfying." In addition, conditioned stimuli may become satisfiers through association and generalization; i.e., they may become stimuli having secondary reinforcing properties through being equated with the primary reward (McGeough and Irion, 1952). If the stutterer blinks his eyes often enough during times when he "breaks through" the block or is experiencing decreasing stuttering, the eye blinking in itself may come to have a satisfying component, or at least it may be regarded as a helpful or magical "starting" device. Yet, of course, stuttering is not simply rewarding. It is punishing too. It elicits societal rejections, and it effaces one's self-image in many different ways.

Of behavior of this kind, Mowrer has this to say:

. . . if an act [such as stuttering] has two consequences—the one rewarding and the other punishing—which would be strictly equal if
simultaneous, the influence of those consequences upon later perform-
ances of that act will vary depending on the *order* in which they
occur. If the punishing consequence [the negative reaction of listen-
ers] comes first and the rewarding one [tension reduction] later, the
difference between the inhibiting and the reinforcing effects will be
in favor of the inhibition. But if the rewarding consequence [tension
reduction] comes first and the punishing one [listener reaction] later,
the difference will be in favor of the reinforcement [of the stuttering].
In either instance the resulting behavior would be non-integrative
(Mowrer, 1950, p. 426).

For instance, John is speaking to a social group. After
a prolonged speech block, he stutters and continues talking.
The tension reduction (rewarding consequence) precedes
the negative audience reaction (punishing consequence).
According to Mowrer's view, the stuttering behavior is reinforced because it has been rewarding and has occurred
prior to the audience reaction.

A related hypothesis is worth mentioning at this point.
Dollard and Miller (1950), in discussing repression in relation to reinforcement theory, state that cessation of anxiety-
arousing thoughts reduces anxiety. Thus, not thinking about
anxiety-arousing ideas becomes a well-learned response.
These authors give the example of a group of persons who
change the topic of discussion because of its anxiety-eliciting
nature. Staats (1957) believes that the same analysis can
be applied to speech; the stopping of speaking may become
a well-learned response. In addition, Staats says, a *confused*
way of speaking (or of thinking) may be anxiety reducing
when it results in a disruption of communication and a consequent diminution of the anxiety-producing subject matter or
of the conversation itself. It is also likely that the disorganized speech elicits behavior from others which is anxiety-
producing, and thus behavior which would avoid this discomfort, in this case the stopping of speaking, would be well
learned.

STUTTERING AS SELF-PERPETUATING

The preceding discussion considered anxiety-reducing stuttering behavior as rewarding. The implication, then, was that the stuttering would be "retained" for its value as a satisfier. This is not a novel notion; Freud maintained that the compulsive repeating of unpleasant activities may very well yield pleasure because of the feeling of mastery that is derived. The stutterer's use of the stuttering as the scapegoat aspect of his behavior has often been discussed in speech therapy. A person is apt to attribute his inadequacies entirely to his stuttering. Often he will be realistic, but many times he will rationalize. He will "blame" the stuttering. Perhaps, having become "adjusted" to the stuttering, he may be less inclined to relinquish it. As Sheehan said, "He may have lived with his stuttering so long that functioning without it involves too radical a change in self-concept to be readily assimilated" (Sheehan, 1954, p. 480). What we are suggesting here is that the stuttering behavior, heretofore regarded as a *symptom,* comes to assume power as a *cause.*

We have said that the personalities of stuttering individuals range along a very broad continuum. In some cases (albeit a minority) stutterers will be as well adjusted as most "normal" nonstuttering persons. Yet, we have maintained that stuttering is caused by feelings of anxiety or fear, depending on the level of consciousness of the impending threats to self-esteem. Now, if this is so, why does the stuttering behavior persist in individuals who do not have more than a "normal amount" of anxiety or fear? We have answered the question partially in declaring that the stuttering speech may persist because of its reward value, because of its scapegoat benefits, and because, perhaps, the person has learned to become "comfortable" with it.

STUTTERING, FUNCTIONAL AUTONOMY, AND PERSEVERATION

At this point, a consideration of G. Allport's *principle of functional autonomy* (1937a; 1937b) is appropriate. This principle involves the concept of contemporaneity of motives. Most simply, it states that given behaviors somehow may free themselves from the original motivating forces and become ends or goals in themselves. Allport maintains that while all adult motives can be traced back to infancy, as the individual matures, the link is severed, the tie being "historical, not functional." As support for this view, Allport cites the mechanism of the "circular reflex," ascribing to it the activity of babbling, for instance. He considers it a basic instance of functional autonomy, "for any situation where the consummation of an act provides adequate stimulation for the repetition of the same act does not require any backward tracing of motives. The act is self-perpetuating until it is inhibited by new activities or fatigue" (Allport, 1937a, p. 198). He also cites experiments which show that "incompleted tasks set up tensions that tend to keep the individual at work until they are resolved. No hypothesis of self-assertion, rivalry, or any other basic need is required. The completion of the task has become a quasi-need with dynamic force of its own (Allport, 1937a, p. 198). Thus, in stuttering, we would have an act which originally occurs because of anxiety, yet when the anxiety is no longer present, the stuttering continues; it resists extinction, even though apparently the "need for stuttering" is no longer present. As a matter of fact, Allport specifically mentions stuttering within the context of functional autonomy, writing:

Why are acquired tics, stammering, sexual perversions, phobias, and anxiety so stubborn . . . ? The reason seems to be that what we usually call "symptoms" are in reality something more. They have set themselves up in their own right as independent systems of motivation. Merely disclosing their roots does not change their independent activity (Allport, 1937a, p. 200).

He adds:

Motives are always a kind of striving for some form of completion; they are unresolved tension, and demand a "closure" to activity under way (Allport, 1937a, p. 204).

An additional question concerning the principle asks whether *all* motives are functionally autonomous. Hall and

Lindzey, in an analysis of Allport's theories, answer in the following fashion:

There are infantilisms and other kinds of motivation that retain their historical links with the early beginnings. However, the extent to which an individual's motivations are autonomous is a measure of the maturity of the individual. The more his present motives are linked to the past and to underlying biological states, the more immature he is and the less he has evolved from a childish state" (Hall and Lindzey, 1957, p. 372).

The condition that increasing maturity tends to correlate with degree of functional autonomy is in keeping with the present authors' viewpoint of stuttering. Theoretically, a completely functionally autonomous person would be one with no anxiety derivatives connected to past stresses. Also, the more anxious a person is, the less functionally autonomous he is, assuming that in some degree the anxiety is linked to earlier developmental frustrations. Continuing this line of theorizing, the more anxious a stutterer is, the less his stuttering is a functionally autonomous behavior. The idea that stuttering as a drive may become inextinguishable due to functional autonomy, however, is an area requiring experimental work. Many presently unanswered issues exist in reference to it. For example, evidence is available (Miller, 1951) that a strong learned drive may appear to be unaffected over long periods of time, yet eventually be extinguished. Criticisms of the principle of functional autonomy are available (Bertocci, 1940; McClelland, 1942; Rethlingschaefer, 1943), pointing up debatable issues.

What could be considered a variation of the principle of functional autonomy, though not so conceptualized by its author, is Eisenson's theory of stuttering as a *perseverative phenomenon* (Berry and Eisenson, 1956; Eisenson and Winslow, 1938). According to this view, perseveration is a tendency for a mental or motor process to continue after the situation which elicited it ceases to be present. Stuttering as a perseverative manifestation occurs whenever the stutterer feels incapable of performing satisfactorily in the speaking situation. Eisenson tested his theory on a small number of stutterers. His findings led him to conclude that stutterers were more resistant than nonstutterers to changes in selected nonspeech activities. Once they made a response, they were more apt to continue (perseverate) making that response even though it was inappropriate for new situations. Some research by King (1953) supports Eisenson's earlier findings. Eisenson says, "If this type of behavior is carried over into speech, as . . . [is] the case with stutterers, an articulatory act which is once initiated would tend to be repeated. If the tendency is inhibited, blocking rather than articulatory repetition would result" (Berry and Eisenson, 1956, p. 268). Eisenson maintains that to determine the cause of stuttering, we would first have to determine the cause or causes of the perseveration phenomenon. He illustrates the universality of the behavior by noting that people cannot easily make rapid adjustments to quickly changing conditions when they are tired; that epileptics, manic depressives, and aphasics reveal clearly observable perseverative behavior; and he adds:

Perseveration may be indicative of a lack of ability due to a temporarily or permanently lowered vitality following mental or physical trauma. . . . Possibly it may constitute an organism's responses when some immediate reaction is called for, but when the complete and adequate reaction has not yet been determined, or cannot be given because of the possible harmful effects on the organism (Berry and Eisenson, 1956, p. 269).

In other words, Eisenson thinks that a multiplicity of causes may be necessary to account for the "psychological phenomenon of perseveration"; etiologies may be constitutional, neuropathological, psychosomatic, and psychopathogical. He does believe, however, that in about half of the stuttering population, the perseveration has an organic basis: ". . . it probably represents a mild amnesic (word finding) disturbance for high-level, propositional language usage. This may arise because of peculiarities of cortical development, competition between cortical and subcortical centers for control of language function, or actual damage to cortical tissue" (Berry and Eisenson, 1956, p. 270). In the "nonorganic" group of stutterers, stuttering may occur initially as imitation and continue because of secondary gains; or it may arise as a consequence of early childhood emotional disturbances.

This perseveration tendency is, indeed, a kind of behavior which is often observed, although the explanations given for the existence of the phenomenon may vary considerably. For example, Murphy (1953), as a portion of a study of frustration in young stuttering and nonstuttering adults, investigated by electroencephalographic (EEG) methods, whether or not any differences existed between the groups in the extent of disruption of cortical equilibrium upon being frustrated and in the rate of recovery of cortical equilibrium following cessation of frustration. It was postulated that the degree and duration of cortical disequilibration (brain-wave rhythm breakdown) were related to a general disruption of psychophysical equilibrium and that the rate of recovery from the frustration to a state of equilibrium was indicative of the subjects' cortically adaptive or integrative capacity. The frustrating stimulus was a 30-second recording of a man and woman speaking different passages concurrently; the male reading was provocative of imagery and feeling, while the female reading was abstract and monotonous. Subjects were required to remember as much as possible of the meaning of what the women said, unaware that the man's voice would be present as a masking-frustrating effect. EEG tracings were taken during resting, stimulation, and recovery, each 30 seconds in duration. EEG records revealed, among other things, that stutterers' cortical disruption during frustration was significantly greater than that of nonstutterers. The most interesting finding, however, in relation to a "perseverative" phenomenon, was the following: Although the nonstutterers, following the cessation of the stimulus, recovered normal brain-wave patterns almost immediately, the cortical behavior of the stutterers during the recovery period corresponded to that found during frustration. It was as though the stutterers were still perceiving the frustrating stimulus. Murphy posits that the lingering effect endures as a consequence of anxiety or tension, noting that anxiety tends to fixate response patterns.

If we add to these findings the considerations of (1) generalizations, (2) reinforcements at various operating levels, and (3) changes from one reinforcing condition to another, to name just a few, we begin to have a conception as to how arduous it would be to determine the degree to which stuttering can be functionally autonomous or "perseverative." We do note that there are research studies available showing that verbal responses, if socially reinforced, increase in frequency (Cohen *et al.* 1954; Talbot, 1954; Verplank, 1955). The condition would appear to be applicable to stuttering verbal behavior.

In discussing reinforcement, Skinner (1953) mentions the value of attention-getting behavior (and stuttering can be included here), stating that gaining the attention of people is reinforcing because it is a necessary condition for other reinforcements from them. If the attention is from an important person (one who is a "satisfier," a reinforcer in many ways, such as the mother), it is a very strong reinforcer. For instance, Mary stutters; her parents immediately and consistently attend to her, perhaps in a sympathetic way. For one reason or another, the stuttering is accomplished with all its accruments. Attention, having been repeatedly and consistently experienced in connection with rewarding circumstances, comes to be capable of stimulating the reinforcing behavior. Mary then stutters to get attention. Although this seems hardly plausible as a full explanation as to why stuttering may be self-perpetuating, it is a contribution in helping to understand why stuttering may persist in the absence of original determinants. An additional secondary gain may occur as a consequence of a possible hostility-satisfaction component (Barbara, 1954) involved in the stuttering, although other dynamics are involved, too. The thinking of Fenichel and Sheehan, for example, is in basic concurrence on this point, as is shown in the following passages:

. . . stuttering may be viewed as serving a dual role: (1) direct expression of hostile feeling through imposing punishment on the audience; (2) expiation of the guilt arising out of the aggression against the audience through imposing punishment on the stutterer himself. At the same time the active audience penalties frustrate the stutterer, who now feels increased resentment at the person who frustrated his communication and made him feel guilty (Sheehan, 1954, p. 480).

Fenichel, discussing stuttering from a psychoanalytical viewpoint, makes statements such as the following one which, though taken from context, shows a surprising similarity to writings of nonanalytic theorists cited throughout the chapter, and which can be compared very directly with the Sheehan statement just cited:

The symptom of stuttering . . . is the result of a conflict between antagonistic tendencies; the patient shows that he wishes to say something and yet does not want to. Since he consciously intends to speak, he must have some unconscious reason for not wanting to speak . . . [for stutterers speaking means] an aggressive act directed against the listener. . . . Quite often [he] begins to stutter when he is particularly eager to prove a point. Behind his apparent zeal he has concealed a hostile or sadistic tendency to destroy his opponent by means of words, and the stuttering is both the blocking of and the punishment for this tendency. Still more often stuttering is exacerbated in the presence of prominent or authoritative persons, that is, of paternal figures against whom the unconscious hostility is most intense. . . . "Words can kill," and stutterers are persons who unconsciously think it necessary to use so dangerous a weapon with care (Fenichel, 1945, pp. 311–13).

Thus far, in attempting to explain why stuttering sometimes persists in the absence of original anxiety or chronic fear states, we have considered (1) the primary reinforcement of tension reduction; (2) the secondary reinforcements involving "scapegoat" benefits, attention-getting techniques, symbolic hostility release, and guilt-masochism processes; (3) the reinforcements of allied complicating factors such as generalization processes; and (4) the operation of the principle of functional autonomy. From another aspect, stuttering may be regarded as an act of compulsive-repetitive proportions, as a highly motivated "habit" which is difficult to modify or extinguish. This calls to mind still another finding from the field of learning theory; namely, that activities which are *overlearned* may be highly resistant to change and hence lead to excessive repetition. The "familiar" is preferred, and the behavior remains stereotyped. It is not far-fetched to regard stuttering, as a consequence of years of existence, as becoming fixated or habituated (overlearned). In fact, "behavior acquired under excessive frustration may become abnormally fixated, and thus resistant to change" (Hilgard, 1956, p. 296).

Probably all these conditions hold in some degree, varying with the individual stutterer, varying themselves in strength as explanatory concepts for the stuttering. Regardless of what unknown configuration constitutes the essential motivating force, the result of that force (the perseveration of the stuttering symptom) is usually sufficient to produce adjustment problems.

STUTTERING REVIEWED

On the basis of the viewpoints and evidence presented in the preceding pages of this book, we may venture to rechart briefly the points of origin and the course of stuttering.

We have maintained that the seeds of stuttering behavior are imbedded in the soil of early socialization experiences and that stuttering's tap roots are intertwined most intimately with the parent-child relationships. When nonverbal or verbal communicative or developmental task breakdowns germinate in these processes, the resulting disruptions to self-differentiation and integration are experienced by the child as feelings of apprehension or dread, termed *anxiety*. These anxieties may occur in relation to specific verbal or nonverbal developmental tasks but, through generalization and similar learning occurrences, become attached to other developmental tasks, both motor and perceptual. Anxieties, while arising as a consequence of introjections, repressions, and guilt reactions to the demands of conscience, come to manifest themselves through other self-defensive processes such as projection. When the strain of attempting to integrate the competing forces—of expressing or repressing feelings and thoughts—becomes too great, a self-disintegration in the form of a self-defensive, oral symptom occurs which is called stuttering. Although the stuttering symptom persists primarily as a consequence of anxiety, in time the person may come to have specific *fears* (conscious awareness) which may confuse and intensify the stuttering dynamics. If and when one of these specific fears becomes a fear of stuttering per se, attention on and attempts to control the stuttering symptom itself occur (secondary stuttering). In time, if the anxiety determinants become resolved, the symptom of their presence (the stuttering) will subside; this improvement will be facilitated by self-insight concerning specific fear processes. The longer a stuttering symptom persists, however, the more the stuttering speech itself becomes self-perpetuating because of a complex combination of determinants or effects: (1) its "rewarding" nature; (2) its attention-getting and "scapegoat" benefits; (3) its satisfaction as a familiar, thus comfortable, self-ingredient; (4) as an "overlearned" and perseverative activity, and (5) because of other secondary gains such as aggression satisfaction and even masochistic values (self-punishment, need for societal disapproval, and the like). All these may be in addition to and quite aside from anxiety promptings.

Stuttering can be defined as "what a person is." It tells us that self-defensive processes are in action, that anxieties or fears of diffused or specific character are operating, that the person is attempting not only to protect himself but to prove and improve himself also. It reveals to us the level of efficiency with which the person has been able to merge outer reality with inner drives and needs. It is an indicator of the individual's past history; of the problem cores around which his present life is revolving, and around which his future life, in some degree, will be centered. Stuttering gives us an idea of what a person thinks of himself, how he feels about himself, and how he thinks others regard him. Stuttering not only coexists with, but is a *result* of, what a person thinks of himself, feels about himself, and of how he believes others perceive him.

Wallen (1959), in a Q-technique study at Boston University of the self-concepts of 30 adolescent stutterers and nonstutterers, developed a Q-sort self-assessment instrument utilizing 100 self-referent statements made by stutterers. The Q-sort was structured into six personality trait areas by five clinicians designated as experts (two speech pathologists and three clinical psychologists). The categories were: (1) self-acceptance; (2) independence; (3) self-rejection; (4) dependence; (5) lack of emotional control, and (6) withdrawal. Each subject was asked to perform three specific self-sorts: (1) the actual-self sort ("how I think I really am"); (2) the ideal-self sort ("how I would like to be"); and (3) the "other"-self sort ("how I think others see me") along a range of "describes me the least" to "describes me the most." A few of the findings can be mentioned.

In comparison to the nonstutterers, the stutterers exhibited responses which, statistically, were significantly *lower* (.01 per cent) in mean score for the personality trait categories of self-acceptance and independence, and significantly *higher* (.01 per cent) in mean score for the categories of self-rejection and lack of emotional control. In all comparisons, the actual-, ideal-, and the other-self sorts of stutterers were significantly lower than those of the nonstutterers. For example, stutterers exhibited a significantly lower actual-self/ideal-self concept relationship than the nonstutterers. (The postulate is that low levels of congruence between actual- and ideal-self concepts reflect high degrees of self-dissatisfaction, and vice versa.) Such findings would appear to increase the validity of postulates expressed earlier concerning the import of disturbed self-processes in stuttering disorders.

The significance of these findings in terms of therapeutic indications, has been implied throughout. Clearly, therapy must be structured so as to cope with the range of verbal and nonverbal dynamics discussed, and although emphasis must be on speech therapy which is psychodynamically based and propelled, nevertheless there is a continuum of therapy procedures just as there is a personality—speech continuum of unique stuttering persons, many of whom will profit by more directive therapies than are considered in this book but which are available elsewhere. In general the sequence of treatment of stuttering persons must move from a prior consideration of the underlying emotional motivations to a focusing on the speech behavior as such. This is especially true with very young stutterers up through the period of preadolescence. In a small number of (unisymptomatic) cases, directive speech therapy alone will be useful. The indication as to "type" or "level" of therapy will vary in accordance with countless variables: the effect of anxiety and fear, the intricacy and rigidity of the stutterer's self-defensive network, the level of frustration tolerance and spontaneity, the age and intelligence of the person, and in addition the training and personality of the clinician. The clinician will need the ability and freedom to identify himself with the stutterer, to coexist with him. He will need to utilize all clues such as voice quality, pitch, and general manner and set up a reverberation of sympathetic responses. He will need to introspect and to analyze as the stuttering person releases his feelings; there should be a coexistence of objective and introspective observations. The clinician will have to be totally acceptant, more permissive, and nonauthoritarian. He will help the person to label his feelings, to differentiate among his reaction tendencies and their motivants, to evaluate the consequences of what he feels and does. These are some of the requirements of the clinician. In addition, knowing that effective therapy is not accidental, the clinician will have a plan of action and materials ready though he will not feel that he must follow the proposed format rigidly. Yet, the plan of action—and a "point of view" may be the best plan in some cases—will give both the clinician and the stutterer a feeling of security. It will prevent aimless wandering by providing general guide lines.

What will be the goal of therapy? Speech fluency? Eventually, yes. But the more basic and immediate aim is simply to extend the realm of consciousness of the stutterer, helping him to release and become cognizant of his feelings which are involved in anxiety and fear, to perceive self and environment realistically and to accept them with positive feelings, to synthesize conscience, basic strivings, and self—in short, *to grow up again.* The closer we can bring the stuttering person to the *fear*-level (i.e., the less the stuttering is *anxiety-*based), the more a combined speech-therapy psychotherapy approach will be indicated. Regardless of what the therapy is "called," i.e., what "system" or "type" is used, it is recognized that all therapeutic approaches may include some psycho-therapy, the most directive or "symptomatic" approaches included. Many times the productive processes in many forms of speech therapy are not those insisted upon by their proponents. They consist of unrecognized elements such as reconditioned social relationships, cathartic experiences, and the fact that probably anything which is said by the clinician has some degree of truth or helpfulness in it. There is thera-peutic effect on the stutterer by the sheer fact that a non-threatening and supportive adult is interested enough in him to set certain times aside for him to use as he wishes.

REFERENCES

ALLPORT, G. W. *Personality: a Psychological Interpretation.* New York: Holt, Rinehart & Winston, Inc., 1937a.

———. "The Functional Autonomy of Motives," *Amer. J. Psychol.,* **50**: 141–56, 1937b.

BARBARA, D. S. *Stuttering.* New York: Julian Press, Inc., 1954.

BERRY, M. F., and EISENSON, J. *Speech Disorders: Principles and Practices of Therapy.* New York: Appleton-Century-Crofts, Inc., 1956.

BERTOCCI, P. A. "A Critique of G. W. Allport's Theory of Motivation," *Psychol. Rev.,* **47**: 501–32, 1940.

BLOODSTEIN, O., and SCHREIBER, L. R. "Obsessive-Compulsive Reac-tions in Stutterers," *J. Speech Hearing Dis.,* **22**: 31–39, 1957.

COHEN, D. J.; KALISH, H. I.; THURSTON, J. R.; and COHEN, E. "Experi-mental Manipulation of Verbal Behavior," *J. Exp. Psychol.,* **47**: 106–10, 1954.

COHEN, M. R., and NAGEL, E. *An Introduction to Logic and Scientific Method.* New York: Harcourt, Brace & Co., Inc., 1934.

CONANT, J. B. *On Understanding Science.* New Haven: Yale Univ. Press, 1947.

DESPERT, J. L. "Psychopathology of Stuttering," *Amer. J. Psychiat.,* **99**: 881–85, 1943a.

———. "Psychosomatic Study of Fifty Stuttering Children," *Amer. J. Orthopsychiat.,* **16**: 100–113, 1946.

DESPERT, J. L. "Stuttering: A Clinical Study," *Amer. J. Orthopsychiat.,* 12: 517–24, 1943b.

DOLLARD, J., and MILLER, N. E. *Personality and Psychotherapy.* New York: McGraw-Hill Book Co., Inc., 1950.

EISENSON, J., and WINSLOW, C. "The Perseverating Tendency in Stutterers in a Perceptual Function," *J. Speech Hearing Dis.,* 3: 195–98, 1938.

FENICHEL, O. *The Psychoanalytic Theory of Neurosis.* New York: W. W. Norton & Co., Inc., 1945.

FREUND, H. "Psychosis and Stuttering," *Folia Phoniatrica,* 7, No. 3: 133–53, 1955.

GLASNER, P. J. "Personality Characteristics and Emotional Problems in Stutterers under the Age of Five," *J. Speech Hearing Dis.,* 14: 135–38, 1949.

GLAUBER, I. P. "Dynamic Therapy for the Stutterer," in *Specialized Techniques in Psychotherapy,* by G. Bychowski, and J. L. Despert. New York: Basic Books, Inc., 1952, pp. 207–38.

HALL, C. S., and LINDZEY, G. *Theories of Personality.* New York: John Wiley & Sons, Inc., 1957.

HANEY, R. H. "Motives Implied by the Act of Stuttering as Revealed by Prolonged Experimental Projection." Unpublished Doctoral dissertation, Univ. of Southern California, 1950.

HILGARD, E. R. *Theories of Learning,* 2d ed. New York: Appleton-Century-Crofts, Inc., 1956.

JOHNSON, W. *Speech Handicapped School Children,* rev. ed. New York: Harper & Bros., 1956.

JOHNSON, W., and AINSWORTH, S. "Studies in the Psychology of Stuttering: Constancy of Loci of Expectancy of Stuttering," *J. Speech Hearing Dis.,* 3: 101–4, 1938.

KING, P. T. "Perseverative Factors in a Stuttering and Non-Stuttering Population." Unpublished Doctoral dissertation, Pennsylvania State Univ., 1953.

KLINE, D. F. "An Experimental Study of the Frequency of Stuttering in Relation to Certain Goal-Activity Drives in Basic Human Behavior." Unpublished Doctoral dissertation, Univ. of Missouri, 1958.

KRUGMAN, M. "Psychosomatic Study of Fifty Stuttering Children," *Amer. J. Orthopsychiat.,* 16: 127–33, 1946.

LEWIN, B. D. "The Body as Phallus," *Psychoanal. Quart.,* No. 2: 24–47, 1933.

McCLELLAND, D. C. "Functional Autonomy of Motives as an Extinction Phenomenon," *Psychol. Rev.,* 49: 272–83, 1942.

McGEOUGH, J. A., and IRION, A. L. *The Psychology of Human Learning,* rev. ed. New York: Longmans, Green & Co., Inc., 1952.

MILLER, N. E. "Learnable Drives and Rewards," in *Handbook of Experimental Psychology*, ed. S. S. Stevens. New York: John Wiley & Sons, Inc., 1951. Chap. xiii, pp. 435–72.

MOWRER, O. H. *Learning Theory and Personality Dynamics*. New York: The Ronald Press Co., 1950.

MURPHY, A. T. "An Electroencephalographic Study of Frustration in Stutterers," *Speech Monogr.*, 20: 148, 1953.

———. "The Speech Handicapped," *Rev. Educational Research*, 29: 519–28, 1959.

NORTHRUP, F. S. C. *Science and First Principles*. New York: The Macmillan Co., 1931.

RETHLINGSCHAEFER, D. "Experimental Evidence for Functional Autonomy of Motives," *Psychol. Rev.*, 50: 397–407, 1943.

SHEEHAN, J. G. "An Integration of Psychotherapy and Speech Therapy Through a Conflict Theory of Stuttering," *J. Speech Hearing Dis.*, 19: 474–82, 1954.

———. "Projection Studies of Stuttering," *J. Speech Hearing Dis.*, 23: 18–25, 1958.

———. "The Modification of Stuttering Through Nonreinforcement," *J. Abnorm. Soc. Psychol.*, 46: 51–63, 1951.

———. "Theory and Treatment of Stuttering as an Approach-Avoidance Conflict," *J. Psychol.*, 36: 27–49, 1953.

SKINNER, B. F. *Science and Human Behavior*. New York: The Macmillan Co., 1953.

SPRING, W. J. "Words and Masses: A Pictorial Contribution to the Psychology of Stammering," *Psychoanal. Quart.*, No. 4: 244–58, 1935.

STAATS, A. W. "Learning Theory and Opposite Speech," *J. Abnorm. Soc. Psychol.*, 55: 268–69, 1957.

TALBOT, E. "The Effect of Note Taking Upon Verbal Responses and Its Implications for the Interview." Unpublished Doctoral dissertation, Univ. of California at Los Angeles, 1954.

TRAVIS, L. E. "The Need for Stuttering," *J. Speech Dis.*, 5: 193–202, 1940.

———. "The Unspeakable Feelings of People with Special Reference to Stuttering," in *Handbook of Speech Pathology*, ed. L. E. Travis. New York: Appleton-Century-Crofts, Inc., 1957. Chap. xix, pp. 916–46.

VERPLANK, W. S. "The Control of the Content of Conversation: Reinforcement of Statements of Opinion," *J. Abnorm. Soc. Psychol.*, 51: 668-76, 1955.

WALLEN, V. "A Q-technique Study of the Self-Concepts of Adolescent Stutterers and Nonstutterers." Unpublished Doctoral dissertation, Boston Univ., 1959.

WISCHNER, G. J. "An Experimental Approach to Expectancy and Anxiety in Stuttering Behavior," *J. Speech Hearing Dis.*, **17**: 139–54, 1952.

——. "Stuttering Behavior and Learning: A Preliminary Theoretical Formulation," *J. Speech Hearing Dis.*, **15**: 324–35, 1950.

WOLPE, Z. "Play Therapy, Psychodrama, and Stuttering," in *Handbook of Speech Pathology*, ed. L. E. Travis. New York: Appleton-Century-Crofts, Inc., 1957. Chap. xxxii, pp. 991–1023.

Part III

Psychodynamic Speech Therapy

Chapter 7

Diagnosis, Evaluation,
and the Evaluator

Not the fact avails, but the use you make of it.——Emerson

The most important diagnostician is the stutterer himself. In the initial interview he tells his story, verbally or non-verbally. In addition to the status of the speech symptom, the clinician is interested in the very broad and often complex configuration of personality dynamics which serves as the operational base for the stuttering. This configuration consists of psychodynamic *processes* which are fluxional and sometimes hardly distinguishable from one another. For ease in verbal handling, we can refer to these dynamics as *factors*. The clinician sets up situations which are designed to tap, identify, and characterize these factors. In addition the character of such factors has implications for improvement in therapy; thus, we may refer to them as *prognostic factors*. The clinician's concern with them is represented by such questions as those that follow. Such questions are not necessarily "asked outright" by the clinician but rather are experienced by him as an attitudinal "set" toward the stutterer, as ideas held in mind and used to structure the diagnostic interview.*

---

* Inasmuch as the validity of the factors in terms of their goodness of predictability or prognostic value is not established, each question should be reformulated in terms of a hypothesis which can be put to test in a variety of ways.

1. What is the age of the person? (The younger the person, the better the prognosis?)
2. What is his general level of intelligence? (The higher the intelligence, the better the prognosis?)
3. What is the impress of environmental factors? (The more strained his situation at home, school, work, or play, the worse the prognosis?)
4. Has there been previous therapy, and if so, what kind and for how long? (What might be the effects of his past therapy structure and experience on future therapy?)
5. What is the level of motivation for therapy? (Was he "forced" to come in by someone who thought he needed help? Or did he come of his own volition?)
6. What is his general attitude toward therapy? (Does he seem to have the ability to establish an effective therapeutic relationship?)
7. What is the general severity of the disorder? (Intensity of the stuttering; presence of associated symptomatology, including not only secondary speech symptoms but also such behaviors as withdrawal, defensiveness, aggressiveness, complacency, and reported somatic symptoms.)
8. What is his level of language usage? (Is it highly intellectual or affectual?)
9. How does he seem to perceive others? (As hostile? Tolerant? Fearful? Does perception of others vary with such factors as the age, sex, independence, or dependence of others?)
10. How does he perceive himself? (As a person of worth? Self-belittling? Dependent? Confused?)
11. What is the nature of his aspirations? (Is his outlook overly optimistic, pessimistic, or realistic in terms of general and speech abilities in the future? Does he wish for more or less than he seems capable of doing?)
12. What is his degree of expressive freedom? (Is he able to verbalize his more basic feelings? Or does he keep his feelings to himself?)
13. What are his general modes of adjustment to frustration or stress?

With such questions as these in mind, it is more easily seen why diagnosis must be an ongoing process, sometimes over a long period of time, and why the phrase *diagnostic therapy* is meaningful, for all therapy is continuingly diagnostic, though often in a very indirect way.

THE PREINTERVIEW FORM

The clinician wants to know about his client's past and present history. A preinterview form is one means to obtain this important historical data. Prior to the initial interview, the client or parent is mailed a preinterview inquiry form, such as that in Fig. 2 which has been used during the past six years at one university speech clinic. The respondent returns the form to the clinic prior to the initial appointment. The form pertains primarily to factual information.

In addition to saving time during the evaluative session, the preinterview inquiry form activates the respondent to do some preinterview introspection. In addition, if the interviewing is to be done by the clinician and if he wishes to establish a beginning relationship which is indirect and unstructured, the preinterview form can be helpful. The form shown in Fig. 2 is a general one and is not designed specifically for stuttering cases.*

In the public school setting, the use of a preinterview form can pose more of a problem. In most cases the parents do not seek out the speech help for their child. The child comes to the attention of the speech clinician through the speech survey or referral by the child's teacher. The clinician initiates the first contact with the child's parents. Some clinicians make the first parent contact by means of a home visit, a telephone call, or a letter. Such communication can acquaint the parents with the services which the school's speech and hearing department offers to the child and his

---

* The mind and the body can never be dichotomized. As a requisite for entrance into therapy, a recent medical examination should be required of every client. Emotional stresses can take their physical tolls. A client may have a history of physical conditions which in themselves may have complicated his adjustment, including his speech adjustment. A copy of a medical report of the physical examination should be obtained on each client in order to clarify his past and present physical status.

BOSTON UNIVERSITY SPEECH AND HEARING CENTER
Preinterview Inquiry Form

Name of client needing diagnosis:

Street Address _____ City _____ State _____ Phone No. ____

Sex: Male ( )   Female ( )   Age: ____ (_____) _____
                                              Date of Birth   Today's Date

Person answering this form: Relationship to client _____

Full Name _____   Age ____ Vocation _____

Father: _____

Mother: _____

Guardian: _____

Brothers: _____
_____
_____

Sisters: _____
_____

---

1. Please describe the speech and/or hearing difficulty.

2. What is the client's occupation?

3. What school does the client attend?

Name of School   Street   City   Grade   Name of Principal

4. Does the client like school? Yes ( ) No ( )

5. Has the client been promoted regularly? Yes ( ) No ( )
   Comments:

6. Do you have a family doctor? Yes ( ) No ( )

Doctor's Name   Street   City   State

7. Who referred the client to the Speech and Hearing Center?

Name   Street   City   State

FIG. 2. A TYPICAL PREINTERVIEW INQUIRY FORM.

Page 2 (for additional space, use reverse side)

8. Did the mother of the client have any accidents, illnesses, or other unusual conditions during pregnancy? If so, please explain.

9. Did the mother of the client have a 9-months pregnancy? If not, please explain.

10. Did the mother of the client have extremely long or extremely short labor? If so, please explain.

11. Conditions of the client immediately following birth:
    a. Did he have convulsions? Yes ( ) No ( )
    b. Did he have difficulties swallowing or sucking?
       Yes ( ) No ( )
    c. Did he have feeding difficulties? Yes ( ) No ( )
    d. Other?

12. At what age did the client learn to walk?

13. If the client had any of the following illnesses, please check the information requested below:

Illness	Yes	No	Age	Mild	Severe
Measles	( )	( )	( )	( )	( )
Mumps	( )	( )	( )	( )	( )
Whooping cough	( )	( )	( )	( )	( )
Scarlet fever	( )	( )	( )	( )	( )
Small pox	( )	( )	( )	( )	( )
Pneumonia	( )	( )	( )	( )	( )
Tonsilitis	( )	( )	( )	( )	( )
Ear diseases	( )	( )	( )	( )	( )
Hay fever	( )	( )	( )	( )	( )
Asthma	( )	( )	( )	( )	( )
Influenza	( )	( )	( )	( )	( )
Pleurisy	( )	( )	( )	( )	( )
Tuberculosis	( )	( )	( )	( )	( )
Appendicitis	( )	( )	( )	( )	( )
Convulsions	( )	( )	( )	( )	( )
Infantile paralysis	( )	( )	( )	( )	( )
Allergies	( )	( )	( )	( )	( )
Frequent colds	( )	( )	( )	( )	( )
Stomach upset	( )	( )	( )	( )	( )
Epilepsy	( )	( )	( )	( )	( )
Gland trouble	( )	( )	( )	( )	( )
Other					

14. Did the client have any aftereffects from the above diseases? If so, please explain.

Page 3 (for additional space, use reverse side)

15. Has the client had any injuries or operations? If so, describe and tell at what age these occurred.

16. Does the client:
    a. Prefer the right or left hand? Right ( ) Left ( )
    b. Have a peculiar walk? Yes ( ) No ( )
    c. Fall or lose his balance easily? Yes ( ) No ( )
    d. Seem awkward and uncoordinated? Yes ( ) No ( )
    e. Have difficulty in chewing and swallowing?
       Yes ( ) No ( )
    f. Have difficulty in grasping objects easily?
       Yes ( ) No ( )
    g. Have cerebral palsy or brain damage? Yes ( ) No ( )
    h. Have a cleft palate or lip? Yes ( ) No ( )

17. If the answer is "Yes" to any of the above, please explain.

18. Please list the names and addresses of the doctors, special teachers, speech or hearing clinicians in public schools, or other clinics to which the client has been for help. Include a statement explaining the kind of help the client received.

19. At what age did the client begin to speak?

20. Have languages other than English been spoken in the home? If yes, which ones?

21. Has any other member of the family (including aunts, uncles, grandparents) had speech and/or hearing difficulties?

22. When and under what circumstances did you first become aware of the client's speech and/or hearing difficulty?

23. Did the client's speech and/or hearing difficulty develop gradually? Yes ( ) No ( )

24. Has the client's speech and/or hearing difficulty remained the same or has it become worse? Same ( ) Worse ( )

25. Is the disorder worse at some times than at others? Yes ( ) No ( ) If yes, please explain.

    Please describe the speech and/or hearing difficulty.

FIG. 2. A TYPICAL PREINTERVIEW INQUIRY FORM (Continued).

Page 4 (for additional space, use reverse side)

26. If the client has expressed any of the following behavior patterns, please check:

	Yes	No		Yes	No
Nervous	( )	( )	Daydreams		
Pities self	( )	( )	excessively	( )	( )
Shy, withdrawn	( )	( )	Jealous	( )	( )
Fears	( )	( )	Lies	( )	( )
Shows off	( )	( )	Steals	( )	( )
Disobedient	( )	( )	Runs away	( )	( )
Whining, cries			Sets fires	( )	( )
easily	( )	( )	Difficult toilet		
Temper tantrums	( )	( )	training	( )	( )
Destructive	( )	( )	Feeding problems	( )	( )
Fights	( )	( )	Sucks thumb	( )	( )
Cruel	( )	( )	Bites nails	( )	( )
Selfish	( )	( )	Constipated	( )	( )
Sleepless	( )	( )	Careless	( )	( )
Nightmares	( )	( )	Perfectionistic	( )	( )
Sleep-walks	( )	( )	Other:		
Wets bed	( )	( )			

27. How does the client get along with
   a. Persons his own age?
   b. Older persons?
   c. Persons at school?

28. What is the client's attitude toward the family or individuals in the family?

29. How does the client feel about his speech and/or hearing difficulty?

30. Does the client avoid speaking situations?

31. Has the speech and/or hearing difficulty had any effect on the client's occupation or education?

32. In what way does the family attempt to help correct the speech and/or hearing difficulty?

(Do Not Write Below This Line)

Recommendations:

parents. The initial interview follows the clinician's introductory contact with the child's parents. It may take place
in the child's home, in the schoolroom, or at the office of
the speech and hearing department. If the clinician contacts
the parents by means of a home visit, the initial interview
may follow immediately. If the clinician writes or phones
the child's parents, the time and place of the initial interview
may be decided on the basis of mutual convenience.

EVALUATION IN THE CLASSROOM

Often the classroom teacher can provide extremely relevant materials as a supplement to the case-history data gath-
ered by the clinician. Teachers have become more "case-
history" minded in recent years. Reports from teachers, such
as that which follows, are not at all unusual. In this instance
the teacher was the referral agent who assumed the responsibility for seeing that his stuttering pupil received speech
therapy. As will be seen, this is actually a report by a "team"
of teachers. Although clinicians cannot expect such detailed
reports from most teachers, because of time factors, experience in giving introductory courses on speech disorders to
over 2,000 New England teachers during the past eight years
indicates that these educators can become capable "clinicians" once they become interested in their stuttering pupils.
The clinician misses a golden opportunity to learn more
about his stuttering children if he does not or cannot tap the
knowledge of the professional who has had the chance to
observe the child in a great variety of activities, the one who
often in a single week interacts with the child more hours
than the clinician does in one year—the classroom teacher.

A Teacher's Report of a Case History.

Early this year, as a result of hearing a talk about speech therapy,
I became interested in a boy who has been in my Art classes for the
past two years. The case history which follows is actually only a
factual report of what I have gleaned in my study of this boy who is
a pupil at a Junior High Training School. He has a noticeable speech

difficulty. I had only a limited opportunity to observe the boy. Because I do not feel qualified, I have made no recommendations. However, I do feel, having made this superficial study, that I have gained an insight into Bob's problem.

Family and Environment. Bob is a 13-year old boy, rather short of stature, but well built and of good appearance. Bob's ethnic group in the medium-sized city in which he lives is small in number and rather loosely knit. Bob's father owns and operates a small repair shop on a street where there are second-class restaurants, taverns, an outmoded hotel, and several cheap rooming houses. Drunks, "bums," and "down-and-outers" frequent the street, and it is their particular hangout. His family lives in one of the numerous "four-decker flats," and although the economic status of the family, consisting of seven children, is better than average, they have little so-called social standing. Bob's father, in bringing up his family, apprenticed the boys to the repair shop, where they performed odd duties and chores. Although the environment was poor, Bob's older brothers and sisters rose above it with one exception, his next older brother, who was crippled by polio. There is evidence of sibling rivalry between him and Bob. Being the "baby" of the family, it is probable that Bob expected more attention from the family than he received, owing to the fact that his crippled brother required more than would normally be the case. The activities of the deformed brother may also have had a poor influence on Bob. In order to gain attention, presumably, from his peers, this brother associated himself with a group of so-called "cats" whose dress (pegged trousers, suede shoes, haircuts, floppy caps, long, loose suitcoats, etc.) caused much unfavorable attention and comment at the time. Many of these "cats" were delinquents of one kind or another, and some became involved in serious offenses. Bob's brother at one time was brought in for questioning, and although he was exonerated, he was the object of much unfavorable comment. These "cat" incidents occurred when Bob was at a very impressionable age, just before he entered Junior High School. They may have had a negative effect on Bob's subsequent attitudes.

Although the mother was employed by a box supply company folding boxes, she managed to do a creditable job of bringing up the girls, who were neat, attractive, and well groomed. All the girls did well in school, and the youngest was in the ninth grade when Bob entered the seventh grade of the same school. She was capable and well thought of by her teachers. Often she seemed embarrassed by her brother's attitude and speech difficulty. She was tall and poised in contrast to her short, ill-at-ease brother. The mother was born and lived her entire life in the city where Bob was born. Attractive, energetic, she took the girls of the family under her tutelage, leaving the boys to the father in the "old country" tradition.

It may be accurately concluded that Bob was subjected to a generally poor environment, as even the elementary school he attended was the poorest in the city in relation to facilities and the segment of population from which it drew its enrollment.

Educational data. In the second grade Bob's teacher prescribed a remedial program in reading which was carried out by a student teacher from the School of Education. The comments of both follow:

SECOND GRADE TEACHER: (1) Poor reader, recommended for special help. (2) Sits and does absolutely nothing. (3) Used flash cards with simple words. (4) In prelesson interview would not participate in discussion of his everyday doings. (5) His classmates laughed at his handicap. It was noticed that he withdrew from the group owing to his fear of their reactions. (6) He took a great deal of time to read, but in his slow word-by-word reading, he would not stutter. However, as soon as he stopped reading and tried to talk to his teacher, he stuttered. (7) Poor home life. (8) Thought a lot of his brother who was in the Navy.

The following information was obtained from available notes in Bob's record folder, which had been made by a *second grade student teacher:* "My first meeting with Bob was quite an experience. He was rather nervous since he had just let the air out of a teacher's tires. He did not know whether or not I would say anything about it to him. I did not, and as we became a little more acquainted, he blurted out the story. We finally straightened things out. Since the previous week had been vacation week, we talked about the fun we had had. Bob is allowed to do as he pleases at home, and he spent nearly the entire week in the theaters. He is fascinated with horror movies. His mind at this point is filled with things such as vampires, science fiction, and ghosts. Bob is not a well boy, physically. He is covered with eczema, and this causes him to be extremely nervous and restless. His rash itches a great deal, and he jumps up and down in his seat continually. No one, as yet, has been able to locate the root of this eczema. I do feel if this can be cleared up, he would be able to do his work better. His eyes seem to be in good condition, as does his hearing. I obtained a book with a story named "Bing." Before starting to read the story I discovered Bob had a dog, a cocker spaniel named "Lady." We talked about tricks "Lady" could do, and with this as background, we decided to read and see if "Bing" were as smart as "Lady." The book was on the first grade level. Bob read very, very slowly, and he failed on a great many words such as "where, is, help, the, good, it." He stuttered a great deal throughout the hour. At first I thought this was due to nervousness, but I discovered he does this most of the time, owing to his present physical condition. As we read about "Bing," I asked several questions to guide his reading. This proved very successful and resulted in good thinking on his part. Although I did not feel Bob did too well in his reading, I have the feeling he was developing the right attitude toward his work, and this is a good point. Bob really enjoyed the story very much, and he was very excited about "Bing." He shows a great deal of interest toward his reading work. His main concern is wanting to be promoted to a higher reading group. He reads with a great deal of expression, and he appears to put himself in place of the characters. He lives the story with them. To me, this is a good symptom of reading enjoyment which has given me encouragement."

After repeating the first grade, Bob's progress in school was regular, if erratic. His marks before coming to Junior High School were average to good, and his attendance excellent. In the Otis Beta EM Test, he scored 19, with CA 12–4, MA 9–8, IQ 82. His mental age and IQ seem to belie his achievement. The first indication of a falling off in his work came in the sixth grade when his spelling achievement dropped from an A to an E while he managed to maintain an average of B in his other work. In grade seven, his work deteriorated to a poor average, with unsatisfactory citizenship and D's in Science, English, Mathematics, and Spelling. Bob's seventh grade home-room teacher, having had training in speech correction methods, was sympathetic to his stuttering difficulties and made the following statements concerning him: (1) serious discipline problem; (2) gum-chewing; (3) talking; (4) unwillingness to conform to group routine; (5) excessive talking, or shouting out; (6) sulkiness; (7) defiant to student teacher when asked to do anything; (8) did not touch pencil to paper first two months of school; (9) would not read or make an oral report; (10) stuttered when asked any question; facial contortion and "full mouth" reaction; unpleasant reaction always to questions. Treatment I have used with Bob: (1) kindness; (2) asked him to do small tasks; (3) interested him in making progress in spelling; (4) praised him. Writing had the same qualities as speech—rather garbled, disjointed quality. Gave him two marks; one for thought, which was all right, and one for expression, which was always expressed in terms of encouragement. Corrected his errors and had him recopy, rather than have him correct his own as others did, because he had no background to make his own corrections. Still writes in a garbled fashion but I feel it necessary to encourage him to express himself. His trouble is, in great part, emotional or protective of self. Talks to his peers without stuttering and gets along with them outside the classroom.

Report of Interview with Bob. I explained to Bob that he would be doing me a favor if he would answer a few questions for me. I assured him he would remain anonymous, and that he need not answer any questions he did not wish to. Our rapport has always been good, and

Bob agreed readily. He talked easily, and I referred to his stuttering only as the "trouble he had when speaking." He replied quickly to my questions, and he did not elaborate on any of the answers.

Briefly, this is the information he gave me. Mother and father are both alive and working. He was the youngest in the family, having three brothers and three sisters. His family treats him well and knows of his speech difficulty, but he seldom, if ever, has difficulty when speaking with his family. Bob stated that he remembered having speech difficulty before going into the first grade. Later he changed that statement and was quite emphatic that I realize the difficulty started when he was in the first grade. He said he got along fine outside school and had no speech difficulty with his friends. School records on file with his permanent records alluded in no way to his stuttering, but he admitted he had had difficulty all the way through school. When asked if anyone had tried to help him with it, he said it had been suggested that he take a deep breath before beginning to speak, also to think of what he was going to say before he said it. Throughout the interview Bob did not stutter or repeat any words. He said his parents know of his difficulty and do not feel he needs help from a speech expert. He has no animosity toward school people even though it is only in school that he experiences his speech difficulty. He does not blame the teachers for this nor does he dislike school particularly. Since Bob's stuttering seems to have its basis in the school problems, his own attitudes, and learning difficulties, I requested further information on Bob later in the year, and I have recorded the gist of it in the ensuing.

SCIENCE TEACHER: "Bob reacts very well to individual attention. During early contacts with him, there seemed to be a wall separating us that he would make no attempt to scale. I went to his father's establishment to see him under other than school circumstances. Although at first he was reluctant to talk, when he realized I wanted to talk to him about his job, he relaxed and we had an interesting conversation. Following this incident I found him to be more outgoing and cooperative in class."

HOME-ROOM TEACHER: "During the second quarter Bob seemed to show improvement both in adjusting and cooperating. However, this spurt did not last long, and he lapsed back to his former inattentiveness. He showed a real desire to improve his penmanship, and he was pleased when complimented on his efforts. It is difficult for him to sit still for any length of time. I have given him the duty of going to the office every day for my mail during the 15-minute home-room period. He has been very reliable, and he takes this responsibility seriously. He chews gum constantly and usually has at least two packages with him. Often, I overlook this because I feel it is an outlet for his nervous tensions. He has received check marks from four of his teachers for not participating in class discussions. This week he appeared with a new pair of blue suede shoes and the swagger that goes with them. Apparently he is imitating an older brother, one of the "cats." There could be a tendency to follow along this line to gain attention. In the home room, at least, he seems to conquer his stuttering somewhat, and I think he feels comfortable and assured here."

SOCIAL STUDIES AND PHYSICAL EDUCATION INSTRUCTOR: "Bob has recently become a target for practical jokers. This was first noticed when he broke off relations with a group who were in trouble with the law. His break away was due to exercise of parental authority when he was forbidden any further association with the group. As a seeming result of this, his stuttering became worse for a while, then it appeared to lessen as he developed new ties. His former associates, by way of retaliation for his shift in loyalties, began to cause Bob's books to disappear. All but one were recovered from such locations as ventilator shafts and work spaces behind urinals. An expensive jacket and a pair of fur-lined leather gloves, prized Christmas gifts, also disappeared. These were not recovered. Later, another jacket was taken, and it was found in a rubbish barrel. During this period of plaguing, his defect was far more pronounced than it had been for several months. Investigation has shown a strong decline in school accomplishment and several instances of infractions of school regulations. As a result of school and home action, which did not turn up the individual responsible but did end the abuse, Bob has begun to respond to school activities again."

In eighth grade mathematics Bob is with the higher of the two groups. His teacher reports on him as follows: (1) requires almost continual individual supervision and direction; (2) often leaves a book or pencil elsewhere when they should be with him; (3) when he volunteers a question, he often speaks clearly and evenly; (4) complies with teacher requests somewhat reluctantly; (5) lately, he has smiled while complying; (6) he might return almost immediately to noncompliance; (7) at beginning of this year, he did nothing; (8) lately, he has been handing in work done at home; (9) seems to have more ability than he shows in a group; (10) gives up easily; (11) does not study independently; (12) appears indolent; (13) finds it irksome to sit in a normal way on a chair at a desk.

ENGLISH TEACHER: "In grade seven Bob was a constant problem, belligerent, uncooperative, sly, anxious to disturb others, never did any written work. As the year progressed, he was influenced to write something. It sounded like his stuttering speech. Gradually, he wrote more on the topic chosen. Then he passed in papers regularly, like the rest of the class, with many misspellings which I corrected, but something about the paper was always praised. He began to do much better in formal spelling work, and he was highly praised."

In grade eight, he has taken his place very well. His class assignment has been with a better-than-average group. I think this has helped his morale. The only time he gives difficulty is for just about three days when we change student teachers. His conduct is noticeable, and there has to be an understanding reached; then all goes well again. Just one thing prevails. He insists on chewing gum. This was not a grade seven trait. His nervousness must be expressing itself this way. He will rid himself of it, but when you look up he is chewing away again, but not with a belligerent or uncooperative attitude. I wonder if the gum offers emotional satisfaction equivalent to thumb-sucking or nail biting. Of late, I have ignored it because the stuttering is much better, and I do not wish to be the cause of a regression. He seems like a happy, adjusted child. He is passing "on his own speed," and we get along amicably. The Rhinehart system of penmanship is used in the school. Although Bob does not know it, he is made an especial exception in relation to penmanship. His writing is extremely small, tight, and pinched. He will copy the exercise over as many times as he is asked, but his efforts to date are not up to the minimum standards of this system. Recently, he attached metal cleats to his shoes which made considerable clatter when he walked. He removed them when he was asked to do so. On a recent paper, he wrote his middle name instead of his first name in what seems to be an attempt to get away from his usual self.

In Art, where I have had an opportunity to observe him, his work is tight and tense even when "scribble" lessons are suggested to provide for freer expression and imagination. His stuttering in my presence has been very infrequent. The principal of our Junior High School, who knows Bob's family, verifies much of the preceding and states that he walks part way home with Bob quite often. During these walks, Bob exhibits little of his stuttering difficulty, but when spoken to by the principal at school he has difficulty frequently.

PHYSICAL HISTORY: Available records of Bob's physical history show no symptom of difficulty. His physical education teacher describes him as slight and wiry. Recently, after having the wind knocked out of him, he spoke evenly when he recovered his breath. This teacher, who has him for social studies, considers him a nonreader, and he feels Bob's inadequacy in this area may be the cause of the frustration which leads to his stuttering.

This year in the eighth grade we have had no discipline difficulty in class at all. He does well in formal spelling, and there is some improvement in his written expression. Outside class I have noticed a very good relationship between him and his sister. They always walked to and from school last year, chatting pleasantly. She has gone to High School now.

I feel Bob is doing well now—good attitude, contributes, does his reading, answers questions, expresses opinions. Attitude of the class is good toward him, and his classmates seem understanding. His writing is beginning to improve definitely. He is straightening out spelling and spelling sense. One noticeable factor is his inability to express himself in the correct tense. He confuses past, present, and future without realizing which is which. This is probably part and parcel of the confusion which causes the speech trouble. I think he needs to feel "accepted as is." Then an expert could take over and straighten out his difficulties. He seems to need help beyond that which is available from an ordinary classroom teacher. Personally, I like Bob, and I am recommending that he attend your clinic.

SOCIOMETRY

Another important source of information from the classroom may be derived from the teacher's administration of sociometric techniques: Hotley (1950); Jennings (1959); Moreno (1934). These test results can be helpful, not only to the teacher as she seeks to improve her teaching through understanding the social structure of her classroom but also to the clinician as he seeks to understand the deeper and broader meanings of the stuttering child's behavior. The basic idea in sociometry is that each child is asked to indicate, in order of preference, three children he wants most to be with for whatever situation the teacher develops (forming an aquarium committee, for example). Past studies have shown that a child's first choice is often for someone more mature who can stand as a guide, model, or a source of support in the specific area in which the chooser may be experiencing trouble. Children's choices are kept confidential. Usually the teacher assures the children that they will be in a group with at least one of their choices. In this way, even the child who is not chosen knows only that he has been given one of his choices, and he feels the right to be in the group. This fact, in itself, may be developmental for such a child. In these situations, it has been found that even least chosen children tend to become more able in using their full capacities (Havighurst, 1953). Highly "acceptable" elementary school children have been differentiated from highly "unacceptable" ones on a sociometric basis in such ways as the following (as determined in conjunction with the paper-and-pencil California Test of Personality and the California Test of Mental Maturity): (1) they smile more frequently; (2) they make more contributions to their groups; (3) they engage in some form of cooperative, voluntary group participation more often; and (4) they are less likely to be alone during activity periods or free play (Bonney and Powell, 1953, p. 490).

One speech clinician, wishing to determine the social positions of stuttering children in regular classroom situations, was able to compare 30 stuttering children with their 708 nonstuttering classmates. McLatchy (1958) utilized 27 classrooms from Kindergarten through grade six, varying her questions in accordance with grade-level requirements. Analysis of individual scores revealed that 19 of the 30 stutterers were in the lowest quartile; 7 were in the second quartile. The percentage of isolates among stuttering children was about twice as high as among other children, while the percentage of "stars," those most highly favored, among the stuttering children was about half the percentage of the nonstuttering ones. The clinician who is able to avail himself of sociometric data compiled by the teacher often finds these data valuable, not only in becoming more aware of forces impinging upon the child but also in working together with the teacher concerning grouping arrangements which may be helpful to the stuttering child.

PSYCHODIAGNOSTICS

In situations in which psychological evaluation is indicated, referral is made, whenever possible, to a clinical psychologist. Even if the clinician is trained in the use of psychodiagnostics, it is preferable, in cases in which he himself is to provide the therapy, that another clinician administer the tests. This is especially so when the therapy is likely to be a relatively permissive, psychotherapeutically oriented one. Certain diagnostic procedures necessitate questioning, leading, and probing actions. The stuttering person may find it difficult in therapy to "take the lead" with a person who tested him and whom he now perceives as the guide or leader. In diagnosis, the person, in essence, is told what to do. In therapy, the person is asked to "tell" *us* what *he* would like to do. Most diagnostic procedures nurture a dependent attitude in the person; he expects to be told and indeed he is told (implicitly or otherwise) what to do. In the therapeutic setting, we wish to promote a more independent attitude.

The psychodiagnostician has a large array of tests or techniques from which to choose. In the area of intelligence, the most commonly used tests are the following: the Stanford-Binet Scales (Terman and Merrill, 1937), the Wechsler-Bellevue Intelligence Scale (Wechsler, 1939, 1946) and the Wechsler Intelligence Scale for Children (Wechsler, 1949). The most commonly used personality and projective tools are: the Rorschach Psychodiagnostic Technique (Rorschach, 1949), the Thematic Apperception Test (Murray, 1943), the Children's Apperception Test (Bellak and Bellak, 1949), the Minnesota Multiphasic Personality Inventory (Hathaway and Meehl, 1951), the Symonds Picture-Story Test (Symonds, 1948), the Machover Draw-a-Person Test (Machover, 1957), Sentence Completion Tests (Rotter and Rafferty, 1950), and the Make a Picture Story (Schneidman, 1947). For those unfamiliar with these tests or techniques, excellent introductory descriptions are available (Thorndike and Hagen, 1955).

Although most speech clinicians are generally untrained in the use of these diagnostic instruments, there appears to be increasing knowledge of such instruments among workers who are not specifically involved in psychodiagnostics. In fact most teachers and clinicians today, by the time they receive the equivalent of a Master's degree, will have had not only a course in general measurements but one in the Stanford-Binet and possibly the Wechsler Intelligence tests. Familiarity and proficiency with the projective and personality instruments usually require special training beyond a Master's degree. Of course some speech clinicians are fully qualified in the use of these instruments. Many of these individuals do much of their own psychological testing. Just as it is desirable for all speech clinicians to become as proficient as possible in the realm of psychodiagnostics in general, it is perhaps now reasonable to *expect* that within the very near future all speech clinicians *should* become familiar with at least the more commonly used tools, such as the Binet, Wechsler, or Draw-a-Person tests. Not that full proficiency in administration is required (though it is desirable), but at least the ability to understand test results or reports should be increased. Some of our most helpful reports of intelligence testing with stuttering persons have been written by student speech clinicians (Master's degree candidates) who were trying to become more able in the realm of psychodiagnostics. Administering such tests to speech-handicapped persons amplifies one's conception of these individuals through seeing them under a variety of "task" conditions. The process seems to increase the clinician's ability to perceive human behavior in a more thoroughly discriminating fashion, an ability so necessary in *therapeutic* interactions. The following report, written by a student speech clinician, while based on the administration of the Binet and Wechsler Intelligence tests, gives something beyond mere intelligence quotients, and reveals the degree to which highly specific functions can be psychodynamically meaningful, if interpreted qualitatively. Perhaps the basic assumption in such an approach is that intellectual functioning, like speech functioning, cannot be divorced from personality structure.

A Clinical Diagnostic Report Based on Intelligence Testing

Background Data. Alan is 8 years and 4 months of age. He was referred by his teacher because of his stuttering, which consisted of mild repetitions; no secondary symptoms observed. Alan's father is an automotive mechanic; nothing else of certainty is known about him. The mother has stuttered since early childhood and impressed the clinician as rigid in her manner and very strict and domineering in her relationship with the boy. She has several nervous manifestations which accompany her stuttering, such as eye twitching and numerous side glances. Alan is the only child. There is no history of other speech or deviant behavior reported in the family or among relatives.

Alan has had whooping cough, mumps, and intermittent sieges of tonsilitis. His general physical appearance is a somewhat lethargic one, with sloping shoulders and wide hips. He has had neither major illnesses nor injuries. He is in the third grade, evidently has difficulty in socializing with others, and when asked how he was doing at school, he just shrugged his shoulders and said nothing. Outside of interest in comic books, no specific interests were ascertained. (Foregoing material collected after administration of tests.)

Behavior During Tests. Alan was rather shy and hesitant at the outset. There were intermittent speech blocks during the examination; such difficulties did not seem to occur in relation to specific types of materials. Verbal responses to the majority of the tests were decidedly meager and spoken rather rapidly, possibly reflective of the underlying anxiety. There was frequent grinning during the test; this usually occurred just prior to answering or responding to items he was uncertain of or plainly was not able to cope with. The feeling was that this was a laugh of embarrassment rather than, for example, a conversion of anxiety energy. There were several indications of verbal aggression which will be considered below. His desire to do well led to an attention sustained throughout the examination procedure.

QUANTITATIVE RESULTS

Binet (L):

Chronological Age (mos.)	87		
Mental Age (mos.)	84	I.Q.	97

Wechsler Intelligence Scale for Children (WISC):

Verbal I.Q.	85		
Performance I.Q.	72	Full Scale I.Q.	77

DISCUSSION OF BINET: The subject achieved a Basal at level VII and spread seven levels, reaching a Terminal at level XII.

1. *Vocabulary* performance was inferior in comparison to the total scale. Responses were extremely brief and the quality was poor. This function agrees in general with the WISC performance.

2. *Memory function* was well above the average of other functions, the subject repeating six digits forward successfully and passing item 4 (memory for sentences) at year XI. However, item 3, (reading and report) at year X was failed. This again seems to be owing somewhat to the highlighting of his symptom which this item necessitated.

3. *Visual-motor analyses and syntheses.* Performance here was in accord with his over-all performance average, the subject doing well with the diamonds, although his drawing of the paper cuts (item IX-9) was rather unusual, the subject drawing the edges of the paper well

within the edges. This might be indicative of an introversial, with-drawn nature. Indications throughout the batteries would appear to verify this trend. His *concentration* appeared to be spasmodic, although good when in use. Only item indicator is seen in (IX-5), Making Change, which he failed.

4. *His judgment and comprehension* seemed to equal his average performance. He did manage to pass item X-2 (picture absurdities), although quality of responses was poor; there were, meanwhile, no other atypical accompaniments. There were no abnormal associations outside of the occasional displays of hostility tendencies. He named a large number of words in the word-meaning item (X-6); nothing irregular observed here. It is difficult to compare the achievement level on the motoric level between the Stanford-Binet and the WISC, mainly because of the smaller percentage of motor performance requirements and the lower level of motor ability tapped by the Binet tests.

DISCUSSION OF WISC: The subject's *general information* ability agrees well with his total score. Responses were average and brief. His *comprehension* score was close to his mean with responses average in quality and quantity, except for items 3 (fight) in which he stated, "I'd hit back" and item 7 (criminals) where the full response, "So they won't kill anybody," seemed to be further indicative of aggressive tendencies. The performance on *arithmetical reasoning* was well below his general mean. There was strict attention to the task, how-ever, which suggested two possibilities for the low achievement level: (1) true deficiency in intelligence in this area and/or (2) the presence of anxieties interfering to an unknown degree with mental function. His best performance was seen in the *memory span for digits* area, which achievement was slightly above his age norm. This implied a reliance on rote memory function, in general, as opposed to more sequential reasoning. The score also reflects a good degree of atten-tion. However, disruption in this function might have been expected if strong anxiety were existent, and the result here appears somewhat inconsistent with other findings. The higher score on *similarities,* ap-proximately second highest level in the battery, is somewhat mislead-ing. There was a poor quality to several of the answers; e.g., 8 (piano-violin): "both music." All responses in this section were extremely brief. His performance on *picture arrangements* was on a par with other motor tasks, although quite well below his age norm. Correct placement was made on several items here, but beyond the time limit to varying extents. He seemed to enjoy this task very much, although there was frustration expressed while manipulating the "train" item. There were no particular motor deviations observed, other than the slowness of performance. In general, his ability to comprehend these situations was adequate. There was a normal amount of trial-

and-error activity. The *perceptual and conceptual abilities* of the subject as revealed on the picture completion test were below the low performance scale average. It was not a case of grasping for unessential details, but rather a combination of actual inability or lack of insight, or immature perceptive ability of a configuration or/plus a suppression of "test-important" areas of one or two of the pictures; for example, item 4 (girl-mouth), ordinarily a fairly obvious lack to be seen at his chronological age, was not obtained until beyond the general time limit. It is interesting that here, the missing part, the mouth, is precisely the focus of his speech irregularity. Most other responses were fairly rapid, whether correct or otherwise. The *block design* performance was slightly above his performance scale, general mean level. Pattern build-up was usually from bottom to top, counterclockwise. Placement was tight and adequately manipulated. The *coding* test performance was on a level with his performance scale average. Writing over lines or fill-ins cost a better score here; most fill-ins were on a diagonal. The *object assembly* performance was also in keeping with the motor area average. There was a good deal of trial-and-error activity and some obvious frustration. He made a special effort to align pieces exactly and lost credits by slow manipulation and exceeding time limits.

General Discussion. It is probable that the best efforts of the subject, considering his present emotional structures, were better seen during the Stanford-Binet, which I.Q. rating lies some 20 points above the full scale WISC I.Q. score. During the first examination, interest was quite well maintained, this being a new experience to him. During the WISC, attention was spasmodic and queries concerning when the test would be over were frequent. It was noted that following the first test administration, several days previously, the mother had acted angrily because the test had taken more than one hour, although she had been informed that it would be "approximately an hour." The subject very possibly felt this anger in the attitude and statements of the mother on the way home that afternoon; this was the indication, at least, as the two left the building. The subject, perhaps, had this in mind during the administration of the second test, although the examiner had attempted to make it clear to both that "we might be a little longer today." At any rate, this "press" seemed evident throughout the WISC administration and very probably impeded his performance. Otherwise, the subject accepted the tasks as a challenge, and, intermittently, would seem to be attempting to excel. This would seem to reflect the effect of coercions in the home situation, especially from a mother who evidently insists rigidly on accomplishment. Her many projections onto the boy and her adverse reaction to components of the boy's personality, which mirrored her own deviations, seemed very obvious. It is conceivable that relief from his emotional involvements would have raised his scores on all levels, especially the motoric, which fell sharply in relation to norms. However, there was consistency of level throughout the performance scale on the WISC, which would lead one to believe that this is merely a generally lower capability area being tested, operating as a function of intelligence, with less import to be placed on the extent of emotional disruption of performance than would be the case if there were greater variations of performance within the motoric category. There appeared to be considerable constriction on vocabulary items; this is probably greatly due to his overconcern with his speech difficulty. The over-all score suffered much from his weak performance here. The ability shown here is probably not truly indicative of his capabilities, considering the possibility of resolution of the emotional conflicts. This view is partially substantiated, it seems, by his time performance on similarities and by adequate responses to the comprehension and information items.

Conclusion. Alan is seen as a boy of low average to average intelligence whose capabilities are being delimited somewhat by emotional involvements which are continually maintained by a poor parental situation. He has a high level of aspiration which is beyond his present capabilities and probably serving further to intensify his frustrations. A change in environment would probably prove beneficial, but this is impractical. It is at least recommended that the boy receive speech therapy in a play therapy structure, pending outcome of full diagnosis. The mother, and thus the boy, indirectly, would benefit from parent counseling. This is highly recommended in order to attempt to provide her with insight into the boy's problem. This will be difficult and, no doubt, will be met with resistance, for such considerations must necessarily strike at her own defenses and general personality configuration, she having the same basic make-up and speech symptom as the boy.

THERAPEUTIC DIAGNOSIS AND DIAGNOSTIC THERAPY

Regardless of the kinds of speech, personality, or intelligence measurements used by the speech clinician during his initial meeting with the client, a primary focus will be on the *interpersonal relationship* which develops. A developmental relationship, one in which the clinician is sincere, interested, acceptant, and supporting, is in reality a therapeutic relationship. Thus the initial interview is a therapeutic interview. From the moment that the client decided to seek out help for his stuttering problem, the treatment facility selected has become a part of his perceptual field. When he crosses the threshold of the clinical setting, it and its personnel are causing him to react affectively in terms of the mental set which he brought with him. How the stuttering person feels about himself and how he feels about the interview become all-important. If a good working relationship is not developed immediately between the client and the clinician, the stuttering person may never return, or if he does, he may fail to keep his appointments after one or two sessions. He will show his resistance to therapy in many ways; for example, being late or being verbally nonproductive, to name but two instances.

In the initial interview, as in the interviews which follow, the emphasis is on the feelings which the client releases as he "tells his story." In the initial interview, the clinician sows the seeds of therapy, creating a beginning relationship which, as the weeks of therapy go by, grows and develops. In settings in which the interviewer will also be the clinician, the structuring of such a feeling-geared relationship is extremely important. This matter can be regarded in another way if we consider that the "diagnosis" does not stop at the end of the diagnosis appointment time. Diagnosis *never* stops (be it on an overt, implicit, or unconscious level). *All therapy is diagnostic therapy.* The shifts in attitudes and actions, in aspiration levels, in motivational strengths, in frustration tolerance, in self-regard, and in self-acceptance demand constant appraisal and reassessment, if not on the part of the clinician then by the other diagnostician, the stuttering person. From another viewpoint, the initial evaluational meeting provides the first materials for support and the development of understanding; i.e., diagnostic materials are the stuttering person's first expressions available to the clinician to "use" in helping (providing therapy for) the person.

To put it even more succinctly, the initial diagnosis may be the first therapy session. The notion is not an inconceivable one if we realize, for example, that seldom does a diagnostic session crystallize the person's problems so that they are completely clear to us in all their dimensions, allowing us to prescribe fully what is needed in a therapeutic program. A diagnosis gives us a supply of reasonable but often ill-defined deductions, hypotheses, or assumptions which we "go for" tentatively. It gives nothing more. Only the combining interaction with the person clarifies (refutes or substantiates) our inklings, leading us, perhaps, to more accurate impressions. When all is said and done, we usually can *predict* very little from the diagnostic session. Time (therapeutic time, for instance) helps us to check on our thinking. As Wolberg stated:

Attempts to evaluate ego strength and to predict the outcome of therapy by means of testing are usually speculative. Where the . . . (clinician) makes predictions as to the quality of change the patient will achieve in psychotherapy, where he estimates definite goals in treatment and indicates the kinds of techniques to which the patient will best respond, he is straining his test materials, attempting to adapt them to areas for which they were never designed.

Prognosis estimates and predictions of what will happen in therapy on the bases of psychologic tests are often fraught with disappointment. While it is possible to determine customary responses to authority, and the habitual interpersonal reactions that emerge in a relationship situation, it is not always possible to guarantee that these responses will develop with the therapist. For therapy involves a special kind of a relationship, the uniqueness of which may prompt latent or new responses. Much, of course, will depend on the therapist, on whether he falls in line with the role the patient expects him to play. Similarly, it is difficult to anticipate the interpersonal potentials of the patient, since we do not know how the therapist will manage the tentative thrusts of the patient toward a different kind of relationship. Finally, it is not easy to predict what the patient will do with insight, whether he can acquire insight or utilize it, once it is evolved, in the direction of change. For these developments, too, are largely contingent on the nature of the therapeutic relationship and the skill of the therapist (Wolberg, 1954, p. 269).

THE EVALUATION PROCESS

The great advantage of observation (in diagnosis or therapy) which is systematic and rigorously controlled is that it yields data that can be scientifically measured and classified. Still the problem arises as to what extent rigid methodology may interfere with situational reality (Murphy, 1960). The standardization of stimuli and situations, such as would be the case in set question-lists or in the use of specific toys in play diagnostics, and the systematic variation of these, may result in valuable comparative data. But standardization can make it difficult to adjust to individual variations and needs, and it can deter the clinician from extensive exploration of an area of potentially great significance that may manifest itself at a given moment with a given person. The more rigorous an evaluative procedure is, the more inadequate is the representation of the phenomena of real life which are propelling the individual. No diagnostic structure has yet been evolved which constitutes a proper sampling of complex, actual life situations.

To varying degrees, then, the evaluation process is an artificial one. Speech pathology appears, as yet, to be at a phase of development in which a primarily *descriptive* level of analysis is indicated. Thus the contemporary task of workers is to collect observable data, tabulate, and describe them; arrange them chronologically or according to some other classification; and abstract the commonalities in accordance with various criteria such as age and subgroupings. Questions concerning what factors determine changes in behavior, the extent and kinds of interactions among the factors, the range of exigency of the factors, and so on, then can be answered with more surety than is possible presently. Before we can discuss the precise reasons for different behaviors which occur in child development or in therapeutic processes, we need to become much more detailed in our descriptions as to *what* actually *does* happen in the evaluation process. As a matter of fact, a great amount of the stuttering research has been descriptive and has been productive in compiling data about observable events. But whether the worker's approach is basically theoretical or empirical, he must be concerned lest he focus his attitudes and procedures on too restricted a segment of human behavior, or lest he generalize too freely on the basis of unvalidated, impressionistic analyses of faulty samples. Of course, to say this is to cite two extremes in approach, and it is not meant to imply that empiricists in speech pathology function with their backs to the theorists, or vice versa. We assume that in most cases the two approaches can interact in a constructive way as we pursue more economical and fruitful measures and procedures in stuttering diagnosis and therapy.

Judging the Judges. What is a clinician doing when he observes a stuttering person in action? In brief, he is making an appraisal of one or more features of this person. Now it is clear that there are differences (1) in the ability of estimators to estimate, and (2) in what might be termed the "estimatability" of those being estimated. In regard to the latter, some stuttering persons are much more difficult to "estimate" than others, and we may assume that generally in assessing certain "kinds" of persons, the degree of correlation among several estimators may be quite low. Although we have no evidence on this point in relation to stuttering individuals, such data exist in relation to nonstuttering persons. Allport, for example, found that introverted persons are the most difficult for judges, even experienced ones, to agree upon (Allport, 1937, p. 443). Allport discussed the "qualifications of a good judge of others." In a summary of several investigations, he presented the following list, given here in an abbreviated fashion:

1. *Experience.* A good judge must be mature and have a rich supply of experience with human nature as well as with all manner of people.
2. *Similarity.* In general, the more *like* the person the judge is, the better able he is to judge that person (also see 4 following).
3. *Intelligence.* By and large, the more intelligent the judge, the more proficient his judgment.
4. *Insight.* The more emotionally stable a person is, the better judge he will be.
5. *Complexity.* Good judges are at least as complex as those

they judge. People have more difficulty understanding others who are more complex or subtle than they.

6. *Detachment.* The best judges tend to be a bit more introverted than the average. They themselves tend to be enigmatic and hard to judge. They may be somewhat asocial, but have the ability to stand aside and "see all" objectively—making more valid judgments.

7. *Esthetic attitude.* The very best judges seem to try to comprehend the inherent harmony of any object or situation that is being attended to, regardless of how trivial it may appear to others.

8. *Social intelligence.* The good judge shows proper tact in human relations (Allport, 1937, pp. 513–16).

EVALUATION TECHNIQUES

Although many different diagnostic techniques are used with persons who stutter, the basic components of any judgment situation inhere in all: the clinician's skill, the complexity of the stuttering person, and the structure chosen to elicit the most significant material. We shall now consider the last mentioned. What does the evaluator wish to accomplish? The answer to this question will indicate the procedures to be followed. He may wish to compile a thoroughly detailed anamnesis in accordance with a prescribed outline which he follows. He may emphasize an analysis and description of the speech act and gather much material concerning early speech behavior and reactions of others to these behaviors. He may have a short outline of topics which he regards as important areas for questioning or discussion. He may follow no specific plan, letting one line of thought lead to another. He may structure a "nondirective" atmosphere, allowing the client to do most of the leading and talking. He may conduct a nonverbal interview (play analysis). Or he may use any combination of these. He may even interview the parents and not see the child at all. He may stress speech behavior; he may stress emotional factors; he may try to consider both. He may have the stuttering person converse, talk extemporaneously, and read aloud. He may have him play with puppets and paints. He may ask for an autobiography. He may use a projective test. He may have the stutterer take a self-administered paper-and-pencil personality test. He may use a drawing projectively. All these approaches are possible, and all occur in different degrees and in different settings. Some of these approaches are described in detail in speech therapy books (Berry and Eisenson, 1956; Irwin, 1953; Johnson, Darley, and Spriestersbach, 1952; Johnson, 1956; Milisen, 1957; Van Riper, 1953; Van Riper, 1954; Van Riper and Gruber, 1957; West, Ansberry, and Carr, 1957). We shall consider briefly a few approaches which have received comparatively little consideration in speech texts—a complete consideration of these diagnostic procedures and materials would require another full volume.

Play Evaluation. One of the most fruitful approaches to a fuller understanding of a child's problems is one which uses the basic "language of childhood"—play. Children tend to mirror their own perceptions and problems in their play dramatizations. Although it is quite possible to overgeneralize from such data (for example, striking a female puppet equals hostility feelings toward the mother), there is general agreement that the free world of play reveals to us as much as any other technique concerning how a child perceives self and world. The fertility of the method derives from its more accurate representation of real-life situations, as well as from the general feeling of freedom which it accords to the playing child.

With children who are four to six years old, a procedure such as the following may be used: The child is invited into the playroom. If he refuses to leave his parents, they may accompany him, remaining near or just outside the door. In the room there is a low table, two or three small chairs, and one large chair and a blackboard and chalk. On the table are three puppets (a male, female, and child), a small lump of clay, a coloring book, several crayons, and a dollhouse with miniature furniture. The child may be told that he is free to play with whatever he wishes and that he may do whatever he likes. Then, again, the clinician may take a more active role. He may speak to the child at greater length, explaining that he wants to help him, and that in order to do this, it would be helpful to know as much about the child as possible, and that the child's doing and saying whatever he felt like would help the clinician to get to know him better. The child is assured that anything he says or does will not be revealed to anyone else, including his parents, unless the child says it is all right. In any case, the clinician observes the child's mode of shaping his play world, his approach to and his choice of material, his constriction or spontaneity, the extent of his verbal output or silence, his reactions to the clinician or to his own behavior, and so on. On the basis of the interview, the clinician has certain impressions which are recorded immediately following the session. When possible, correlation with the reactions of a second observer (through a one-way viewing window, for instance) is made. Any conclusions made at this time would be no more than speculations to be checked against subsequent events.

Here is a brief description of a play interview with a stuttering six year old. Bill entered the playroom hesitantly and stood motionless looking at the objects on the table, picking at his fingers. After a minute, the clinician stated that sometimes it is very difficult to say or do anything in a new place with a new person, but that this was all right—he could do whatever he wished. Bill touched the clay gingerly, then quietly and slowly he handled the furniture in the dollhouse, looking at each piece before replacing it in its original position. This lasted five minutes. Then he turned the pages of the coloring book, but he did not use the crayons (three minutes). He picked up the female puppet, took the piece of clay and rubbed it slightly on the puppet's nose. He looked at the clinician; getting no reaction, he rubbed harder. He put the puppet on the table and pressed the clay onto the face of the puppet with the palm of his hand, completely obliterating the face. His own facial expression had not changed. He kept glancing at the clinician, who verbalized what was being done but made no comments or evaluations. Then Billy stuffed the puppet into the bathroom of the doll house and turned the house around so that the opening was against the wall. He got the color book and began coloring vigorously in short, rapid strokes.

Billy's behavior obviously suggested feelings of aggression toward female figures (later, in therapy, the strong feelings of repressed hostility felt by Billy toward his perfectionistic, demanding mother were revealed quite clearly). In this interview, although no speech occurred, the rigid and withdrawn behavior observed provided clues as to the nature of the speech therapy required to meet Billy's needs. In addition, the play interview gave the clinician an idea as to how Billy would react in treatment if he were assigned to a play-therapy structure.

It is to be emphasized that such an interview is not an evaluative end in itself. It is but one way of gathering more information about the child which, in the light of all other available data, will contribute to a more productive therapy program.* Play evaluations contribute a global picturization of the child and a clarification of his *uniqueness*. They indicate the general quality of the child's adjustment abilities, his expressiveness or rigidity, his social maturity, his general level of anxiety, his perception of his universe, and his self-perceptions. These, together with more specific and quantitative evaluations of speech and general behavior, enable us to "see" the stuttering person, not just the stuttering speech. We see "what and who the stuttering child is."

Rating. The necessity for discriminating observation on the part of the clinician in such activities is clear. Not only must he see and hear "all" and decide which features are most vital, but he must be attuned to the more formalistic and motivational aspects of behavior; i.e., not only must he

---

* The reader is referred to Van Riper's accounts of two diagnostic play interviews (1953) and to Chapter 8 in the present book, which includes several verbatim reports of play interviews.

CLIENT BEHAVIOR EVALUATION SHEET

Client: _____ Address: _____ Tel. No. _____

Age: _____ Birthdate: _____ Speech Problem: _____

(Check √ those that apply to this person)

Evaluator's Initials

Date of Evaluation

A. Speech and Language
    Behavior

    1. Fluency

        a. repeats . . . .

        b. blocks . . . .

        c. secondary symptoms . . .

    2. Articulation

        a. accurate . . . .

        b. inaccurate . . . .

    3. Volume

        a. adequate . . . .

        b. inadequate . . . .

        c. too much intensity . . . .

    4. Pitch

        a. too high . . . .

        b. no variety of pitch . . . .

        c. too low . . . .

    5. Verbal Output

        a. adequate . . . .

        b. limited . . . .

        c. excessive . . . .

FIG. 3. A SAMPLE CLIENT BEHAVIOR CHECK SHEET FOR STUDENTS.
This evaluation sheet is to be checked by the clinician after the initial
interview as well as periodically as therapy progresses. It can be used
with a child, adolescent, or adult who is involved in either individual
or group therapy. Base your evaluation of this client's behavior on
your observations, recording his behavior as it appears to you.

Client's Name:

    6. Attitude Toward Oral
       Contributions

      a. volunteers easily ......

      b. never volunteers ......

      c. volunteers occasionally .

    7. Motivated to Improve ....

B. Some Indications of Anxiety

    1. Avoids Eye Contact ......

    2. Bites Fingernails ....

    3. Blinks Eyes ....

    4. Clears Throat ....

    5. Displays Dominating
       Behavior ....

    6. Feeling Tone

      a. overtly bland ....

      b. overtly neutral ....

      c. overtly aggressive .....

    7. Palms Sweating ....

    8. Picks at Fingernails ......

    9. Relates to Inanimate Objects
       (in reference to children) .

    10. Tics ....

    11. Displays Withdrawing
       Behavior ....

    12. Other ....

C. Defensive Processes

    1. Compensation ....

    2. Denial ....

    3. Displacement ....

    4. Fantasy ....

    5. Identification ....

    6. Introjection ....

    7. Projection ....

    8. Rationalization ....

FIG. 3. A SAMPLE CLIENT BEHAVIOR CHECK SHEET FOR STUDENTS
(*Continued*).

Client's Name:

    9. Reaction Formation ......
   10. Sublimation ....
   11. Withdrawal ....

D. Attitude Toward Self
    1. Lacks Self-confidence .....
    2. Self-confident ....
    3. Self-critical ....
    4. Makes Many Self-references
    5. Self-aspiration Level
       a. too high ....
       b. too low ....
       c. realistic ....

E. Attitude Toward Clinician
    1. Aggressive ....
    2. Anxious ....
    3. Dependent ....
    4. Negativistic ....
    5. Overly Anxious to Please ..
    6. Passive ....
    7. Positive ....
    8. Spontaneous ....
    9. Withdrawn ....
   10. Resistant ....

F. Attitude in Group Interaction
    1. Aggressive ....
    2. Anxious ....
    3. Competitive ....
    4. Hostile ....
    5. Negativistic ....
    6. Placid ....
    7. A Follower ....
    8. A Leader ....
    9. A Nonparticipant ....

describe *what* happened, but often more importantly, he must try to explain *how* it happened and sometimes *why* it happened. He must ask himself *why* he describes what he experienced in the way that he does. With student clinicians, we have found that one way to improve their sensitivity to such dynamics is to utilize a client-behavior check sheet such as is shown in Fig. 3. Such a list serves best, it appears, not primarily as a "valid diagnostic indication" but rather as a way of helping beginning clinicians to look for essential behaviors in *therapy*. The assumption is that, in time, a discriminating perceptual "set" will become more or less second nature to the clinician.

Self-Reports. Any evaluative procedure which relies upon information consciously provided by the subject may be regarded as self-reporting. The questionnaire and standard interview are those in most common usage. Questionnaires are suspect when comparatively nonspecific information, such as attitudes and feelings, is being sought; i.e., paper-and-pencil personality lists. The questionnaire is more valuable for the gathering of unambiguous data, but even in this respect reliability checks are necessary to offset incorrect or "halo-effect" responses. Interviews may be rigid or informal. The former produce more quantitatively manipulable material but generally less rapport and "uniqueness," while the latter are more qualitatively productive and are more akin to a dynamic therapeutic interaction.

Another source of information is the autobiography or diary which, though subject to "tailoring" and questionable in authenticity, can be revealing in terms of the stuttering person's perceptual and defensive modes. For example, a 14-year-old girl, in response to the suggestion that she "write about the low and high points of her life, if she wished," may write two sentences, both scratched out to the point of intelligibility (as happened in an actual case). An adult who has been stuttering since early childhood may write a 350-page autobiography. In both cases there is meaning, but only if viewed in the light of all other known information.

The *New York Times* carried an article about one of the world's known and admired stutterers, Somerset Maugham. The article discussed Maugham's masterpiece, *Of Human Bondage,* which he admits is autobiographical. The central figure in the book, of course, is a young man with a club foot, rather than a stutter. Maugham stated: "The book did for me what I wanted, and when it was issued to the world . . . I found myself free forever of those pains and unhappy recollections. I put into it everything I knew and, having at last finished it, prepared to make a new start" (Beavan, 1959, p. 34).

Reactions to Self-Referent Statements. In one variation of the sociometric method, the Q-sort (Stephenson, 1953), the subjects rate themselves as to how they think others will rate them. The subjects categorize statements about themselves along a continuum in accordance with specified criteria. In a study at Boston University, Wallen (1959) selected approximately 300 raw items which were taken from published and unpublished studies and reports as well as from interview and therapy sessions of stuttering adolescents. Each item is a self-descriptive statement of a personality characteristic. For example:

1. I prefer to be alone.
2. Sometimes when I'm nervous I can just about breathe.
3. I usually try to hide my feelings.
4. I am self-conscious.
5. At times I have felt that life was not worth living.
6. Sometimes I think I pity myself.
7. I feel that other people don't understand me.
8. I am very close to my mother.
9. I can be depended upon.
10. Sometimes I feel inferior.
11. I feel equal to my friends in intelligence and emotion.
12. My speech irritates me.
13. I tend to withdraw from conversations.

Each valid item is placed on an individual card. The stutterers are asked to sort the statement population in three

different ways: first, in terms of how he perceives himself
to be; second, in terms of the kind of person he would like to
be; and third, in terms of the kind of person he thinks others
perceive him to be. In a forced-choice technique, items are
sorted along a range from "most characteristic of me" to "not
characteristic of me. (See pages 172–73, Chapter 6.)

The interesting aspect of data derived in this fashion is
that they are not measures of global traits or of elicited
stimuli. They are measures of *perceptions*, for which there
can be no independent correlative measures. The basic issue
relates to the degree to which the subject's reports of perceptions correlate with actual perceptions. Yet, such considerations are not unique to Q-sort methodology at all. For example, in questioning parents concerning the early and recent
history of their child's stuttering, to what extent does what
they say or report correlate with actual fact? The tendency
for parents to perceive their relationships with their children
in a more favorable light and to convey this more idealistic
impression to others, such as clinicians, is well recognized.

THE CLINICIAN AS AN ARTIST

The majority of data that are derived from diagnostic
procedures eventuate as concepts or generalizations. It is
true that testings and appraisals can provide helpful information in clarifying etiological factors, in estimating current
functioning, in unfolding relevant hypotheses, in formulating a tentative therapeutic structure, and in referral considerations. Diagnostics can also be security-building to both
client and clinician. Too often, however, the diagnostics
result in the stuttering person's being depicted as a profile of
speech and personality "scores." It is as though the stuttering individual were to be regarded as an entity completely
different from the clinician, as someone to be measured,
anatomized, and compared in order to derive "laws" of a
clearly conceptual nature. At times, in the past, diagnostic
relationships with stuttering persons have been of this kind.
Although we are able to see and hear the stutterer's overt

behavior, and indeed to perceive it through the other sensory modalities, we are not able to touch, hear, or smell his *essential being*, his *uniqueness*. Uniqueness is not the sum of what is heard plus what is seen. It cannot be comprehended through analysis. It can be understood fully only through *intuition.** It is through intuition that the clinician arrives at his initial understanding of the individual who seeks his help. The clinician has little idea (unless he treats each client in exactly the same way) as to how he will conduct the interview or the therapy until he begins to get some notion as to what manner of person confronts him. To do this, he intuits. If he does *not* intuit (i.e., if he relies more or less solely on conceptual dissection), he fails to use a most sensitive diagnostic and therapeutic tool—himself.

This viewpoint does not and obviously should not justify dogmatic claims, nor need it desensitize one to the pitfalls of speculative thinking. It does assert, however, that a successful clinician has the ability to react appropriately to the essential, unitary nature of the stuttering individual. Like social scientists, speech clinicians find themselves functioning in a collectively oriented society and in subgroups of similar character. These groups put a high price upon systematization and group action, whereas the clinician must be guided by unique impressions. He must act and set goals in a unique way. It is plain to see that the clinician must be a singular person. In our efforts to develop speech pathology as a science, we may forget that its practitioners, to be fully effective as clinicians, must by nature, be artists (Murphy, 1960).

REFERENCES

ALLPORT, G. W. *Personality: a Psychological Interpretation.* New York: Holt, Rinehart & Winston, Inc., 1937.

BEAVAN, J. "Maugham: A Free Man at 85," *The New York Times Magazine* (January 25, 1959), 14, 34, 37.

* For a most thought-provoking discussion of inference, empathy, and intuition, the reader is referred to Allport's brilliant treatment (Allport, 1937, pp. 523–48).

BELLAK, L., and BELLAK, S. S. *Children's Apperception Test.* Rev. ed. New York: C. P. S. Co., 1949.

BERRY, M. F., and EISENSON, J. *Speech Disorders.* New York: Appleton-Century-Crofts, Inc., 1956.

BONNEY, M. E., and POWELL, J. "Differences in Social Behavior Between Sociometrically High and Sociometrically Low Children," *J. Educ. Research,* **46**: 481–90, 1953.

HATHAWAY, S. R., and MEEHL, P. E. *An Atlas for the Clinical Use of the MMPI.* Minneapolis: Univ. Minn. Press, 1951.

HAVIGHURST, R. J. *Human Development and Education.* New York: Longmans, Green & Co., Inc., 1953.

HOTLEY, D. C. "How to Give Your Class a Social Analysis," *Clearing House* (1950), pp. 24, 403.

IRWIN, R. B. *Speech and Hearing Therapy.* Englewood Cliffs, N. J.: Prentice-Hall, Inc., 1953.

JENNINGS, H. H. *Sociometry in Group Relations.* 2d ed. Washington, D. C.: American Council on Education, 1959.

JOHNSON, W. (ed.). *Speech Handicapped School Children,* rev. ed. New York: Harper & Bros., 1956.

JOHNSON, W.; DARLEY, F. L.; and SPRIESTERSBACH, D. C. *Diagnostic Manual in Speech Correction.* New York: Harper & Bros., 1952.

MACHOVER, K. *Personality Projection in the Drawing of the Human Figure.* Springfield, Ill.: Charles C. Thomas, Publisher, 1957.

McLATCHY, M. R. "A Sociometric Study of Thirty Stutterers in Regular Classroom Situations," Unpublished M. Ed. thesis, Boston Univ., 1958.

MILISEN, R. "Methods of Evaluation and Diagnosis of Speech Disorders," in *Handbook of Speech Pathology,* ed. L. E. Travis. New York: Appleton-Century-Crofts, Inc., 1957. Pp. 267–309.

MORENO, J. L. *Who Shall Survive?* New York: Nervous & Mental Disease Publishing Co., 1934.

MURPHY, A. T. "Objectivity, Subjectivity, and Research," *Exceptional Children,* **26**: 454–57, May, 1960.

MURRAY, H. A. *Thematic Apperception Test.* Cambridge: Harvard Univ. Press, 1943.

RORSCHACH, H. *Psychodiagnosis,* 4th ed. New York: Grune & Stratton, Inc., 1949.

ROTTER, J. B., and RAFFERTY, J. E. *The Rotter Incomplete Sentences Blank.* New York: Psychological Corp., 1950.

SCHNEIDMAN, E. S. *Make a Picture Story.* New York: Psychological Corp., 1947.

STEPHENSON, W. *The Study of Behavior.* Chicago: Univ. of Chicago Press, 1953.

SYMONDS, P. M. *Symonds Picture Story Test.* New York: Teachers College, Columbia Univ., 1948.

TERMAN, L. M., and MERRILL, M. A. *Revised Stanford-Binet Scale.* Boston: Houghton Mifflin Co., 1937.

THORNDIKE, R. L., and HAGEN, E. *Measurement and Evaluation in Psychology and Education.* New York: John Wiley & Sons, Inc., 1955.

VAN RIPER, C. *Case Book in Speech Therapy.* Englewood Cliffs, N. J.: Prentice-Hall, Inc., 1953.

———. *Speech Correction,* 3d ed. Englewood Cliffs, N. J.: Prentice-Hall, Inc., 1954.

VAN RIPER, C., and GRUBER, L. *A Casebook in Stuttering.* New York: Harper & Bros., 1957.

WALLEN, V. "A Q-sort Analysis of the Self-Perceptions of Stuttering Adolescents." Unpublished D. Ed. thesis, Boston Univ., 1959.

WECHSLER, D. *Wechsler Intelligence Scale for Children.* New York: Psychological Corp., 1949.

———. *Wechsler-Bellevue Intelligence Scale.* New York: Psychological Corp., 1939, 1946.

WEST, R.; ANSBERRY, M.; and CARR, A. *The Rehabilitation of Speech.* New York: Harper & Bros., 1957.

WOLBERG, L. R. *The Technique of Psychotherapy.* New York: Grune & Stratton, Inc., 1954.

Chapter 8

Play Therapy in
Individual Settings

*Every playing child behaves like a poet, creating his own
world.*——S. Freud

Stuttering has been referred to as "what a person is." In
play therapy, the child is able to show what he is to a clinician who responds with sensitivity. He learns what he is and
finds the self-strength to chart a better integrated personality.
The clinician responds to the child's emotional dynamics
with feelings of acceptance and respect that are deeply and
genuinely felt and communicated. The following *case notes*
about child-stutterers bear out this dynamic emphasis.

1. It has been six months since Connie (age 6) began therapy,
eight months since her transfer from the institution (for orphans) to
her present home. The anxiety has gone, and spontaneity is unfolding. Today while finger painting she said, "I got a new mother, a new
father, a new name, a new house, new dresses, new books, a new
school, a new teacher . . . I'm a new kid (very softly), a new kid."

2. Janie's activities revolved completely around oral activities. She
made a salad of clay, sand, and green paint and proceeded to "eat" it,
saying "Ugh-pooh" every time she raised the spoon to her lips. She
followed this with protrusions of lips and tongue and with nose
wrinkling. This continued for 30 minutes and was thoroughly enjoyed. Continue to structure therapy so as to allow for oral indulgence.
Her stuttering is decreasing, and she is eating a bit more lately. [Janie
(age 7) has been a severe eating "problem" for several years and a
stutterer since she was 6.]

3. Today Henry (age 7) did the same thing over and over for the
entire period. He places the doll on the toy sailboat, making it sail

along the floor. As the boat travels along, he says, "I guess everyone will be sorry that they were mean to him when he goes away." Will allow for continued release of his rejection feelings. . . .

4. Fred is beginning to release feelings verbally. Our little "conformist" sat with a xylophone, beating it at a fast tempo and yelling loudly over and over, "You noisy thing, be quiet! You noisy thing! BE QUIET!"

5. . . . Tommy puts the family figures in the truck, then abruptly he overturns the truck, spilling out the occupants. This happened 8 or 10 times. It seems to be a good reflection of how he feels about the new situation. (His parents had separated the week before.)

6. Wally (a very bright 6 year old) continues to verbalize his needs to be more infantile (his parents had rushed him from one developmental accomplishment to the other, literally from "stool to school"). Late in the session he informed me: "I'm going to take an early pill. I'll turn back the years," whereupon he picked up the nursing bottle and sucked on the nipple. . . .

PLAY THERAPY: A BRIEF OVERVIEW

Directive Therapies. The term *directive* implies that, while the treatment process is geared to the emotional processes which are related to the person's behavior symptoms, the clinician *may* interpret, ask questions, suggest answers, and evaluate in relation to emotional forces and behavior. Freudian or analytic therapy comes to mind when one considers directive therapies. In 1909, Freud (1925), in his paper "Analysis of a Phobia in a Five Year Old Boy," made an indirect application of play and drawing as treatment supplements. But it was his daughter, Anna Freud, who made the first dynamic imprint in the area of child therapy.

In her early work in child analysis, Anna Freud (1928) divided her treatment plan into three phases: (1) the preanalytic phase, a period which was devoted to the building of a positive relationship with the child; (2) the analytic phase, which utilized four techniques, case-history taking, dream interpretation, daydream interpretation, and the analysis of the child's drawings; (3) the postanalytic phase, during which time the parents were guided by the therapist regarding the optimal methods of reacting to their child and his newly acquired behavior. Anna Freud's views and methodology vary with those of Melanie Klein (1937, 1955), a leader in the English school of psychoanalysis. Klein emphasized play as a substitute for free association, and she gives deep verbal interpretations to the child concerning the symbolic meanings of his play. Of the two, Anna Freud's influence is more apparent in child psychotherapy in the United States.

With the work of Anna Freud and Melanie Klein to serve as bases, many variant approaches and viewpoints have developed in child therapy. Lowenfeld (1939), a British therapist, employs psychoanalytic principles but does not conform completely to orthodox psychoanalytic thought. For example, she uses a sand tray on which the child depicts his world through his play activities. Jackson and Todd, both English workers, perceive the child's play as a means for understanding unconscious conflicts. They state that play is analogous to the conversation and free association of adults (1950). Slavson discusses play as a substitute for inadequacy in child communicative ability, stating:

Play therapy has been devised for young children because of the inadequacy of language as a medium of expression. When the child is supplied with appropriate materials, he conveys symbolically his phantasies and preoccupations (Slavson, 1952, p. 145).

David Levy's (1938, 1939a, 1939b, 1940) *release therapy* is distinguished by its emphasis upon the child's acting out of his anxieties and problems through play. Release therapy has been recommended for use with children from two to ten years of age. Levy limited the application of release therapy by these criteria:

1. The child's problem should be a definite symptom which was precipitated by a specific traumatizing event.
2. The child's fears and anxieties should not be of long standing.
3. The child's problem should be rooted in his past rather than in his present experiences.

Lippman, using the psychiatric team approach to therapy, applies psychoanalytic principles and treatment methods in his work with children who present various neurotic and behavior problems. Once again the saliency of the therapeutic relationship is stressed. Lippman asserts:

> Basic to all therapeutic work with conflicted children is a strong, positive, warm relationship between the child and therapist, which assures the child that he is accepted and respected as an individual, that the therapist believes he can help him, and that he can help himself (Lippman, 1956, p. 283).

Hamilton applied a dynamic, psychiatrically oriented frame of reference to child therapy in case work practice. She, too, emphasizes the importance of the relationship in play therapy:

> It is not the play which is therapy; it is the relationship which the child experiences. The child uses play to communicate with the therapist. The child creates his own environment, and as he manipulates his environment, the therapist through participation, guides him—the play roles themselves being often the chief means of interpretation (Hamilton, 1947, p. 183).

Basic to the development of the important therapeutic relationship is acceptance. Beata Rank, a psychoanalytic child therapist, underscores acceptance as the most vital attribute in the whole child therapy process:

> We emphasized the necessary element of restitution through acceptance of the child on whatever level or levels of emotional development he may be, regardless of chronological age (Rank, 1952, p. 132).

And finally, Pollak extends diagnostic and therapeutic planning so that it includes the child's total family, emphasizing "the importance of a situational approach to the problems of diagnoses and therapy" (Pollak, 1956, p. 5). Play therapy, parent counseling, and teacher counseling are practical applications of this premise to which Pollak holds.

Nondirective or Client-Centered Therapies. As Sigmund Freud (1925) is the progenitor of directive child analysis, Otto Rank (1945) is the forefather of nondirective child therapy. Rankian principles and practices were adumbrant to the thinkings and therapies of Taft (1933), Allen (1942), Rogers (1942), Axline (1947), Dorfman (1952), and Moustakas (1953). In nondirective play therapy, there is theoretically no manipulation by the clinician of the child's behavior or of the materials the child is using. Interpretations, probing questioning, and the analysis of resistances are avoided. The clinician, maintaining a consistent respect for the integrity and basically positive nature of the child's personality, sets up a permissive setting in which he is warmly acceptant of the child's actions, reflects emotional content, tries to understand and empathize with the child in his mode of perceiving self and world, and attempts to aid the child toward a more positive self-regard and eventual fullest self-actualization.

Taft (1933), a pioneer child therapist, emphasized that the focus in therapy must be on what a client can be helped to achieve rather than on what can be done to or for a client. Allen shared the Rankian percepts with Taft. He developed a relationship psychotherapy which stressed that therapy is a positive growth experience for the child as well as a relationship in which a child is helped to help himself. Allen stated that:

The therapeutic relationship is conceived as an immediate experience. The therapist begins where the patient is and seeks to help him to draw on his own capacities toward a more creative acceptance and use of the self he has. While maintaining an interest in understanding what has been wrong, the therapeutic focus is on what the individual can begin to do about what was, and more important, [what] still is wrong. Therapy emerges then from an experience in living not in isolation but within a relationship with another from whom the patient can eventually differentiate himself as he comes to perceive and accept his own self as separate and distinct (Allen, 1942, p. 49).

Client-centered methodology holds much in common with Rank, Taft, and Allen, focusing upon acceptance, reflection of feeling, and the child's responsibility for self-direction. Carl Rogers conceived play therapy as an experience in which "there is complete freedom to express any type of feeling, but certain broad limits to action" (Rogers, 1942, p. 89). But the direct application of client-centered principles to play therapy has been made explicitly by Axline, who stated:

Play therapy is based upon the fact that play is the child's natural medium of self-expression. It is an opportunity which is given to the child to "play out" his feelings and problems just as in certain types of adult therapy an individual "talks out" his difficulties (Axline, 1947, p. 9).

Dorfman, another client-centered child therapist, contended that the aim of the client-centered play therapist is "to see things through the child's eyes in order verbally to clarify the child's expressed feelings" (Dorfman, 1952, p. 276). Moustakas, also of client-centered orientation, accented the therapeutic values which are inherent in the child-therapist relationship as well as the supportive, nonpunitive atmosphere of therapy. Moustakas commented that the therapeutic process "becomes possible in a therapeutic relationship where the therapist responds in constant sensitivity to the child's feelings; accepts the child's attitudes; and conveys a consistent and sincere belief in the child and respect for him" (Moustakas, 1953, p. 9).

For readers interested in additional source materials regarding various points of view, Caplan (1955) and Witmer (1946) have presented omnibus surveys of theories and therapies by workers who represent a heterogeneity of both background and philosophy. Caplan's compendium presented diagnostic, therapeutic, and preventive research as well as clinical material which is international in scope and cross-sectional in orientation. Witmer, who writes from a psychiatric orientation, provided the reader with clinical records of eight therapists who represent many theoretical systems.

PLAY THERAPY: PROCESS, SETTING, AND MATERIALS

When a stuttering child enters the play-therapy situation for the first time, we can be reasonably sure that he brings at least one fear with him—the fear of his harsh conscience (the internalized parents). He is quite apt to mistrust the clinician, to believe that the clinician is on his parents' side. This occurs primarily because of two reasons: (1) the child who has been hurt emotionally by his parents tends to generalize, i.e. to equate or to associate all adults with his parents, perceiving other adults as he has learned to perceive his parents; and (2) because the parents (or teachers) have caused him to come to this therapy situation, the child has every right to assume that the awaiting clinician is working together with his elders. Immediately, then, the clinician who offers the child such a truly unique experience as play therapy's permissiveness affords, may be mistrusted.

One of the clinician's prime tasks is to estimate how the child is perceiving self, parents, and world as well as how much he is distorting, misperceiving, and misinterpreting. In order to do this, the clinician must provide situations and materials which will give the child the opportunities to *externalize* and project his deeper feelings. Play's therapeutic value lies in giving the child a chance to communicate some aspects of his inner world to an understanding adult, to re-evaluate his perceptions and confusions; in short, to integrate. The clinician enters the child's world by allowing him to speak his own language, often a highly nonverbal, symbolic, esoteric one. The child will express his needs to be aggressive; to be infantile; to suck; to mess; to do what he wants and needs to do. The child's formerly suppressed and derogated behavior will be reacted to differently by the clinician whose role is one of "new parents." The clinician submits and resubmits the child's fears, desires, hostilities, condemned wants, and wishes to the child's self or conscious awareness for relearning and resocialization, for differentiation and integration of self.

To accomplish this catharsis, re-evaluation, and reformulation of perceptions and attitudes, the materials of play therapy must be of a kind which will extract such behavior. The child is provided with a smaller, more manageable world —a world of toys, a world which can be manipulated more easily than the world outside therapy. Some of these materials may be quite unstructured or ambiguous; clay, finger paints, and cloth, for example, are materials which can be projected upon (individually interpreted) easily. Others will be more structured (more definite); toy animals, puppets, trucks, and dolls, or materials which will encourage the expression of displacement activity in which the child can express toward nonhuman objects his feelings and reactions about humans. Some children will not be able to express deep feelings about or with persons (in group situations, or to the clinician), but they will do so with dolls or toy animals. A few may find it difficult to express conscience-dominated urges even with dolls and toy animals. For such children, these materials are too similar to humans, and thus they induce anxiety when unacceptable urges are felt. Such children may release their feelings only with unstructured materials, such as water, paint, or clay.

As the child uses the play-therapy materials under the therapeutic relationship, he may retrench any psychosocial deprivations of his nursery years. He may retrace the psychosocial steps which he took during the course of his growth in object relations. He may relive and experience once again anal, oral, or urethral gratifications with an adult who communicates a consummate feeling of faith and trust in him. The variety of play materials provide many opportunities for increased sensory and motor differentiation and integration. The colors of materials provide visual-perceptual experiences. The shapes and textures as they are manipulated supply varied tactual experiences. The sounds of the toys as they are blown, beaten, hammered, scraped, splashed, squeezed, and torn enrich and provide differentiating experiences in the auditory realm.

There are two common approaches which are used in the organization of toys in play therapy: (1) a structural grouping in which specific toys which reflect specific problem areas for the child are therapist-prearranged; (2) an unstructured placement in which some or all the toys in the playroom are available for self-selection by the child.

The following check lists contain suggestions for toys and equipment useful in play therapy, as well as desirable characteristics of the physical setting for therapy. The toys and equipment listed are the items which were available for use by the children whose play therapy sessions are reported later in this chapter. For a discussion of the kinds of toys used in play therapy and the play therapy room, see the writings of Axline (1947) and Moustakas (1953). Since finger paints are used extensively in play therapy and commercially prepared products are expensive, we have also included several recipes for serviceable homemade paints.

SUGGESTED TOYS AND EQUIPMENT FOR SPEECH-PLAY THERAPY

General

† airplanes, assorted types and sizes
aluminum pie plates
† animals (farm and jungle)
† baby doll with plastic skin
† balloons
* balls
Bang-a-ball
* bean bags
* blackboard
blocks
cash register, toy
* chalk, white and colored
chimes
craft set (for older children)
* crayons
dart set
doctor set
doll house with doll furniture
dolls, assorted sizes, both sexes
driftwood, assorted sizes and shapes
drum
easel for painting
Easter basket grass
† fire engines, assorted sizes
flashlight
† little boats and cars
† little trucks
maracas
nurse's set
* paint: finger, poster, and water

* paint brushes
paint jars
* paper: bogus, manila, and newsprint
* pencils
piano, toy
piece of plastic hose
† pipe cleaners
† plastic and rubber guns and knives
† plastic nursing bottles and rubber nipples
plastic stand-up, punching figure
* plasticine, clay
pounding bench and hammer
pull toys
† puppets: hand, string, and stick
† rag dolls, assorted sizes
rags
rattle, push
† rattles, plastic
* rhythm band instruments
round and square block stacks
† rubber animals
† rubber ball
sand
sand box
sand pails and shovels
* scissors
shells, assorted
sponges, assorted
string, cotton and plastic

tape (mystic, adhesive, scotch, etc.)
† toy dishes
† toy Indians
† toy knives, forks, and spoons
† toy money
† toy soldiers
toy store
† toy telephone
* water and † watering cans
whistles
wrist bells

Anal Gratification

* clay, plasticine
  finger paints

sand, paper, cloth

Oral Gratification

† balloons
† plastic nursing bottles and rubber nipples
† puppets: hand, string, and stick
whistles

Tactile Gratification

hard, soft, dry, wet, smooth, and rough materials of different kinds
† plastic skin doll
plush toys (animals)
† rubber animals
† sponge animals, cut-out

Urethral Gratification

* water

---

* This is equipment which may be available for the general instructional program in the public school setting. Such equipment may be collected and stored in each school which is on the clinician's schedule. A carton will serve as an adequate storage receptacle. A book room, a closet, or the corner of a room can be convenient storage places.

† This is equipment which will be needed as supplements to the "public school staples" which are mentioned in the above reference. These are the toys which will be transported from school to school. A carton, a plastic bag, or a suitcase can serve as an adequate conveyance for the transportation of the toys.

RECIPES FOR MAKING FINGER PAINT

I

1½ cups laundry starch
1 qt. boiling water
4 tablespoons powdered paint

1½ cup soap flakes
½ cup talcum (may be omitted)

Mix the starch with cold water to form creamy paste. Add boiling water and cook until mixture becomes transparent or glassy looking. Stir constantly. Add talcum. Let mixture cool a bit; then add soap flakes, stirring until evenly distributed. Let cool and pour into 8 jars with screw tops. Stir into each jar ½ tablespoon powdered paint.

RECIPES FOR MAKING FINGER PAINT (*Continued*).

II

1 cup Linit starch   3 cups boiling water
½ cup Ivory Snow

Cook until smooth and thick. Put in jars. Paint need not be added directly to the jars but may be sprinkled on the paper at the time of using it.

III

To wallpaper paste add cool water until thick smooth paste is formed.
Note: Glycerine may be added to any finger-paint mixture to retard drying. A few drops of oil of wintergreen or formaldehyde will aid in keeping the mixture from spoiling and giving off an offensive odor.

DESIRABLE PHYSICAL FEATURES FOR SPEECH-PLAY THERAPY

Size of the Room:	adequate space for "motor activity"
Some Features of the Room:	1. washable walls (if possible) * 2. soundproofing * 3. one-way-vision mirror
General Furnishings:	1. round, hardwood table with a 42″ diameter † 2. two 12″ chairs 3. one 10″ chair 4. one 15″ chair

---

* These features are the ideal. A room of any size which can be made free from trespass can be adapted for each therapy session for the weekly or biweekly session conducted in the public school setting.

† A library table and three chairs or three desk-chair units lend themselves for use in play therapy in the public school speech-therapy setting. Ideal for public school speech-play therapy use is a hollow box table, 22″ x 44″ x 25½″, which provides for storage as well as for conversion into a four room, box-type doll house. One 12″ chair and one 16″ chair would make this an adaptable unit for play therapy in the public school speech-therapy program.

PLAY THERAPY GOALS

In working with adults and adolescents who stutter, a very important aspect of the relationship involves the working together of stutterer and clinician in the selection of treatment goals; i.e., the stutterer contributes to the therapeutic process by working out goal patterns in conjunction with the clinician. The same process exists in child therapy, though on a more nonverbal level. The child contributes to the therapy plan by revealing his pressing needs. The more he is given the opportunity to reveal his deeper wishes, self-estimates, and drives, the more he "helps" the clinician to understand his needs. Thus he helps to formulate and re-formulate the treatment structure and goals.

In this sense, to a large extent the child tells us what to do. The clinician contributes most importantly to the process by giving it some kind of *organization,* a plan or framework within which therapeutic interaction is to occur. This treat-ment plan is in the mind of the clinician only. He helps the child to think and feel realistically. But, this occurs only in relation to the child's "leads"—his unique need expressions. The clinician's plan will incorporate the consideration of the time to be invested, the materials to be made available and techniques to be used, the roles to be played, the principles to be followed, and the goals to be sought. The child is usually not aware of and he does not verbalize or symbolize his very own supreme goals, namely, fullest development of self or maximum self-actualization. This is the eventual goal which the clinician sets. He patterns the activity so as to move along through to this goal structure. The clinician is always prepared to alter the process according to changes which occur as therapy progresses. He formulates the activ-ity in the light of estimates which he makes concerning the paths they will follow. In this sense, the tentative nature of initial diagnostics is recognized. As therapy moves along, greater knowledge of the person and his dynamics accrues. It is then that diagnosis becomes more accurate. In a very real sense, then, therapy goals are seldom fixed marks. They are like moving targets at which we aim our process, mostly striking close to the child's need centers, sometimes missing altogether, sometimes scoring a direct hit on need revelation and need satisfaction.

Oftentimes these goals will be striven for and met first in therapy, then in relation to family figures, and finally in rela-tion to social situations. Though recognizing that therapy goals are more easily defined than attained and that they are likely to be value judgments rather than safely proven points of reference, the following goal structure, though varying with the stutterer's age, symptom severity, and other factors, recurs in play-therapy planning:

1. Spontaneous and pliable motor and verbal behavior (the former having to precede the latter, especially with young children).
2. Motor and verbal catharsis (an emotional giving of self).
3. Supportive experience through feelings of acceptance and belonging.
4. Reduction of anxiety, fears, and guilt feelings.
5. Understanding and relinquishing of infantile, defensive speech and nonverbal behavior.
6. Increased awareness (consciousness) and objectivity in the perception of self and others.
7. Increase in positively toned verbal self-references (acceptance of self) and attitudes toward others.
8. Introjection and comfortable utilization (greater tolerance) of desirable social standards.
9. Greater independence and discrimination in communicating and in decision making.
10. Heightened ability for speech-reality testing and vocal fluency as psychological equilibrium is attained and self-integration is accomplished.
11. In sum, the development of greater personal and speech *comfort* through increased self-awareness and the reduction of anxiety—the harmonious synthesis of inner drives with outer social reality plus the restoration in the stutterer of *faith* in his own general and speech future.

As these goals are met, partially or completely, more specific speech derivatives will become apparent. In general, there will be (1) greater oral communicative confidence, pliability, and spontaneity; (2) associations of increasing pleasure in the speaking process; (3) lessening of respiratory deviations; (4) the dissolution of "secondary" symptoms; (5) more affective, inflective, rhythmic speech usage; and (6) a healthy consistency in speech content and pattern.

Behind all these goals, far in the recesses of therapeutic interaction, lies one momentous wellspring—the desire of the child stutterer to communicate with the clinician. To accomplish this, he must relinquish those defensive reactions which have stood by him for so long. As one student has suggested, "He must set out for himself, a veritable pioneer in the world of speech." This giving up of defenses and these direct attempts to communicate basic feelings are filled with great anxiety; yet the child dares because (1) he has been able to develop in the therapeutic relationship a warm association of complete faith, and (2) he has been confronted by the clinician with an image of himself which is so favorable that he finds himself imbued with more self-confidence than he has ever before experienced. So strengthened, he can experiment with more normal speech and general adjustive attempts. But his efforts would perish if he were not to receive the reinforcement associated with the acceptant responses which are given him by the clinician. Unsuccessful tries are not of major import. More important is the fact that the child feels the very deep wish to make the attempts. He is motivated to try because: (1) he wishes to communicate with the person who gives him love, tenderness, and acceptance—the clinician; (2) he wishes to do all he can to please the clinician—this includes improving his speech; (3) he wants to identify with the clinician—*be* like him and *speak* like him; and (4) he wants to live up to the idealized picture of himself which the clinician has been holding up indirectly for his contemplation since the very first moment of their being together in therapy.

These processes can be translated easily into the terminologies of other theoretical systems. For example, we have here not only simple stimulus and response, motivation and reward, but conditioning and reconditioning, too. But, in addition, there is no punishment for lack of learning, for plateaus, for relapses; there is no reliance upon anxiety or guilt as means of provoking learning; the desire to communicate with and be like the clinician is all the motivation the child will need for a great while. The feeling that he is not succeeding is all the punishment he will need, whereas the successful learning of a task is, by and large, all the reward he will need (assuming adequate social recognition occurs). As therapy progresses, situations which will necessitate the continuing reinforcement of improved speech fluency will need to be re-experienced, assimilated, and differentiated, made an integral part of the total functioning person. But the drive for all of this will come primarily from within the child.

ROLE OF THE CLINICIAN IN SPEECH-PLAY THERAPY

The *interpersonal relationship* between clinician and child is the foundation upon which the detailed and intricate process of therapy is developed, maintained, and worked through to its end point. In comparison to more highly formal speech therapy, the clinician's attitude here is more permissive rather than directive; feeling-oriented rather than content-oriented; and acceptant rather than regulative. The clinician is truly nondemanding and nonjudgmental. He respects the child's "right to stutter," his right to express previously forbidden attitudes, his right to resist the therapeutic plan, his right to help chart his course of treatment. The clinician builds a relationship which is fundamentally kind and tender. He focuses on basic feelings and reaction patterns as they may be linked to symptomatic expressions. He tries to perceive as the child perceives; to empathize profoundly with the child; to regard the child as the axis around which treatment revolves. He concentrates on the child's feelings as the child experiences them; he avoids the use of prestige, persuasion, pressure, or intellectual reassurance. Examples of such techniques are displayed in the following:

PRESTIGE: "I want you to try to make more oral contributions. I know that you can do it. Be willing to stutter. I'll feel so happy and proud of you if you can tell me next time that you are contributing more to your class discussions, Andy."

PERSUASION: "You are a very bright boy. You can make contributions to your class discussions that are really worth while.

Use that good intelligence that you have. Just give it a chance to show. Share your thoughts. You can do it, Bill. Don't be afraid."

PRESSURE: "You'll have to apply yourself more. There are other little boys who want to try but they have to wait to come here until you have learned to overcome stuttering. You want to help them, too, don't you? Then you must try."

REASSURANCE: "You're afraid to talk, but you don't have to be. People can understand what you say even when you do stutter, David. You talk without stuttering more times than you talk with stuttering. You'll have less fear if you face up to your stuttering."

The clinician very often encourages nonverbally, always accepts completely, and clarifies understandingly the feelings which the child releases. He tries to help the child understand why he feels and acts as he does. Above all, perhaps, the clinician is a tolerant, democratic individual—tolerant of the feelings and attitudes of others, and most of all, of his own. He believes that play can be the child's main mode of expression and communication with his world. The clinician believes that there are realistic limitations which must be set in working with stuttering children. He believes that release of feelings increases the state of comfort of the child through anxiety reduction. He holds that within the child lies the potential for eventual, full self-actualization if the necessary conditions in therapy can be provided. All these basics are felt and communicated by the clinician to the child, mostly in nonverbal ways—his accepting, nodding, his facial expression; in sum, his general manner. Even the clinician's voice reveals his beliefs and his operating principles. A gentle voice, warm and responsive to feelings, binds the child volitionally to his clinician, facilitating identification and a positive, therapeutic relationship. Such a voice reaches out to the child and penetrates perceptually. The child experiences the feeling of hearing his own conceptions accepted and clarified by an adult who responds to him affectively and vocally with a voice which reflects amiability, benignity, and respect. Such is the voice of therapy.

Of all the attributes of a clinician, that of complete acceptance is among the most crucial. It is this *unmeasured acceptance* that is the rudiment of the child-clinician relationship. All-pervasive acceptance is emotionally absolving, emotionally emancipating, and emotionally enriching to the child stutterer as it is communicated to him verbally and nonverbally by the clinician, and as the communicated acceptance is perceived and experienced by the child. The importance of acceptance is emphasized meaningfully in the guide, *Health Supervision of Young Children,* which states:

In recent literature two words which seem to crop up often are "accepting," "permissive," and of these, "accepting" is probably the most important in the entire list. There is no synonym for it. It conveys in one word most of the ideas of all the words in the "non" list (noncritical, nonpunishing, nonmoralizing, noncoercive, nonjudgmental, noncondemning) and is, in a sense, a part of the meaning of all the other words, too, for without an accepting attitude none of them (warm, kind, gracious, patient, friendly, sympathetic, tolerant, understanding, interested, sensitive) will work (1955, p. 32).

The need for positive confirmation of self as a person and as a person who stutters is requisite in the child stutterer. His hesitations, repetitions, verbal vacillations, oral circumlocutions, and acute blockings make the child who stutters more than ordinarily prone to debilitating feelings of emotional-social exile and to feelings of self-inadequacy, retrenching his development both as a person and as a speaker.

Total acceptance does *not* mean, however, that there are absolutely no boundaries, no limits to set for the child in play therapy. Limits will vary depending upon specific therapy settings. In no case is the child allowed to behave so that moral or physical harm of any sort may occur. Permissiveness is to be taken as *permissiveness within realistic limits.* For example, one of the goals of therapy is to help the child to accept and utilize comfortably the requirements society decrees. Chapter 4 pointed out that conscience is introjected parentally and then expressed as the child's own. But for conscience to develop, *something* must be *available* to be introjected. The child must be able to experience these as external limitations before they can be made a wholesome part of his own internal frame of reference. This is an important reason for avoiding therapy which is completely, unqualifiedly, and passively permissive, i.e., therapy which fails to place realistic limits on the child's behavior. If the child is to learn and accept *reasonable* amounts of conformity to societal demands, therapy must be geared so that it moves toward the societal standards. The child needs to know which way the wind is blowing. If he has no signposts, no guide or standard of socially acceptable behavior, he is likely to remain confused and anxious. A *total* absence of externally imposed limits places too great a challenge upon the immature child to develop desirable goals through self-actuated behavior.

TRANSCRIPTS OF INDIVIDUAL PLAY-THERAPY SESSIONS

In the pages that follow are summaries of the case studies of five child stutterers, transcripts of their play-therapy sessions, and for each a commentary which discusses each play therapy session from the point of view of both content and form. A notation regarding parental involvement in parent counseling appears at the close of each case study summary. The transcripts show the form in which each stuttering child utilized the play-therapy structure and relationship to express his anxieties, aggressions, aspirations, conflicts, frustrations, hostilities, projections, and regressions. In each the child contributes to the design of his own play-therapy experiences so that he gains for himself an understanding of the "what" and the "why" of his internal, psychic environment, as well as of his external environments of family, school, and compeers.

The transcripts show how the play-therapy experience can become the child's sanctuary where he feels secure—where he feels free to expose his anomolous self with its emotive and communicative inadequacies, inconsistencies, and instabilities. Each of these children makes his own personal use of his therapy hour in keeping with his pressing emotional privations and problems. Many persons have noted that the child's perception of himself in regard to his world is communicated most poignantly in the language of play. The following transcripts should help us to appreciate the above statements.

Lonnie. This boy is an only child in a family constellation which consists of father, mother, and Lonnie, aged six and one-half years. The socio-economic status is lower middle class. Lonnie is a tall, somewhat obese, second grade pupil in a public school. He is the youngest pupil in his room as well as the tallest and heaviest.

Lonnie's chief problems are school and speech difficulties, underachievement, an articulation problem, and stuttering which is characterized by blocks and repetitions. In the first grade, Lonnie was administered the Stanford-Binet, Form L, which yielded an I.Q. of 119.

Lonnie was bottle-fed on a flexible schedule. He was always held for feeding. He was weaned to the cup at one year. Toilet training was implemented at an early age, five months. Bowel training was completed at the age of 14 months. Bladder functioning remains a problem in the form of nocturnal enuresis. Developmentally, Lonnie was well ahead of normal, having sat up at five months, walked at ten months, and spoken his first words at nine months. His stuttering manifested itself first when Lonnie was around four years of age, and it has fluctuated from mild to severe since that time. Presently, the stuttering is characterized by repetitions and some blocking. Lonnie remains a thumb sucker in spite of the application of physical (slapping) and verbal pressures by his parents. He was hospitalized for a period of one week for a hernia operation at the age of six months. His history of childhood illnesses show the occurrence of measles at the age of four and chicken pox at the age of six years.

Lonnie's father, a factory foreman, works nights, and he

has contacts with Lonnie each afternoon and week end. Both mother and father are completely in agreement concerning the necessity for being "strict with Lonnie so that he won't become spoiled."

Both parents share an expectation for mature, self-disciplined behavior. Lonnie is a mature-looking boy whose chronological age contrasts markedly with his physical maturity and development. As a result, a high level of performance is expected of Lonnie by his parents and people in general, including his peers.

Lonnie has an incessant need for food, doting on cake, candy, and cookies. Presently he is on a diet which was prescribed for him by his family physician, who found Lonnie to be in good physical condition with the exception of his obesity. Lonnie is inclined to be shy with strangers and those who show a lack of acceptance of his stuttering. He is also prone to frequent crying. He is inclined to be destructive with his toys, plays "hard," and "throws himself right into his play," his mother reports. His history suggests that his problems are symptomatic of psychological deficits. He has many problems of an oral nature: thumb sucking, eating, and stuttering. Each suggests possible frustration, confusion, and general nondifferentiation in early developmental task experiences.

Lonnie's problems reflect his parents' rigid, demanding conceptions concerning child behavior. Coercion and control are the means which they employ in their discipline and training. Still, both mother and father show very high motivation in their desire to work toward the goal of elimination of Lonnie's stuttering speech. Evidence of high parental motivation is seen in the regularity with which Lonnie's parents attend a series of joint parent-counseling sessions.

Lonnie's First Therapy Session. Lonnie enters the playroom, his eyes scanning the contents of the playroom. The clinician greets Lonnie at the door, stating that he may come to play each week, that he may play with the toys or not as he wishes. Lonnie responds as though incredulous that such an arrangement could ever be a reality.

L. 1: You mean, I can do what I want? That I can play? I don't believe it; I just don't believe it (slapping his right side with his right arm). I just don't believe it (shaking his head). I just don't believe it!

CL. 1: It's hard for you to believe that you can play or not, as you want to, Lonnie.

L. 2: (Going to the tom-tom, beating the tom-tom moderately, softly, then increasing in intensity.) I'm an Indian. Ya-hoo, Yahoo.

CL. 2: You're an Indian.

L. 3: (Taking plasticine, and breaking it into lumps, hitting the tom-tom with each ball of clay.) I'm going to hit this tom-tom.

CL. 3: You're going to hit the tom-tom with the clay balls.

L. 4: (Hitting the tom-tom with force.) Go, go, go, clay. Oh, I missed that!

CL. 4: Missed that one.

L. 5: Go, clay, go. That one made a loud pop. Good boy.

CL. 5: That was a loud one.

L. 6: The clay is getting all over the floor (looks at clinician).

CL. 6: You may play as you want to, Lonnie.

L. 7: (Picking up the clay.) I'm going to make something. (Sitting down at a table across from the clinican.) This clay smells. It smells like a puppy dog—like a puppy mutt—like a puppy hound.

CL. 7: The clay smells, like a puppy.

L. 8: I'm going to make a hot dog. I've got the hot dog all ready—a real long one (rolling the clay between his hands, then pretending to eat the hot dog). I did eat a hot dog once that was a foot and a half long—mile long hot dogs they call them. It was good too. I ate every bit of it too. I'm putting relish and mustard on this. (Calling out) Relish, mustard, relish, mustard. Red clay for a hot dog. I have eaten a hot dog raw. It tastes better than a cooked hot dog. My mother didn't want me to eat it but I did. I ate a raw hot dog—a raw hot dog.

CL. 8: Even though your mother didn't want you to, you ate it.

L. 9: Yup, but I ate it—raw.

CL. 9: Uh huh.

L. 10: I'm going to make a yo-yo (making a long string of clay with a clay ball attached to it). Hey Yo-yo, Hey Yo-yo, I'm going to make a farm—a farmee, a farmee. That's what I'm going to make. I'll use these animals and make a farmee, a big—little farmee.

CL. 10: That's what you're going to do.

L. 11: (Taking a billy goat and putting it behind a clay fence which he made.) Billy goats make a funny noise "Baa -a-a-a, baa -a-a-a." Billy goats like to eat. (Laughing) They eat everything—paper, food, tin cans, everything. My mother says I'm a billy goat—always eating. I'm on a diet, and I don't like it. I don't like it one bit.

CL. 11: You really don't like it.

L. 12: Sometimes I s-s-sneak things to eat.

CL. 12: You sneak things.

L. 13: Yup, sometimes. (Putting a clay rope around the billy goat's neck and attaching the clay rope to a toy truck, humming a made-up little tune all the while.) Here comes Mr. Alligator. He's going to bite the rope—(making smacking lip noises) m-m-m-m! This clay smells funny (putting the clay near his nose). This clay smells like a B - B - B-1. Just like a B-1. It sure smells funny (laughing).

CL. 13: The clay smells funny—like a B-1.

L. 14: (Taking the alligator, having him break the clay rope with his mouth, singing) the walls of Jericho come tumbling down. I'm going to separate the alligator from the billy goat. The billy goat can get out and get something to eat. He can eat some paper (moving the billy goat near some paper on the table). He can eat paper. I eat paper.

CL. 14: That's what happens.

L. 15: Yup, sometimes I eat paper. People say, "Look at that old billy goat."

CL. 15: So you're a billy goat.

L. 16: Yup, my mother gets mad at me and Mrs. Boone, she's my teacher, she gets mad at me 'cuz I chew paper in school.

CL. 16: They both get mad when you chew paper.

L. 17: Yup. I threw some spit balls—three of them—but Mrs. Boone didn't see me throw them. (Snickering as an artful smile creeps across his face.) But she caught me chewing the paper, though.

Cl. 17: You got away with one thing and she caught you on the other.

L. 18: Yup. Boy, was she mad! She was ripping, ripping, *ripping* mad.

Cl. 18: *Really* mad.

L. 19: My teacher is a poop-deck, a poop-poop-poop deck.

Cl. 19: Uh hmm.

L. 20: She makes me sick—always crabbing and hollering—do this, don't do that, do, do, do, do, do; don't, don't, don't, don't. She gets me nervous. Bossy old thing. I'd like to tell her to shut up.

Cl. 20: That's the way she makes you feel—and you'd like to tell her to shut up.

L. 21: I'd like to, but I don't.

Cl. 21: I see.

L. 22: Last year, I did better in school. I got all "S-es" on my report. But this year, it's U, U, U, U, U all over.

Cl. 22: Not doing as well this year.

L. 23: I hate school—I just hate it.

Cl. 23: You really don't like it much at all.

L. 24: (Working with the toy animals and making clay fences around them.) Animals are lucky; they don't have to go to school. I hate school.

Cl. 24: Just hate it. You're not able to do what the animals do.

L. 25: (Leaving the clay and the animals, going to the drawing paper and the crayons, drawing a picture, singing softly every so often.) Stinky, stinky school. Stinky, stinky, stinky Mrs. Boone. I wish I never had to go to school.

Cl. 25: You don't like it at all.

L. 26: I sure do hate school. I hate it, hate it, hate it.

Cl. 26: Uh huh.

L. 27: But you have to go to school.

Cl. 27: Have to.

L. 28: (Drawing) Stinky roof, stinky door, stinky windows, stinky bricks, stinky school, stinky school, everything about school is stinky.

Cl. 28: M-m-m. You have five more minutes left, Lonnie—five more minutes to play.

L. 29: I'll finish my picture. (Increasing speed of his coloring, turning paper over, lettering on the paper.) This is a good joke.

CL. 29: You're making a joke.

L. 30: A funny joke—wait till I finish it; you'll see.

CL. 30: When you're through, I'll see it.

L. 31: See! (holding picture up [see Fig. 1, Appendix] showing first one side and then the other). I told you that it would be a good joke, didn't I?

CL. 31: You told me all right.

L. 32: Will you keep it for me till next time?

CL. 32: You want me to keep it for you. Yes, I'll keep it, Lonnie.

L. 33: Be sure now.

CL. 33: You want me to be very sure to keep it.

L. 34: Yup. Hey, don't show it to Mrs. Boone!

CL. 34: You're afraid she might see it.

L. 35: I don't want her to see it! You bet I DON'T!

CL. 35: O.K. I won't show it to anyone. What you play and do in the playroom is just between you and me. All right? Private.

L. 36: (Another artful smile crosses Lonnie's face.) Just between (pointing) you and (pointing to himself) me.

CL. 36: Just between you and me. I see that your time is up now, Lonnie. I'll see you next week; all right?

L. 37: O.K. I'll see you next week. Bye.

CL. 37: See you next week, Lonnie. Good-bye.

Commentary. Lonnie's initial play-therapy session is interesting from several aspects. His stuttering is characterized by repetitions and some blocking. However, he stutters infrequently during this initial play interview. He stutters (L1) as he expresses his incredulity concerning therapy's permissiveness, and also in L6 as his anxiety is activated by his anticipatory fears concerning negative reactions to his dropping of the clay on the floor.

His initial reaction to the permissiveness of play therapy (L1) and his testing of its permissiveness by means of motor activity (L2, L3, L4, L5) are particularly noteworthy. In L6 Lonnie projects his past experiences with his authoritarian mother, showing some anxiety when he felt certain that he must have exceeded the limits of acceptable behavior. His feelings in this regard are accepted and reflected. He is able to feel secure enough to test the permissiveness and the acceptance again. In L7 his description of his clay dog ranges from the usual "puppy dog" to the more socially unacceptable "puppy mutt." When these bits of unorthodoxy are accepted, Lonnie moves on, feeling free to indulge in a social taboo, i.e., in reference to feces (L13).

Throughout the session there are many references to orality or references that reflect orality, i.e., his running verbal commentary concerning each action, the verbalisms that appear to spill out of Lonnie's mouth, verbiage that gives him satisfactions as he repeats words and as he engages in the oral play of verbal and oral repetitions (L18, L19, L20, L28) as well as his use of the diminutive; for example, his coinage of "farmee" in L10. Lonnie's many references to eating, diet, food, and chewing (L8, L9, L11, L12, L13, L14, L15, L16, L17) are indications that oral dynamics are permeating factors.

Lonnie projects his feelings of hostility concerning his mother onto his teacher (L19, L20, L22). He indicates that school is failing to contribute to his feelings of success and achievement (L22 and L23). In L25 he turns from verbal release of feeling to graphic release. In L29 he uses the safety device of a joke to test reactions to his release of negative feelings concerning his teacher. In L31 and L32 Lonnie gives proof positive that a child-clinician relationship which is built upon trust has evolved; his sharing of the picture with the clinician and his placing of the picture in the custody of the clinician. A relationship which has its basis in trust, acceptance, faith, respect, and understanding is emerging out of this first play session which moved progressively and positively throughout its 50 minutes.

Joel. This four-year-old boy is the older child in an upper middle-class family consisting of his father (an optometrist), his mother, and a 37-month old brother. Joel is a thin, handsome child with dark brown eyes which have a bold, inquiring look. Joel's chief symptoms are stuttering, which is characterized by numerous repetitions of initial consonants, and head banging.

Joel's birth was at term. Presentation was vertex, but labor was prolonged 8 hours. His birth weight was 7½ pounds. He was breast-fed for a period of one month, following which he was bottle-fed on demand. His mother stated that she had strong self-recriminations concerning her inability to continue with breast feeding, and because of this, she had always insisted on holding Joel during feeding. Joel responded well and continued to progress throughout infancy. His developmental schedule was well within normal limits. Joel said his first words at 10 months. When he was 11 months of age his mother gave birth to another boy. During the period of his mother's confinement, Joel was cared for by his paternal grandparents in their home. His grandmother is reported to have favored the "schedule" type of baby care and training. Joel's mother stated that when she returned from the hospital Joel was visibly irritable and fussy. Joel's weaning was accomplished during the period of the mother's hospitalization. Joel's health history is conspicuously devoid of illness. He was hospitalized at the age of three for a tonsillectomy. He was prepared for this separation and this experience appeared to leave him without imprint of trauma.

Joel is reported to cry easily and often. When he is frustrated he bangs his head, behavior which causes his parents much consternation. It appears to be a most formidable weapon with which he can activate frustration reactions by his parents. During the daytime he will bang his head on the toilet seat. At bedtime he uses the headboard of his bed for this purpose. Because of the nearness in ages of the two brothers, Joel's mother handles both her sons as babies, thereby reducing the individual attention which could have met the needs of each somewhat more satisfactorily. Joel is said to be "defiantly disobedient." His mother often finds it necessary to tell him to do something she doesn't wish him to do, in anticipation of what she calls his "consistent obstinacy." Joel's father is inclined to be directive and compelling with Joel. When Joel is told to do something by his father, he will do so, after an almost undiscernible flicker of hesitating noncompliance. All the children in the immediate neighborhood are of school age, leaving Joel without playmates. Joel's brother is inclined to wander away from the yard. For this reason he is kept in a play pen or tied in the yard. Joel gives vent to his sibling jealousy feelings by teasing his brother, causing him to cry and scream. This leads to maternal interjections of a verbal or physical nature.

Both parents have involved themselves in joint counseling on a weekly basis. Recently, the parents, in speaking to their pediatrician, were advised that Joel was in good physical health but that they should relax in regard to Joel's problems. The pediatrician advised them to secure speech therapy for Joel and to investigate nursery school placement for him. Joel will attend nursery school this coming fall.

Joel's First Therapy Session. When the clinician came out of the office for Joel, he was being admonished for his refusal to sit quietly. Joel's mother introduced the clinician as "someone who will play with you." Joel acknowledged the introduction with a "Hi" as he ran around his mother. He walked readily with the clinician, leaving his mother without a backward glance. As Joel and the clinician walked together, the clinician explained that they were going to a room in which there were some toys, and that he could play with the toys or not as he wished. Joel entered the play room and assumed a kneeling position on the floor. He located himself near a variety of toys, picking up a rubber turtle and squeaking it three times. He threw the turtle down and picked up a rubber bunny. He squeaked the bunny softly, more loudly, and very loudly.

J. 1: (Holding up the rabbit) What's this? I know; it's a rabbit. I can make him hop.
CL. 1: You can make the rabbit hop.
J. 2: (Throwing the rabbit down and picking up the poodle dog.) What's this? (Answering himself) I know. It's a doggie. Bow-wow, doggie. I know what the doggie says, "Bow-wow."

CL. 2: You know that the doggie says "Bow-wow."

J. 3: (Throwing the poodle down and picking up a rubber knife and tapping it on the floor.) What's this? I know. A knife. (Tapping the knife on the floor with fast taps and slow taps.) I slap it.

CL. 3: You slap the knife.

J. 4: (Picking up a gun.) I show you. I show you how to do it. Bang, bang, bang!

CL. 4: You're showing me how the gun works.

J. 5: Oh, wait a minute! Something's the matter. Here it is! I show you. Bang, bang, bang!

CL. 5: You fixed the gun.

J. 6: (Picking up the knife and bending it.) I can do this. (Putting the knife into the nozzle of the gun and holding the gun as he dragged the knife along the floor—leaving the gun and climbing on a chair.) My mother says I'm too big to climb on a chair.

CL. 6: Your mother doesn't want you to climb on the chair.

J. 7: (Continuing to climb on the chair.) She says that I get the chairs all dirty.

CL. 7: You get the chairs dirty.

CL. 8: (Continuing to climb up and down the chair for about 5 minutes.) Where do you live? Do you live here? Do you have a Mummy? Do you have a Daddy? Do you have a little boy?

CL. 8: You want to know all about me.

J. 9: (Running to a fire engine pull toy.) Oh, I have one of these at home (pulling on the fire engine and causing it to speed along the floor) R-r-r, R-r-r, R-r-r (making a fire siren noise).

CL. 9: You have a fire engine like that one at home.

J. 10: (Going to a chair, appraising the clinician, banging his head on the back of a chair.) I bang my head.

CL. 10: You bang your head, just like now.

J. 11: (Continuing to bang his head.) Just like this.

CL. 11: (very calmly) Like that.

J. 12: (Leaving the chair and taking up the knife.) I hit the bunny.

CL. 12: Yes.

J. 13: (Hitting the dog.) And the doggie!

CL. 13: The doggie, too!

J. 14: (Going along the shelf hitting the animals as they appear on the shelf.) And the moo-cow.

CL. 14: You hit the moo-cow.

J. 15: And the duck (laughing).

CL. 15: You hit the duck—you like to.

J. 16: The Kitty. Meow-meow.

CL. 16: You hit the Kitty and then the Kitty said, "Meow-meow."

J. 17: And the horsie, a big fat horsie.

CL. 17: You really hit him.

J. 18: I guess I go for a ride. (Holding the stuffed horse between his legs, holding it by the neck with his two hands.) Go; go; go; go; go. (Galloping around the room rapidly.) Did you see how fast my horsie goes?

CL. 18: Your horsie goes fast.

J. 19: (Out of breath) Puff, puff.

CL. 19: You're out of breath.

J. 20: I'm tired. I'm going to sleep in my house (crawling under a table, curling up, and closing his eyes).

CL. 20: You're so tired, and you're going to go to sleep in your house.

J. 21: (Snoring)
(Pause)

J. 22: (Snoring some more) I'm snoring.

CL. 22: Uh huh.

J. 23: (Getting up and going to the nursing bottle.) Jay-Jay has these. Jay-Jay is my little baby.

CL. 23: Jay-Jay is your baby and he has bottles like these.

J. 24: Me, baby Joel (sucking on the nipple).

CL. 24: You feel like a baby.

J. 25: (Taking the bottle and going under the table, stretching out under the table, sucking on the bottle.) Me, baby Joel.

CL. 25: You're baby Joel.

J. 26: (Spending approximately 10 minutes under the table sucking and chewing on the bottle.) I chew it.

CL. 26: You chew on it just like a baby.

J. 27: (Chewing vigorously) I chew hard.

CL. 27: You chew on it very hard.

J. 28: (Getting up when the bottle is empty, holding on to empty bottle.) Jay-Jay has a play pen. I teach Jay-Jay. I say, "Be a good boy Jay-Jay."

CL. 28: You tell Jay what to do.

J. 29: (Putting bottle on table and going to the wastebasket, sitting in wastebasket, almost doubled up, moving the basket from side to side until it falls over to the right.) Rub-a-dub-dub. I ride in the tub.

CL. 29: You ride in the tub like the people in the story, Rub-a-dub-dub.

J. 30: It's tight (meaning inside the wastebasket).

CL. 30: It feels tight on you. You have only a little while more to play, Joel—five more minutes.

J. 31: Five minutes—you tell me.

CL. 31: Five minutes more.

J. 32: (Taking the bottle, climbing on a chair, filling the bottle with water, bringing the bottle and the nipple to the clinician, extending the nipple and the bottle.) Here, fix.

CL. 32: (Taking the bottle and nipple, securing the nipple.) You want me to fix it.

J. 33: (Sucking the bottle.) Me, baby Joel.

CL. 33: You're baby Joel—a real baby.

J. 34: (Taking a loud, very long sip.)

CL. 34: M-m-m. It's time for us to go now, Joel. I'll see you next Monday. We'll go out to where your Mummy is. (As the clinician and Joel approach Joel's mother, the clinician bids them good-bye. Joel responds with a series of short, little waves and a succession of "bye-byes." Joel's mother asks "Did you have fun?" In response to this query, Joel extends his lower lip and begins to pluck it with his first three fingers.)

Commentary. Joel is a "primary" stutterer. His non-fluency pattern consists of repetitions of initial consonants. Joel stutters as he greets the clinician, perhaps reflecting a generalized anxiety in relation to therapy. In J3, he stutters on the word "knife" (an instrument of aggression). He stutters as he speaks the word "show" in J5, as well as when he discusses his mother's evaluation that he is too big a boy to climb on a chair (J6). In J7 the word "dirty" is accompanied by much stuttering, possibly reflecting the culturally taboo associations which this word holds for him. Interestingly, he does not stutter as he becomes aggressive in action or word.

Joel tests therapy's freedom by means of his manipulation of the rubber toy animals. He sounds each animal in progressively louder squeaks. In J1, J2, J3, his feelings of inadequacy motivate him to ask questions for which he can supply the answers immediately and accurately. He receives complete acceptance from the clinician in Cl1, Cl2, and Cl3. In J4, Joel reveals once again his need to prove his adequacy by exposing his knowledge. In J6, Joel verbalizes about the negative judgment which his mother made concerning his behavior. He uses therapy's permissiveness to experience that which he is denied by reality, i.e., climbing up on a chair (J6, J7, and J8). The clinician's acceptance and therapy's freedom yield him validation as a person in Cl6, Cl7, and Cl8. In J8, Joel endeavors to ascertain qualifying, descriptive data about the clinician. In Cl8, the clinician makes what can be called an interpretation concerning the personal questions, avoiding the supplying of the information requested, at least at this time. The direct giving of advice at this early meeting could leave the implication that the clinician is one who provides "answers," rather than a person who is a "blank sheet" upon whom the child can project as he wishes and needs. In addition, direct answering by the clinician of Joel's questions would approximate too closely the actual mother-child relationship and precipitate his reacting to the clinician as he does to his mother, i.e., defensively.

In J10, Joel introduces his problem of head banging, appearing to await the customary reactions which his performance elicits from adults. In Cl10, Joel's recital concerning his head banging as well as the head banging itself are accepted completely. In J11, he tests this acceptance by his continuation of the head banging. Once again, the head banging is accepted and permitted (Cl11). Joel voluntarily relinquishes banging and becomes aggressive, hitting the toy bunny, testing the clinician's acceptance. This testing continues in J13, J14, J15, J16, and J17. His aggressive behavior is accepted completely during this time. His testing stops, perhaps because he finds the acceptance and permissiveness to be absolute. In J17, his response changes. He indulges in motoric release, i.e., hard, fast galloping about the play room. In J20 his behavior becomes regressive as he rests under a table. In J21, he engages in pretended snoring. This is accepted completely (Cl21) and Joel continues with his regressive behavior, which takes the form of handling the nursing bottle (J23). He makes mention of his younger brother. Sibling rivalrous feelings erupt to the surface and he engages in more regressive behavior as he calls himself "Baby Joel," acting out his longing to assume the position of preference which he perceives to be his baby brother's. His regressive behavior is accepted in Cl23. In J24, there is oral activity, i.e., sucking on the nursing bottle. This is accepted (Cl24). In J25, Joel calls himself a baby once again as he seeks out the security of regression. He indulges in sucking (oral gratification) as well as chewing (oral aggression) for an extended period. The freedom of therapy is Joel's and his regressive behavior has been accepted completely, as in Cl26. There is more oral aggression in J27; this meets with complete acceptance (Cl27).

In J28, Joel relinquishes his regressive role of baby and implicitly suggests his method of coping with his feelings of sibling rivalry. His big brother role allows him to give vent to his aggressive feelings which he masks by overreaction. Joel is accorded complete acceptance in Cl28. In J29, he becomes more spontaneous, motorically and verbally, as he rocks in the wastebasket and calls out a nursery rhyme. In Cl31, the time limit in therapy is introduced, following which Joel returns to a regressive activity, water play with the nursing bottle. He asks the clinician's help with the bottle nipple, giving a hint of the beginning of his perception of the clinician as a helper and fixer. In Cl32, the clinician reflects and complies with Joel's request. In J33 there is regressive reversal of roles with his baby brother once again. In Cl34, this therapy hour was terminated. Joel's anxiety mounts when he returns to his mother, indicating again that maximum therapeutic success accrues when parent and child are involved jointly in the therapeutic program—play therapy for the child and counseling for the parent.

Jonathan. This middle-class family consists of father, mother, an older sister, age 15, Jonathan, age 8, and a younger sister age 4½. Jonathan is controlled in speech, countenance, and response, appearing to hold hostility in check so that it will never escape his defensive "floodgates." Jonathan's presenting problems are stuttering speech, an articulation problem consisting of a sound substitution of [w] for [r] and a school problem—retarded school progress. Jonathan was retained for two years in the first grade. He spent one year in grade two. His promotion to grade three was questionable, and presently he is faced with a repetition in grade three. In the first grade he was administered a Stanford-Binet, Form L, and an I.Q. of 87 was obtained, which, in the opinion of the examiner, was to be considered as a minimal I.Q.

Jonathan's birth was a normal one. His infancy and early childhood were turbulent. From the age of three to six months, he experienced many high fevers, with German measles at three months, a purulent ear condition at four months, and a severe case of bronchitis at six months. He was bottle-fed on demand and weaned to the cup at nine months. He showed a normal developmental schedule in everything but speech. He spoke his first word at approximately 15 months. The use of propositional speech came at approximately 3½ years.

Jonathan is reported to be very sensitive, crying frequently and easily. His frustration tolerance is very low in the familial environment. In school he keeps his feelings tightly encompassed within himself. He is anxious to have friends but he stands on the periphery of activity at school and in his peer relationships. Jonathan is unable to make a successful adjustment at school, home, or play. His parents are very concerned about his lack of adjustment and by the ensuing problems which he presents in all life spheres. The mother stated that her first suspicion concerning his "difference" came when she and Jonathan were guests at a friend's birthday gathering, Jonathan's first party. At this time, he was three years old. She stated that his "differences" were revealed as she observed and compared Jonathan's behavior to that of the other three-year olds—his lack of spontaneity and responsiveness, his lack of speech, and his peripheral status in social relationships.

When Jonathan entered the first grade and failed to make a satisfactory adjustment, parental anxiety concerning his differences deepened.

The parents feel grossly inadequate, and Jonathan has become a symbol of their own inadequacies as parents. They have never become sensitive to their son's needs because they have been unable to see beyond their own needs; needs to be adequate, successful parents of an adequate, successful son in whom resides the enhancement or derogation of the family name. Incidentally, both daughters are above average in intelligence and both appear to introject parental attitudes and aspirations. The sisters are critical of Jonathan and verbally abusive. In this family constellation the "pecking order" prevails, and Jonathan appears to be perceived as of the lowest order. In his family milieu it appears to be Jonathan and his inadequacies against mother, father, and his two sisters. In his school environment, it appears to be Jonathan and his inadequacies against academic work in which he is unsuccessful. Nonaccepting teachers who find Jonathan, his stuttering, and his academic failure threatening, plus peer nonacceptance and rejection, add fuel to the fire.

Jonathan's parents participated in joint counseling sessions on a voluntary attendance basis coincidental with Jonathan's initial play-therapy sessions. His parents were quick in their follow-up of the clinician's request that Jonathan have a medical examination prior to the initial play-therapy experience. The pediatrician indicated that Jonathan was physically normal but seven pounds underweight, for which a daily intake of multivitamins was prescribed. Thus, with the involvement of mother, father, and son in the counseling process, Jonathan's problems should diminish as attitudinal and behavioral changes emerge and spark additional positive changes within the *total* family milieu.

Jonathan's First Therapy Session. Jonathan entered the playroom with the clinician, who noticed the rigidity of his over-all posture, especially the wooden stiffness with which he held his head. The clinician explained that Jonathan could come to play each Wednesday. The freedom and the limits of the play therapy structure were discussed. Jonathan was silent and remained silent throughout this first session.

When the clinician had finished speaking, Jonathan examined the toys cautiously, and then squatted near some of them. He remained in this position throughout the period. He selected a place which allowed him to have his back to the clinician, seeking quietly and cautiously those toys within arm's reach. He picked up a zebra and looked it over, putting it down immediately. He selected some animals, setting them up in a row: a pig, a goat, a chick, and a zebra. He picked up an alligator and made it hop on the pig, goat, chick, and zebra. The animals fell over. As each one fell, he put it back in a standing position. He picked up the alligator and looked it over carefully and completely. After this inspection, he placed the alligator near the animals. He sucked his thumb and looked at the animals. He picked up a boy Flagg doll * and put it down. He sucked on the tips of his four fingers. Next, he took the alligator and placed it on a nearby chair. He moved the pig, the goat, the chick, and the zebra around; after which he placed his thumb in his mouth and sucked on it. Then he sucked his finger tips. He then moved the alligator around the animals which stood in a row. When any animal tipped over, Jonathan righted it immediately. He put his hands together and picked at his left thumb nail. While so doing, he looked at the clinician, who remained accepting and permissive. Soon Jonathan took a plastic-skin baby doll that was dressed in diapers. He fingered the alligator; he put the alligator on the baby doll. Then he removed the alligator and placed the baby

* The Flagg doll house flexible dolls are washable, soft plastic dolls whose clothes are removable. The Flagg dolls come in a family constellation of father, mother, sister, brother, and baby, etc., available from Creative Playthings, New York, N.Y.

doll in a sitting position. He looked at a baby doll that was sitting in a toy high chair, picking at the skin on his lips as he did so.

Next Jonathan picked up some A, B, C, blocks. He turned each block around, speaking the letter name of each block as he silently moved his lips. His perusal of each side of the block was done with studied intent. At this point, the clinician mentioned that there were five minutes left. Jonathan uttered his only verbalism of the session, a whispered "O.K." Jonathan picked up a dry paint brush, ignoring the jars of water that stood next to the paint boxes. He rubbed the dry brush along the dry water colors; picked up the alligator and moved it along the floor. Then he placed his fingers in his mouth. He put his hands into his pockets, crackling a piece of cellophane. As the hour came to its close, the clinician walked to the door with Jonathan, bidding him good-bye. Jonathan replied with another "O.K.," and he walked down the corridor in his wooden, expressionless, puppet-like way.

Commentary. Jonathan's first play-therapy interview is interesting in itself as well as interesting when viewed as the initial session in a series of the three play sequences presented here. Jonathan's verbal communication is limited to an "O.K." His nonverbal communication, however, is surcharged with significance. The basics which child-centered play therapy offers—acceptance, permissiveness, and understanding—are little known quantities to Jonathan. He reacts to the therapy situation with personal and affective rigidity in communication, gesture, and posture. He derives autoerotic pleasure from his thumb sucking and his finger-tip sucking. He is not yet ready to use therapy's freedom for release of his deeper feelings; rather, he turns his aggression inward, picking at the skin on his thumb and at his lips. In this first play session, Jonathan gives classic examples of blamavoidance, i.e., avoiding blame by being well behaved and obedient. Throughout, he keeps his psychological distance. He needs time to experience at a deep level the permissiveness of the therapy as well as the clinician's tolerance and affective compatibility. He needs time for his fears to be reconditioned.

Jonathan's Second Session. Jonathan entered the therapy room guardedly. The clinician greeted him. He responded with a subdued "Hello." The clinician believed that he needed the support to be derived from a reiteration of the conditions and the limits which prevail in the play-therapy hour. These were recapped for him.

Jonathan picked out a wolf puppet, put it over his right hand, and somewhat passively made the head and arms move slowly. He sucked contentedly on his left thumb as he manipulated the puppet on his right hand. He put the puppet down and picked up a donkey puppet and moved its head up and down: first to the right, then to the left. He sought out, manipulated, and discarded in turn a bird puppet, a dog puppet, a cat puppet, and a bear puppet. All this was done without verbalization. Each puppet was placed down with care. He moved on to a rubber French poodle toy, causing the poodle to turn around and to move backward and forward. He picked up a rubber elephant, Dumbo. The elephant made a loud, robust "squawk." Jonathan made a wry face as the noise reverberated throughout the room. He picked up a rubber bear, turtle, fox, and duck, squeezing each of these to make a noise. He lined up the elephant, the bear, the frog, the turtle, the fox, and the duck, effecting a sound from each animal. He picked up a rubber girl doll and made it squeak. He moved on to the rabbit, the bear, the frog, the turtle, the fox, and the duck, producing five noises from each animal. After that cacophony, Jonathan advanced down the line of animals and made each animal sound its noise 10 to 12 times. He picked up the animals and threw them gently on the floor.

Jonathan took two toy boats and made them crash. As this happened, he said very softly, "kr—sh, kr—sh." He took some toy airplanes and placed them on the floor. He sat on the floor. His movements were becoming less rigid, less controlled, and more rapid. He sat on the floor with his legs in a sprawled out position. He put the boats in position and placed the planes in formation. He flew the airplanes over the boats and landed them. This activity continued for ten minutes, whereupon he moved on to a piano book. He started to play the piano book, running his fingers over the keys. He picked out the nursery rhymes "Twinkle, Twinkle," "Mary, Mary, Will You Get Up?" and "Merrily We Roll Along" (the notes to these songs were numbered). He played a music box, turning the handle slowly, then quickly. He sat cross-legged on the floor. He arose and sat at a table with a piece of drawing paper and a box of crayons, drawing a picture of a red brick building with prison-like bars on every window (Jonathan's school is constructed of brick). The hour was coming to an end, and the clinician commented that five minutes remained. To this Jonathan said in a soft voice, "O.K." He turned his drawing paper over and made a sad-faced clown figure that had tears falling from its eyes (see Fig. 2, Appendix). The clinician mentioned that the time was over, saying, "Your time is up now, Jonathan; I'll see you next week." Jonathan said "Good-bye," talking on in a very soft voice, "See you Wednesday." Jonathan's walk down the corridor was more elastic, and his posture was losing some of its rigidity.

Commentary. Jonathan enters his second play therapy session, greeting the clinician guardedly. The clinician gives Jonathan the support of a restructuring of play therapy's attributes and limits. Jonathan selects an animal puppet (a wolf) manipulating it without verbalization. He continues to derive pleasure from his thumb sucking. He concentrates on the operation of the puppets—still without verbal communication. He activates the toy elephant Dumbo, causing it to produce a strong squawk. As in the first session, this inadvertently provided a test of the permissiveness of the therapy hour. The noise was accepted, just as a verbalization would have been, enabling Jonathan to perceive what words were unable to convey, the *permissiveness of therapy.* He feels the freedom so that he becomes able to experiment with the sound-producing toy animals. He concentrates on the toy animals, making sounds and noises from many of the animals. He leaves the animals and moves on to aggressive motoric release. He utilizes a speech sound (K-K-K-K) several times as he simulates a bombing of the toy airplanes. His rigidity is easing; his manner becomes less fastidious as he sits in cross-legged informality on the floor of the therapy room. His newly acquired spontaneity is reflected in his next choice, picking out familiar nursery rhymes on the toy piano book. Again his developing spontaneity reveals itself as he plays a hand-turned music box rapidly. Jonathan turns to a nonverbal medium in which to release his feelings, i.e., crayon drawings which reveal his rigid defenses, his constraining control as well as his general unhappiness.

Jonathan's Third Session. Jonathan enters the playroom, responding to the clinician's greeting with a soft "Hello." He picks up a large rubber beach ball and spins it around, holding the ends of it with fingers arched. He watches it revolve as he turns it about slowly and then quickly. He changes the direction of the ball's rotation, and in the process, he drops the ball. The ball rolls and bumps into some toys, knocking them onto the floor. Jonathan goes quickly to the ball, and as he does so, he steps on the rubber animals, setting off a discordant confusion of sound.

J. 1: (Jonathan steps on a plastic dish and it cracks. A look of apprehension floods his face as he picks up the two pieces of the dish.) I broke it.
CL. 1: You stepped on the dish and it cracked.
J. 2: The ball bumped into the toys.
CL. 2: Just landed there.
J. 3: (Picking up the toys and putting them on a shelf.) I like this ball.
CL. 3: You like that one.
J. 4: (Bouncing the ball and counting.) I can bounce it up to 10.
CL. 4: Up to 10.
J. 5: (Bouncing the ball. The ball slips and knocks the toys over. He picks up the ball and leaves the toys on the floor

where they fell.) One, two, three (increasing the speed of the bounce of the ball). See how fast it goes.

CL. 5: It's really going fast.

J. 6: (The ball rolls to the side and knocks into some plastic animals, causing them to fall onto the floor. In the melee, a plastic rabbit and a plastic dog become cracked. Jonathan rushes over.) They got broken.

CL. 6: The rabbit and the dog got cracked.

J. 7: The bunny's tail is cracked and the dog's head is cracked. They're no good now.

CL. 7: Both cracked. You don't think they're good now.

J. 8: They're no good to play with now.

CL. 8: No good now.

J. 9: I'd like to smash them good with my heels.

CL. 9: That's what you'd really like to do.

J. 10: I like to break things.

CL. 10: Uh huh.

J. 11: (Grinding the toys into the floor with his heels.) I like to smash and break things.

CL. 11. You really enjoy that.

J. 12: (With a smile creeping over his face.) There. They're all smashed now.

CL. 12. You've smashed all of them now and you feel good about it.

J. 13: (Picking up an almost life-size, boy rag doll, flinging it on the floor, dragging it along the floor to the sink.) I'm going to wet him.

CL. 13: Uh huh.

J. 14: (Wetting the doll, doubling it up in the sink), saying: You shouldn't have taken a bath. (Laughing) You're all wet—You're all wet. April Showers bring May flowers, ha, ha, ha. (Pulling the doll out of the sink, dripping water on the floor, throwing the wet doll with a thud on the floor, stepping on the doll's face.) I pushed his face in.

CL. 14: He's all wet and you pushed his face in.

J. 15: (Jumping on the wet doll, kicking him in the face, causing the cotton to push out from a torn hole on the doll's face.) I'm knocking the stuffing out of him.

CL. 15: You are really beating him up.

J. 16: (Kicking and jumping on the doll.) Take that; take that, and that, and that. I beat him up, all right.

Cl. 16: You sure beat him up.

J. 17: (A smile on his face.) I sure beat him up.

Cl. 17: You really did beat him up.

J. 18: (Picking up a rubber sword, putting it into the rag doll's side.) I got ya, I got ya.

Cl. 18: You got him.

J. 19: I'm going to set up the toys and try to hit them with my sword.

Cl. 19: I see.

J. 20: (Placing a toy reindeer on the stool, aiming and throwing the sword.) I missed him.

Cl. 20: Missed.

J. 21: I'll get you. I'll get you. I'm going to hunt all the animals with my sword and hunt them down.

Cl. 21: Find them all with your sword.

J. 22: (Placing a rubber lion on the stool. The lion was difficult to place in a standing position.) You lazy thing, stand up there, I told you.

Cl. 22: The lion doesn't do what you want him to and you're mad.

J. 23: He's a no good lazy thing.

Cl. 23: No good and lazy.

J. 24: Here goes. I got him! I got him! (Smiling)

Cl. 24: You really got him.

J. 25: I'm going to pick up some more animals and set them up. Here a cow, bear, lion, giraffe, elephant, and a rabbit. I hits them with my magic sword. I hits them, and they dies.

Cl. 25: They all die.

J. 26: Here goes. I got him. You stinky cow.

Cl. 26: You got the cow.

J. 27: Ready, aim, fire. You stinky lion. I got you.

Cl. 27: You got the lion.

J. 28: Four more to go. I don't like bears. They're stupid. Watch out, stupid bear. I got him.

Cl. 28: You got the stupid bear.

J. 29: Three to go. Three to go. I missed (aiming at the giraffe).

Cl. 29: You missed the giraffe.

J. 30: I'll get him. I'll get him. Watch out, you stinker.

Cl. 30: You'll get him.

J. 31: (Aiming carefully and throwing the sword forcefully.) I got them, I got them all, the giraffe, the elephant, and the rabbit. I got them all (laughing).

CL. 31: You got them all with one throw. You really got them all. Oh, the time is almost up, Jonathan, you have five more minutes left.

J. 32: (Looking at the clinician.) You know. I hate school.

CL. 32: You hate it.

J. 33: School is junky. It's so junky. It stinks.

CL. 33: That's how you feel about school.

J. 34: It stinks—plain stinks. I'd like to dig a ditch near my house. The bus would go in the ditch and it wouldn't get out and it couldn't take me to school.

CL. 34: You wish that you didn't have to go to school.

J. 35: But I do. Sometimes I make believe that I'm sick. I lie. Sometimes my mother lets me stay home. But most times she doesn't.

CL. 35: Sometimes you make believe that you're sick so you can stay home from school. And sometimes you do. Uh huh. Well, I see that our time is up. We can talk about how you feel about school next week if you'd like, Jonathan. I'll see you next Wednesday afternoon. O.K.?

J. 36. (Walking out the door, raising right hand to right eyebrow in wavelike salute.) Good-bye. See you next week.

Commentary. Jonathan's stuttering consists of some blocking and some repetitions. He stutters practically not at all during this play session. His stuttering became evident while he discussed breaking the plastic dish (J1) and while he talked about the broken plastic toy bunny and dog (J6). Jonathan becomes anxious (J1) after he breaks some of the toys. He anticipates an upbraiding but receives acceptance (Cl1 and 2). In J2, he becomes defensive, projecting the blame on the ball, "the ball did it." In J3 he states "I like this ball." Can it be that Jonathan likes therapy with its acceptance and permissiveness? Is he using the ball as a symbol for the therapy hour itself? In J4, feelings of increased self-adequacy are sprouting from the roots of self-strength which are growing in therapy's soil of acceptance

and permissiveness. Jonathan's self-system is strong enough
for him to verbalize about his achievement, i.e., bouncing the
ball ten times.

In J5, Jonathan shows that he understands therapy's permissiveness. He retrieves the ball without anxiety and without rearranging the topsy-turvy toys. In J5, his increased
spontaneity reveals itself in the speed of the ball's rotations.
In J6 there is some apprehension concerning the damage
that was inflicted on the plastic animals as the ball was recovered. This anxiety is met with complete acceptance.
In J7 and J8, this acceptance frees Jonathan so that he is
able to give a description of the damage inflicted on the two
toys. In J9 he shows once again that he feels secure in relation to therapy's unqualified permissiveness and acceptance.
He feels free enough to let his aggressive feelings break
through as he verbalizes that he'd like to smash the damaged
toys "good." Again in Cl9 and Cl10 his aggressive strivings
meet with acceptance. In J11 he grinds the toys into the
floor, releasing additional pent-up, repressed aggression.
In J12, a smile on his face is a nonverbal communicator which
reveals the reduction in tension which he feels as he expresses
his aggressive urges. In J13 more aggression is unleashed.
In J14 there is increased motor and verbal spontaneity as he
engages in water dripping, throwing the doll on the floor,
as well as stepping on the doll's face.

In J14 through J24, the freedom that therapy holds for
Jonathan is in evidence. He becomes more aggressive verbally as he announces "I pushed his face in," combining
motor with verbal release. In J25 his increasing spontaneity
is shown by his ungrammatical, unorthodox, "I hits them,
and they dies." In J26 through J31 Jonathan becomes more
able to use verbalization as a vehicle for his release of deeper
feelings: ("stinker," "stinky," "lazy," "no good," "stupid,"
"stinks," and "plain stinks," etc.). In Cl31, his motor and
verbal aggression is accepted again completely. The clinician
introduces the time limit as the therapy hour draws near its
close. In J32, Jonathan is able to express his feelings by talking about them. His freedom of expression bespeaks well

of the strong relationship which has developed between him and his clinician during the three play-therapy sessions which have transpired.

Jonathan's feelings are accepted in Cl32, and he is able to move on to release more aggressive feelings in J33. Again, his feelings are accepted (Cl33). He abreacts, reducing the guilt which his phantasy concerning the avoidance of school attendance has activated. His abreaction is accepted (Cl34). The reality factor involved in school attendance is recognized. He releases guilt feelings which revolve about a conflict between self and conscience concerning his pretense of illness. In Cl35, the focus is on future exploration of feelings during the next therapy hours. It is interesting to note that as Jonathan purges himself of some of his aggression, his posture and gait yielded their stiffness and constraint.

Jonathan has found in these surroundings a release which will soon enable him to develop a continuously more comfortable spontaneity and freedom, including greater speaking release and autonomy.

Diane. An only child in an upper middle-class family consisting of mother, father, Diane, and the paternal grandmother, Diane is an attractive, well-scrubbed girl of six years whose waist-long hair is plaited into tight braids, tied with ribbon which matches or complements her freshly starched frocks. She is socially poised and loquacious. This latter trait appears to be a verbal façade, a reaction formation to a basic insecurity about herself and her interrelationships.

Diane's presenting problem is unisymptomatic, i.e., repetitive stuttering. She ranks in the ninetieth percentile on her Reading Readiness test, and functions in the first reading group in her first grade class. Diane's birth history is normal. During a previous pregnancy, the mother lost prematurely a male abortus. Presently the mother is looking forward to a new arrival due in three months.

Diane's infancy and childhood were free from crisis. Her developmental schedule was in advance of the normative pattern. She was bottle-fed, and weaning began at an early age, five months. Her mother remarked, "Diane was weaned from the bottle early as she seemed to have no attachment to the bottle and enjoyed drinking out of a glass." Toilet training was initiated early, too, at five months. It was accomplished at the age of one and one-half years, for both bowel and bladder control. Diane was sitting up at five months, talking and walking began at nine months. She spoke fluently and extensively at 19 months. Her stuttering, which was noticed first by the mother when Diane was about three years of age, has varied from time to time since. With her entrance into the first grade—Diane had no nursery school or kindergarten experience—the stuttering became increasingly evident.

The presence of the paternal grandmother in the home is a complicating factor. There is a negative relationship between the mother and her mother-in-law, both women tending to be dominating and controlling. The mother expects and gets conforming, mature behavior from Diane at the toll of provoking within the girl basic anxiety and feelings of insecurity which are translated outwardly in the stuttering symptom. The grandmother is very kindly disposed toward Diane in both thought and deed. Diane and her grandmother play house, games, and read books together in the grandmother's room. This relationship is a source of frustration to the mother. Actually, the mother has some warm, positive feelings toward Diane, but her own psychic needs, which cause her to pressure Diane for perfectionistic behavior and attainments, constitute an adverse factor in the emotional and social development. Diane is very fond of a pet cat (which her mother dislikes) and her grandmother's parakeet. The mother has threatened Diane with the banishment of cat, grandmother, and parakeet if she isn't "a good, little girl." The mother is extremely anxious about Diane's physical health, and whisks her off to the family physician at the slightest provocation. The pediatrician has advised the mother of Diane's excellent physical health and has suggested to her that she be less anxious concerning Diane's health and her stuttering. The mother has a strong motivation to control and dominate. This is apparent in the joint counseling sessions which she and her husband attend on a voluntary attendance basis. Through her play-therapy experiences, Diane will be able to redefine herself in relation to others and to lose her psychogenic motive of blamavoidance, i.e., avoiding blame by being well behaved and obedient. The reduction in overcontrol should also reveal itself in reduced stuttering.

Diane's Fifth Play Session. Upon her entrance to the playroom, Diane went directly to the nursing bottle and then to the sink. She filled the bottle almost to the top, placed the nipple on the bottle top securely, and began to suck, holding the water in her mouth, gargling and spitting the water into the sink.

D. 1: This time I'm going to take a long drink (filling the water bottle to the top).

Cl. 1: A long drink.

D. 2: (Coming to the clinician, handing the bottle to the clinician.) You hold it for me—just like a baby (snuggling up and placing her head in the clinician's lap).

Cl. 2: It's just like being a baby.

D. 3: (Taking long drinks—smacking her lips—trying to make bubbles.) It's all gone.

Cl. 3: All gone.

D. 4: (Getting up and biting the nipple from the bottle, and putting the bottle down, spitting the nipple into the sink.) I guess I'll finger paint (taking some paper and wetting it under the running faucet).

Cl. 4: O.K.

D. 5: (Pouring out little piles of powdered paint from the paint boxes.) Hey, look! Rainbow colors. They look pretty even without the water.

Cl. 5: Look good this way too.

D. 6: (Being very generous with both paint and water.) Here we go. Now to get busy. It's pretty now. Look, just like mahogony. Ugh—now I'm getting dirty—but dirty. Look.

Cl. 6: Really messy.

D. 7: Now some more red. Now a mite more water. Just a teeny weeny bit more red. (Smoothing it around the paper with the palms of her hands.) Ugh, it looks just like blood—red, red, red blood. Yipes! I think I'll wash my hands (goes to sink and rinses her hands). I'll put some blue in it. It's purple now—real purple. (Singing an original rhythmic little "da, da, da" melody.) This is nice and gooey —nice purple goo. Oh—oh, I goofed. It doesn't matter when you goof when you finger paint, you can rub it right out.

CL. 7: You can make a mistake and rub it right out and it's all right.

D. 8: When you finger paint, it doesn't matter. But at home and at school when you make a mistake, crash, bang, crash.

CL. 8: It really matters there. People let you know.

D. 9: My mother blows her top when I don't do things right.

CL. 9: She gets angry if you don't do what she wants you to do.

D. 10: Sometimes she makes me sit on a chair and she sends me up to my room.

CL. 10: She punishes you sometimes.

D. 11: (Swirling her hands around in the paint on the paper.) Oh boy, this is fun. This is nice. I'm going to make a fish (taking a metal fish and making an impression of the fish on the paper). I made a fish. See my fish.

CL. 11: Yes sir—a fish.

D. 12: One, two, three, four, five—a million—all over my paper little fishy—wishy.

CL. 12: Your paper is covered with fish.

D. 13. I'm going to print my name (smearing the fish and rubbing the paper so the paint is smooth). (Getting the A, B, C blocks.)

CL. 14: Uh hm.

D. 15: Where's the D? Here it is. (Placing the D block down on the paper with some force.) Where's the I? Where the heck is the A? Oh, here it is, and here's the N right beside it. Now I need an E. Where is it? Oh, here. (Placing D, I, A, N, and E blocks down on the paper.) Here's my name, Diane. (Placing the paper on the floor.) Now that can dry. (Going for the ball.) Let's play ball.

CL. 14: Now you'd like to do this.

D. 15: Catch.

CL. 15: You want me to play ball too.

D. 16: (Throwing of the ball back and forth between Diane and clinician. One throw doesn't reach the clinician and the ball stalls midway between them.) Go get it.

CL. 16: You want me to get the ball (walking and picking the ball up, smiling). You like to tell me what to do.

D. 17: (The ball game continues for a few more throws.) I think I'm going to learn a song (going to the piano book).

CL. 17: Uh huh.

D. 18: Not Jingle Bells—that's too long. I'm going to pick a short song. I bet I can't play it right.

CL. 18: You think you may not do it right.

D. 19: (Playing the numbers on the piano keys.) Oh—oh—I goofed. I'll begin again. I knew that I'd goof. I'm going to skip that one and play "Twinkle Twinkle"—that's an easy one.

CL. 19: You made a mistake so now you'll play an easier one.

D. 20: It's easy, but I'm going to make it hard.

CL. 20: Make it even harder.

D. 21: I'm going to see if I can play "Twinkle Twinkle" without looking at the numbers. I'll close the book and do it from memory. That is really hard.

CL. 21: It's very hard to do it that way.

D. 22: I don't know if I c-c-can do it. Here goes.

CL. 22: You're going to try anyway.

D. 23: (With a very intent, serious look upon her face and the book closed. Playing "Twinkle Twinkle" without an error.) I did it!

CL. 23: You played it—and just right, too!

D. 24: Now, I'm going to do it again. But this time I'll make it really, really hard. I'll play it much faster.

CL. 24: Even harder this time.

D. 25: Now, here is a most famous piano player, the most famous piano player in the world. The most famous piano player in the world will play Twinkle Twinkle the fastest that it has ever been played before, without looking at a single note. (Plays the tune with both speed and accuracy.) (To the clinician) Clap, clap!

CL. 25: (The clinician claps as directed and Diane bows as the applause sounds. The time limit is mentioned), Well, you have five minutes left now, Diane.

D. 26: I'm going to make something—I'll just have time. Close your eyes and don't look. You better turn around—all around.

CL. 26: You like to make me do things—things that you tell me to do.

D. 27: I'm making something. Don't peek. (Singing a little, happy made-up tune.)

CL. 27: You're making something that you don't want me to see. You feel happy. You feel happy so you're singing.

D. 28: I *am* happy.

CL. 28: You *do* feel happy.

D. 29: (Little noises that come from fingers at work with scissors, crayons, and paper are audible.) Open your eyes. Quickly. Here! (Holds a large cut-out, large size card in front of the clinician.) Here, this is for you. Here.

CL. 29: You made it just for me.

D. 30: I made it for you.

CL. 30: And you made this just for me. (Holding the card and looking intently and appreciatively at the card.) You want me to have this, to keep it. And I will. O.K. That's fine. Well, I see that our time is up now, Diane. I'll see you next Thursday. Good-bye for now.

D. 31: Good-bye. I'll see you later—on Thursday. See you Thursday. Good-bye, now. (Waving.)

Commentary. Diane's stuttering is characterized by some blocks and repetitions. She reacts to these with an overt show of frustration, i.e., a twisting of her mouth to the right side as she works to gather verbal momentum. As the therapy progresses and Diane's spontaneity increases, her blocks and repetitions disappear. She stutters as she discusses making a mistake (D7) and her mother's anger and the resultant punishment (D9), but outside of these moments, there is no stuttering.

Diane is now perceiving therapy with a confidence and faith strong enough to allow her full expression of formerly blocked feelings. In D1 she indulges in regressive behavior with much oral activity, i.e., sucking on the nursing bottle. In D2 the regressive behavior continues. She shows her trust as she casts the clinician in the role of a ministering mother-substitute. She engages in more oral activity in D3, smacking her lips and making bubbles. There is some oral aggression as Diane bites on the nipple and expels the water into the sink (D4). She moves on to another regressive activity, i.e., messing with the finger paints and water. In D5 and D6, she shows that she accepts the freedom therapy offers her, and her spontaneity is evidenced by her generosity with paint, water, and movements. Her reactions to the mahogany color shows anal components, and her disgust reflects cultural conditioning (D6). Her messing activities afford her release for aggression and satisfaction of socially unacceptable behavior.

Diane is allowed to pace her therapeutic direction; anxiety is not generated by interpretation which could motivate the use of denial or precipitate other defensive withdrawals. Her freedom is evidenced by her singing of her rhythmic, original song—freedom resulting in creativity. Diane refers to her "error" as "goofing"; she feels sure enough to accept her error without the activation of anxiety. In D8, by implication, she contrasts the acceptance of therapy with the nonacceptance of mistakes and errors in other situations. In Cl8 there is acceptance and some interpretation of the outcome of mistakes and errors in home or school environments.

In D11, Diane experiences the freedom of the therapy hour to its very fullest—motorically and verbally. She realizes greater self-actualization, self-realization. In D13 Diane reflects this evolving, stronger self as she imprints her name. In D16, Diane assumes an authoritarian role, controlling the clinician. In Cl16, the clinician accepts the directions and interprets Diane's assumption of the omnipotent authoritative role. In D18, her feelings of inadequacy rear themselves. Anxiety interferes with her achievement in D19. She selects an easy task for herself in order to ensure successful accomplishment. In Cl19, the clinician reflects the anxious feeling which disrupted Diane temporarily. In D20 and D21 Diane sets her aspiration level higher. In D22, apprehension arises again, but Diane is free to deal with it more positively. In D23, her more positive attitude is reflected in successful achievement which she set for herself. In D24, she sets her level of aspiration still higher. In D25, her introjected perfectionistic strivings are activated and ventilated. She assumes her authoritarian role in directing the clinician (D25 and D26). In Cl25, the clinician accepts Diane's authoritarian behavior, interpreting this in Cl26. In D27, Diane's feelings of omnipotence and well-being are reflected again in creativity, the singing of a happy little tune and work on an art activity. In Cl27, the clinician interprets this happiness which seems to pervade Diane's whole being. In D28, Diane reacts positively to this interpretation. The positive child-clinician relationship is seen in its fullest affective and tangible fruition, i.e., the giving to the clinician of a material token of love, her art product which bespeaks of the warm affective interchange in this relationship.

Lee. This polite, somewhat guarded eight-year-old boy is the elder child in a middle-class family constellation which consists of father, mother, Lee, and a six-year-old brother who is presently recuperating from rheumatic fever. Lee is a tall, heavy-set boy with straw-colored, crew-cut hair. His large gray eyes hold a hint of the anxiety and feelings of insecurity which encompass him. His manner is slow in both speech and movement. Stolid is a word which the superficial observer could use to characterize him.

The chief complaints are underachievement in school and stuttering, consisting of effortless repetitions with eye blinking. His mother reported that she was in excellent health during the pregnancy and the birth was at term. Presentation was breech, and labor was prolonged. Lee was breast-fed for the first month, after which he was given the bottle. He was held during feeding. His mother stated that Lee was an easy infant to care for, eating and sleeping well, crying but little. She also declared that she is inclined to be nondemonstrative and perfectionistic with the children. Lee was weaned from the bottle to the cup at the age of one year without difficulty. Toilet training, begun at six months, was reacted to with strong, steady resistance by Lee. (Cleanliness is of great importance to Lee's mother.) Lee was completely trained for bowel and bladder control, day and night, at the age of 20 months. Lee sucked his thumb when he was tired, sleepy, or hungry. This source of gratification was blocked when his mother soaked the thumb in "bitters." Lee also had sleeping problems. He would wake up during the night, crying that he was afraid of some big tigers. These incidents have ceased. There have been neither serious injuries, operations, nor illnesses other than those usual in childhood.

Lee began to use words at the age of one year, and he was speaking fluently at two. His stuttering became noticeable upon Lee's entrance into the first grade. Presently his stuttering consists of mild repetitions and some eye blinking and is most severe when he is in his mother's presence.

It is important to both parents that Lee be obedient and that he respond with maturity in thought and action. Both parents are demanding and conscientious concerning their roles as parents. His mother is the more stern and demanding. Lee shows a competitive attitude toward his younger brother. His attitude has become increasingly hostile and competitive since his brother has been ill and the recipient of much parental concern and care. Lee regards his brother as "different," and he perceives the extra health and hygienic precautions and care that his mother takes as favoritism. The brother is a poor eater as a result of his illness, and the mother prepares special dishes for him.

In informal play settings, Lee is able to get along well with one chum only. In an unorganized group of three or more children, he often projects his sibling rivalrous feelings. He seems to enjoy more an organized group structure such as Cub Scouts and Sunday School. His grade two, Stanford-Binet, Form L, I.Q. was 112. Lee has made normal educational progress; however, his all-pervasive feelings of anxiety and insecurity interfere with achievement at his highest potential. Lee projects the insecurity that he feels regarding his relationship with his mother onto his teacher relationships, perceiving teachers as demanding, nonsympathetic, and critical.

Lee, then, is an affection-starved, apprehensive little fellow who displays strong feelings of self-inadequacy. He is inclined to be compulsive about cleanliness and order, i.e., the arrangement of his toys, closets, and drawers. His mother made the statement, "Even as the smallest child, Lee lacked confidence in his own ability." This statement was not accompanied by insight. Under the areas of parent-child conflict, these notes appear in the clinician's counseling record:

1. High levels of aspiration and achievement.
2. Early needs and training experiences supplied by anxious, tense person with perfectionistic strivings.
3. Mother feels that she must prod Lee in order to secure obedience and achievement.
4. Lee's low frustration tolerance, i.e., easily elicited temper tantrums and oral aggressions, meet with parental counter-aggression, especially from his mother.
5. Sibling rivalry pervasive.

Lee's mother attends parent-group counseling sessions. Intellectually, she has been aware of the psychological variances which are in operation in her family. Through counseling, she may be able to clear away many of the emotional obstacles and feelings which prevent her from her own self-actualization and the healthy satisfaction of Lee's needs.

Lee's Sixth Session. Lee comes into the playroom and picks up the ball, bouncing it up and down.

L. 1: You know, I have a cat, and her name is Fluffy. She's a beautiful cat. I love her.

CL. 1: You love Fluffy.

L. 2: My brother yaps about the cat—all the time. But when I come home the cat is in his room and he's talking to Fluffy as nice as can be. He's sick. He calls Fluffy "stupid" when I'm around. But he's always playing and talking sweet talk to her when he thinks I'm not around. He's sick, but he makes me sick.

CL. 2: He's sick but he makes you feel mad. You feel mad about the way he acts.

L. 3: (Continuing to bounce the ball; then walking around the room while he bounces the ball.) A couple of nights ago, my father let me sleep in his bed. I felt something very soft and warm under the blanket. Do you want to know what it was? It was Fluffy (laughing). I didn't tell my father where Fluffy was and do you know what happened? Fluffy jumped out of the bed onto the bureau. She knocked over a perfume bottle that belonged to my mother. Phew, did it stink! All that stinky perfume that my mother uses! Phew! Fluffy must have liked the color of the bottle. My mother was so mad. My father was mad too. My mother said, "Three days—no T.V." My father chips off a dime from my allowance each day that I'm bad. I was so angry. I didn't do it, but I got punished.

CL. 3: They felt angry and you were punished and you were angry.

L. 4: (Going to the sink and filling the nursing bottles, squirting water from one bottle to another bottle.) It's raining. (Sprinkling water on the ball as he rotates the ball around in his left hand.) It's raining on top of the world. It's raining on top of the whole world. (This goes on about five minutes.) The whole world is crying big tears and little tears.

CL. 4: The whole world is . . .

L. 5: (Interrupting) My brother is a haunt, nothing but a haunt. He pesters me. He keeps insisting on doing everything his way.

CL. 5: You feel that your brother pesters you and always wants things his way.

L. 6: I don't like him sometimes.

CL. 6: Sometimes you don't.

L. 7: (Going to the table and taking the clay, making it into little balls.) Sometimes I hate him and sometimes he's O.K.

CL. 7: It changes.

L. 8: (Taking the pipe cleaners and inserting the pipe cleaners into the clay balls.) These are bombs.

CL. 8: Uh huh.

L. 9: (Throwing the bombs against the wall.) I got into trouble yesterday.

CL. 9: Uh huh.

L. 10: I went to the brook. I went fishing. My father and

mother don't want me to go to the brook. They're afraid that
I'll get drowned. The water isn't even deep. But they keep
saying so. It's so silly. The brook is out of bounds for me,
my mother and father say.

CL. 10: You're not supposed to go but you went.

L. 11: I was at the brook all afternoon after school. Last night
my father went down to the basement to get something. He
smelled my clothes. They smelled fishy. He knew where I
was. He was so mad. He screamed at my mother because I
went. My mother got mad and whipped me. She sent me
to bed. I cried.

CL. 11: You were punished because you disobeyed them. You
got whipped. You cried.

L. 12: It seems like I get punished all the time.

CL. 12: Like it happens a lot to you.

L. 13: (Working on his bombs.) It's either at home or at school
—sometimes both places.

CL. 13: You get it at both places. Getting punished, you mean.

L. 14: People get mad with me when I don't do what I should.

CL. 14: You get into trouble.

L. 15: I'm writing my nickname. You didn't know that my nickname was "Scotty" did you?

CL. 15: Scotty, eh? and you're going to write it on the board.

L. 16: (Writing Scotty in regular size letters.) Scotty, that's
me. (Writing Scotty in huge letters that extend from the
top frame to the bottom ledge of the blackboard.) That's a
big Scotty.

CL. 16: A real big Scotty.

L. 17: A big name for a big fellow.

CL. 17: That's Scotty. A big fellow.

L. 18: I'm not a baby any more.

CL. 18: You feel that you're big now.

L. 19: I grow out of my clothes and my shoes. I'm growing fast.

CL. 19: Really big.

L. 20: There's a kid in my room. He's big. His name is Charles.
He's a smart kid, too. He gets his work done all the time,
and it's always right too. He's a smart kid. I'm just as big
as he is now.

CL. 20: You're just as big. It's good to be like Charles.

L. 21: The teacher likes Charles. The kids like him too.

CL. 21: It's nice to have everybody like you.

L. 22: I'm going to ask my mother if I can invite Charles to lunch.

CL. 22: You'd like to have him with you.

L. 23: My mother doesn't know Charles but she'd like him.

CL. 23: Um.

L. 24: Charles does everything right; my mother likes that.

CL. 24: She likes to have things done just right.

L. 25: (Erasing the board.) I'm going to cover the board this time from top to bottom and from side to side. I'm going to make my name really big this time—the biggest you've ever seen.

CL. 25: You want to make it *really* big.

L. 26: Watch (Stepping on a chair, lettering his nickname and calling out each letter) S-C-O-T-T-Y. (Stepping back to survey his name) That's a big "Scotty" all right.

CL. 26: That's really a big Scotty.

L. 27: Wow!

CL. 27: Really big. Well, our time is up, Scotty. I'll be seeing you next Friday.

L. 28: (Erasing his name from the board in large, free, wavelike motions and translating his freedom into gliding motions as he walks rapidly to the door.) I like you to call me Scotty. Good-bye. See you—Friday.

Commentary. In this interview the child places a heavy emphasis upon verbal release. Lee's stuttering occurs in L2 as he talks about his brother's illness; in L3, as he discusses the cat incident and again as he discusses his brother (L5). He becomes fluent; then stuttering reappears in L11 as he discusses his father and mother and in L13 as he talks about punishment. There is an absence of stuttering for the remainder of this session.

Lee shows a strong identification with his pet, and he appears to displace some of his retained or unused love onto his pet cat, Fluffy. He moves into the problem of sibling rivalry in L2, indicating the insecurity with which he perceives his status in his family, especially with his parents. In L2, his description of his brother's provocative acts demonstrates that both brothers engage in mutually aggressive acts, reflecting the insecurity which both feel regarding parental standing. Lee verbalizes his hostile feelings towards his brother. In L3, among other things, he is critical of his mother and the unfairness of punishment inflicted by his parents.

In L4, Lee's perception of his world as a sad, unpleasant place is recorded symbolically by the ball world upon which tears of rain fall. He returns to his rivalrous feelings concerning his brother as he calls his brother a name and discusses his brother's domination. In L6 Lee reveals his mixed feelings concerning his brother. In L7 he explores his ambivalence concerning his brother. He works out some of his aggressive feelings in his clay work, i.e., making bombs in L8 and L9 and throwing bombs against the wall. He releases verbally his feelings about getting into trouble with his parents and about disobedience. In L11 his verbal release continues as he reveals his world to be one in which his parents act as detectives who are to be outwitted whenever possible and who meter out punishment strictly and authoritatively. In L12 and L13 he reveals that school and home are places of nonacceptance. In L14 his guilt and some limited insight appear as he reasons that people get "mad at me when I don't do as I should."

In L15 and L16 there is motor and verbal activity as he concentrates on writing his nickname in various sizes. L17 shows strivings for independence and autonomy as he comments, "a big name for a big boy." In L18 Lee appears to wish to put immaturity with its parental dependence and supervision behind him as he says, "I'm not a baby any more." In Cl.18 the clinician focuses on this feeling, restating the feelings for the purpose of clarification. Lee introduces a tangible confirmation of his growth as he discusses outgrowing his clothing in L19. Growing up is so important to Lee and is so clouded by uncertainty that he needs to reassure himself of its reality. He verbalizes concerning his self-ideal. However, the actions of this self-ideal, Charlie, appear to be somewhat chafing to Lee's superego as evidenced by his remark that he matches this boy physically (L20). In L21 Lee comments concerning teacher and peer approval of

Charlie, the paragon. In L22, he appears to be trying to identify with Charlie as he speaks of his plans to invite Charlie to lunch. In L23, his feelings of self-inadequacy and his feelings of maternal nonacceptance are not verbalized. However, they are present in Lee's feelings as he does verbalize that he knows that his mother would approve of his classmate Charlie. In L24 Lee evaluates correctly his mother as one who sets a high level of aspiration and achievement and as one who gives her acceptance only to those who conform to her preconceived conceptions of what constitutes acceptable achievement and behavior.

In L25 Lee goes to the board once again and produces in a graphic representation his inner strivings for increased maturity as he writes his nickname in extra-large size letters. Lee becomes directive in L26 as he tells the clinician to watch, remarking on the enormity of the name he is writing. That Lee is impressed with what he is writing is evidenced by his use of an expletive during his graphic expression. The ease and fluidity of motion which Lee displays as he erases the name from the blackboard and as he walks out the door is evidence of the lessening of his feeling burden which has occurred during his therapy hour. His directing of the clinician to call him by his nickname, Scotty, is meaningful. His assumption of the new name to fit the new grown-up boy indicates that Lee is trying to leave behind him the immature boy whose name is Lee. The clinician has been nondirective, accepting and verbalizing feelings as Lee experienced the freedom to express them. The purpose was to help Lee to gain insight into and control of his feelings as well as to give him the perceptual experience of feeling and living acceptance.

Ex Post Facto. Emily Dickinson wrote:

> A word is dead
> When it is said
> Some say.
> I say it just
> Begins to live
> that day.

So it is with play therapy. Its end is a beginning. The child stutterer parts company with his therapy as a person and a speaker of greater self-adequacy and self-realization, more capable of influencing self and others more positively. He goes forth able to extend to self and others the acceptance, respect, and trust which he himself felt and lived during play therapy—hour after hour. Thus, such dynamic consequences, like those of the spoken word, endure.

REFERENCES

ALLEN, F. H. *Psychotherapy with Children.* New York: W. W. Norton & Co., Inc., 1942.

AXLINE, V. *Play Therapy.* Boston: Houghton Mifflin Co., 1947.

CAPLAN, G. (ed.). *Emotional Problems of Early Childhood.* New York: Basic Books, Inc., 1955.

DORFMAN, E. "Play Therapy," in *Client-centered Therapy,* ed. C. Rogers. Boston: Houghton Mifflin Co., 1951, pp. 235–77.

FREUD, A. "Introduction to the Technique of Child Analysis," *Nervous and Mental Disease Monograph Series,* No. 48. New York: Nervous & Mental Disease Publishing Co., 1928.

FREUD, S. "Analysis of a Phobia in a Five Year Old Boy," in *Collected Papers,* vol. 3. London: Hogarth Press, Ltd., 1925.

HAMILTON, G. *Psychotherapy in Child Guidance.* New York: Columbia Univ. Press, 1947.

Health Supervision of Young Children. New York: The American Public Health Association, Inc., 1955.

JACKSON, L., and TODD, K. *Child Treatment and the Therapy of Play,* 2d ed. New York: The Ronald Press Co., 1950.

KLEIN, M. *The Psycho-Analysis of Children.* London: Hogarth Press, Ltd., 1937.

KLEIN, M., HERMANN, P., and MONEY-KYRL, R. *New Directions in Psychoanalysis.* New York: Basic Books, Inc., 1955.

LEVY, D. "Psychotherapy and Childhood," *Amer. J. Orthopsychiat.,* **10:** 905–11, 1940.

———. "Release Therapy," *Amer. J. Orthopsychiat.* **9:** 713–37, 1939a.

———. "Release Therapy in Young Children," *Child Study,* 16: 141–43, 1939a.

———. "Release Therapy in Young Children," *Psychiat.,* 1: 387–90, 1938.

LIPPMAN, H. *Treatment of the Child in Emotional Conflict.* New York: Blakiston Division, McGraw-Hill Book Co., Inc., 1956.

LOWENFELD, M. "The World Pictures of Children: A Method of Recording and Studying Them," *Brit. J. Med. Psychol.*, 18: 65–101, 1939.

MOUSTAKAS, C. *Children in Play Therapy.* New York: McGraw-Hill Book Co., Inc., 1953.

POLLAK, O. *Integrating Sociological and Psychoanalytic Concepts.* New York: Russell Sage Foundation, 1956.

RANK, B. "Adaptation of the Psychoanalytic Technique for the Treatment of Young Children with Atypical Development," in *Specialized Techniques in Psychotherapy*, eds. C. Bychowski and J. Despert. New York: Basic Books, Inc., 1952, pp. 119–34.

RANK, O. *Will Therapy; and Truth and Reality.* New York: Alfred A. Knopf, Inc., 1945.

ROGERS, C. *Counseling and Psychotherapy.* Boston: Houghton Mifflin Co., 1942.

SLAVSON, S. *Child Psychotherapy.* New York: Columbia Univ. Press, 1952.

TAFT, J. *The Dynamics of Therapy in a Controlled Relationship.* New York: The Macmillan Co., 1933.

WITMER, H. (ed.). *Psychiatric Interviews with Children.* New York: Commonwealth Fund, 1946.

Chapter 9

Play Therapy in a
Group Setting

The great source of terror in infancy is solitude.——William
James

Self-actualization is achieved when the stutterer is able to
enter into happy and socially productive interpersonal relations with others. To accomplish this, the stutterer must
perceive himself realistically, recognize and accept his own
role. He has to recognize and accept the roles of others.
He must be able to give of himself emotionally and to control
or sublimate impulsive strivings. He must cooperate. The
degree to which he achieves self-differentiation and self-
integration will be determined in great part by his early
relationships with groups, beginning with his family group.
Attitudes evolved in family living are transferred to subsequent group settings. It is becoming increasingly evident
that stuttering problems derive from the individual's relations with groups. It is becoming clear, also, that groups
may be employed effectively in speech therapy situations.

The social relationships of stutterers tend to be imperiled
for a number of reasons. The stuttering child often has felt
the verbal sting of ridicule and rejection because of his stuttering. He probably can remember the impatient looks of
listeners as his communicative attempts were disrupted,
either by his stuttering or by the interruptions of others.
He may have experienced feelings of isolation as a consequence of the side glances or averted heads of listeners as

he struggled to speak. Stuttering is not only a symptom of past disturbed interpersonal relationships; it may also be an instigator of additional interpersonal disturbances. The stuttering, initially an effect, becomes an effector. Stuttering is, then, both an end and a beginning—an end result of interpersonal disruption, and a beginning determinant of other breaches in human relations. Stuttering is a breakdown in interpersonal communications. More than most, the stutterer needs opportunities for multiple interpersonal experiences which are positive; i.e., which enable him to have gratifying, self-enhancing social experiences. A move in this direction is taken in a therapeutic setting which is capable of nurturing this healthy reformulation of interpersonal dynamics, viz., group therapy (Ali, 1957; Axline, 1947, 1955; Backus and Beasley, 1951; Backus, 1957; Rosenthal and Garfinkel, 1957; Slavson, 1956).

Backus and Beasley advanced the application of the group therapy structure in speech therapy when they wrote:

Speech therapy shares with other fields of human relations the goal of helping each individual to change behavior in interpersonal relationships to the extent that he can function in such relationships with greater relative adequacy in terms of satisfactions and security (Backus and Beasley, 1951, pp. 7–8).

DYNAMICS OF GROUP-PLAY THERAPY

There is but one inflexible rule regarding group therapy and its organization, viz., that the group structure should *never* be selected solely in terms of limited time or weighty case load. The group therapy structure has much to offer child stutterers in its own right. In group therapy, the child who stutters has opportunities to adapt himself socially in activities which approximate the adult-peer social interactions which he encounters daily. In addition, the structure provides the child stutterer with experiences in living social relationships under a nonthreatening, nonjudgmental therapeutic relationship, hour after hour. For children in the latency years of nine through twelve, group-play therapy holds considerable therapeutic adequacy. It is during these childhood years that the group assumes ascendancy in its appeal and prominence. Group play therapy with its social-therapeutic interchanges and interplays can serve the social-emotional-communicative needs of many stutterers:

1. The child stutterer who stands at the circumference of a group, delineating himself from the group constellation, and who needs feelings of belonging and status.
2. The child stutterer who has found himself to be the lowest member in the "pecking order" regarding self and speech with parents, peers, and other persons of major or minor significance, and who needs increased self-esteem.
3. The child stutterer who copes with his disorganized self-process by means of verbal or physical aggression or other defensive processes.
4. The child stutterer who perceives his stuttering and every communicative interchange with fear reactions which approximate those stipulated by Johnson when he defined stuttering as "an anticipatory, apprehensive, hypertonic avoidance reaction" (Johnson, 1956, pp. 216–17).
5. The child stutterer who has a sense of self-isolation because of his stuttering speech.

A 12-year-old stutterer is speaking during a private interview after his second group play therapy session:

When the kids are standing around or playing together, I can't seem to join in. I don't go over—much as I want to. I know that I'd stutter, and I don't like to have the kids hear me and see me. Another thing, I don't like to be "nosey" either. So I move on, or I keep on doing whatever I am doing. But that works against me. The kids think that I think I'm too good for them. ME think I'M too good for THEM! That kills me! Me with my mushy talk. I know that I only make things more tough for myself, but I can't seem to push myself. I think if I wasn't so afraid of stuttering, I know that I could push myself. I hang back just like a "stupe." I know that if I didn't talk with such mush-mouth stuttering that I would act more friendly. When kids do act friendly with me, I feel so good—a kind of easy, velvet feeling runs all over me—like soft, little goose pimples—and I feel really good. I don't talk so mushy-mouthed, either, and my stuttering isn't so bad then. (Deep sigh.) But that doesn't happen very often—not often enough.

Group treatment goals are identical with those listed for individual play situations. In addition the group participants are helped to identify with others in the same group and to introject and utilize desirable social standards. In general, the over-all goal is to positively recondition the young stutterer's social relationships through the transfer of group-therapy learnings. Group therapy with its social structure, its opportunities for group interactions, and its experiences in social learnings can provide the young stutterer with a renascence in personality, speaking ability, communicative freedom, and improved social adjustment.

The group constellation may consist of two to five children. Into the group-play therapy process each group member interpolates his needs and his projections in the light of his past experiences. Thus, during group therapy, there are many affective claims placed upon the clinician as he is called upon to accept, reflect, and clarify the irregular feelings, actions, and attitudes of two, three, four, or five children. It is necessary for the group-play clinician to have an abundance of inner emotional stability and elasticity so that each group member may have his emotional demands met adequately and therapeutically. The child-clinician relationship is the positive growth nucleus in group play therapy just as it is in individual play therapy. It is the therapeutic relationship which offers each child something which he has never received enough of, something which is crucial to his emotional equilibrium, i.e., acceptance that is not provisional or problematical but acceptance that is positive and permanent, come what may. This therapeutic soil of acceptance enables each child to dig into his defensive system as deeply as he wishes, weeding out, when he is ready, his maladaptive behavioral functionings; transplanting within himself a more integrated self-system; and cultivating more satisfactory adult and peer relationships, first within the confines of each therapy hour and ultimately within the greater terminus of his daily social intercourse.

An able group clinician is a responsive and sensitive person who establishes relationships that abound in therapeutic sufficiency (Kotkov, 1956). His relations with children are responsive in their warmth and understanding. He knows that:

1. An effective play clinician may be all things to all group members.
2. The group-play clinician communicates with each child not by word alone.
3. Full acceptance of each group member is critical.
4. In group-play therapy, relationships are complex in emotional stratifications as well as in quantity.
5. Emotional exploitation of a group member or the clinician is often a factor to be worked through in the group play therapy structure.
6. The feeling of safety which a good therapeutic relationship provides is conducive to cathartic verbal and motoric release and ultimately to vitalized emotional-social learnings.
7. Clarification of cathartic expression—oral or motoric—must be *accurate* in terms of its feeling tone as well as in terms of its verbal content.
8. The clinician's faith is placed in the child's ability to draw upon the therapeutic relationship so that he is able to design his individual, psychic alterations and modifications in his own way, at his own rate, as he struggles for self-differentiation and self-integration.

In brief, the group-play clinician provides support; recognizes, stimulates, and provides sublimation and reality-testing opportunities; helps the group set goals; accepts not only suggestions but criticisms; and pervasively accepts and tries to clarify the feelings being experienced.

The initial perception of the clinician by the youngsters will vary a great deal. Of course if Johnny has been with the clinician in individual therapy—and this is usually desirable prior to group activity—the relationship "ice" has been broken. (All the children discussed in this chapter's reports of therapy had been seen previously for at least several hours individually by the group clinician.) The children will variously regard the clinician as an advice-giver, as another teacher, as someone akin to a "Doctor" who gives prescriptions or probes, or (sometimes immediately) as a self-ideal. The perception by the youngsters of one another will soon be revealed as the group experience unfolds. Rivalry, often for the clinician's attention, is so extremely common that it is almost universal. Jimmy will be fearful; Nancy, silent; Carl, hostile; Barbara, tattling; George, clowning; Ted, competitive; Helen, jealous; Paul, withdrawn; Tom, advice-giving; Jean, bossy; and so on.

Rather common among stutterers, especially as we near the preadolescent years, is the monopolist, the one who does most of the talking. He is apt to be quite skilled verbally, sometimes to an obsessional degree. Yet, he is the child who is inclined to be in more or less constant conflict—submissive trends being confused with dominating actions—verbal overactivity as reaction formation to feelings of inadequacy.

With preadolescent stutterers there appears to be a tendency toward discussion of the speech symptom per se, and the clinician finds it may take a little longer to bring the group focus within the feeling-oriented framework desired. This is one reason for trying to ensure that the group composition is a somewhat heterogeneous one in terms of selection criteria like severity, age, socioeconomic background, and sex; however, the relative efficacy of homogeneous as compared to heterogeneous groupings is yet a debatable issue (Leopold, 1957).

TRANSCRIPTS OF GROUP-THERAPY SESSIONS

Excerpts from five group-play therapy sessions with three boy stutterers follow. They give a practical indication of: (1) the structuring procedure; (2) the handling of limits; (3) the action of continuing release and acceptance in developing a group synthesis; (4) the process of working through to thresholds of insight; and (5) technique in terminating therapy. In general, it will be seen that the group action moved from more or less cautious, deliberate, and discreet conduct which was lacking in group unity to behavior which reveals increased motoric and verbal spontaneity and mutual

acceptance. Finally, group cohesion became manifest, showing an increase of positive responses, insight development,
and self-actualization.

A commentary for each group-play therapy excerpt is not
provided as was done in the previous chapter. The purpose
of this omission is to provide the reader with opportunities
to educe for himself the motivational determinants which are
being revealed within the behavioral samplings.

Case History Summaries. *Bruce*, a shy, self-conscious,
fourth grade pupil, is the oldest child in a middle-class family
consisting of father, mother, Bruce, a five-year-old sister, and
a three-year-old sister. Bruce is a tall, brown-haired boy
whose attractiveness is marred by an extreme overbite. The
chief complaint is stuttering, which is characterized by mild
repetitions, shyness, and passivity.

Bruce's birth history was normal. He was bottle-fed on a
schedule, and he is reported to have responded well to his
formula. He sucks his thumb despite prohibitions in the
form of parental criticisms and applications of foul-tasting
substances to the thumb. His developmental schedule was
advanced; he sat alone at six months; walked at eight months;
and spoke his first word at nine months. He was weaned
from the bottle to the cup at the early age of five months.
Toilet training was initiated at six months. His mother reported that Bruce was very possessive concerning his bowel
movements. He would cry when he was taken from the
stool. Hospitalization for an appendectomy at the age of
five years was without complication. At age four, Bruce was
bitten by a dog on the arm. The bite had to be cauterized,
and Bruce retains a fear of dogs. When he entered the first
grade, the travel to and from school imposed a problem
because of the fear engendered in him as dogs crossed his
path. In addition to his general timidity and fear of dogs,
he is also fearful of class recitations and the possibility that
he may get into fights with the other boys. Bruce's educational progress has been normal. His third grade Stanford-
Binet (L) I.Q. was 109. The richness of the vocabulary

which Bruce uses is indicative of a higher intelligence potential.

Bruce's father, a sales manager, is absent from the home frequently. When he is at home, most of his time is spent working on reports, leaving little time available for companionship with his son. Bruce's sisters are mentally alert and well behaved, both displaying an aptitude for ballet, an activity which brings them much recognition. The mother assumes a dominant role, making most of the decisions for the family. She is inclined to be overly strict, rigid, and demanding. For example, Bruce finds an outlet for expression in drawing and painting, and he has expressed a desire to attend a children's art class which meets each Saturday morning. But Bruce's mother does not approve of art school and "painters"; consequently, she has denied this outlet to Bruce.

Recently, Bruce was encouraged to join the Cub Scouts. His den mother is a psychologically sophisticated, warm, accepting person who recognizes his problems. She structured the Cub Scout activities so that some of Bruce's needs are being satisfied. He enjoys this group and looks forward to joining the Boy Scouts when he's older. At the speech clinician's suggestion he was given a full medical examination which was essentially negative, but as a result, orthodontic treatment was arranged for the malocclusion.

Francis is a friendly, talkative, fourth grade pupil in a parochial school. He is the next to the youngest child in a middle-class family of nine children, ranging in age from 25 to 6 years. Francis is a tall, well-built boy whose glasses (for strabismus) give his face a somewhat owlish look. The chief complaint is "secondary" stuttering, which is characterized by blocking, wild arm swinging, and facial grimaces.

Francis' birth history was normal. He was breast-fed on a schedule. At three months, bottle feeding was used as a supplement. Breast feeding ceased at six months. At one year he was weaned from the bottle to the cup. His developmental schedule was within normal limits. He spoke his first word at ten months. Toilet training was initiated when he was six months old. The mother reported that it was a very easy project which Francis implemented himself, imitating his brothers and sisters. Francis' health history has been typical, and at present his health is good.

His educational advancement has been normal although he works two to three hours each night on his homework in order to keep up. Francis is amenable to authority, coping by means of reaction formation. He is reported by his mother to be the easiest of all her children "to handle."

Francis' father, employed as a meat department manager in a chain store supermarket, is older than the average father of a nine-year-old boy, i.e., 52 years of age. His interests center in work and a fraternal religious organization. His manner is quiet and courteous. Francis' mother is 48 years of age. Her interests are her family, her home, and a church women's club. Many demands are placed upon her by such a large family. She tends to be dominating in her relationships with her children. Her motivations are positive, however. She does only what she thinks and feels is best for her children. Her very high goals and aspirations as a mother reveal the misinterpretation in her orientation. Francis' position is complicated not only by maternal domination but also by sibling interaction in which correction and criticism are assigned to him without stint by his three older brothers and four older sisters. It was impossible to arrange weekly parent-counseling sessions, but the mother is seen at intervals.

Jack, a ten-year-old fourth grader, is an only child in a middle-class family. He is a tall, attractive blond who is usually meticulously groomed in white shirt, tie, and duck trousers, quite a contrast to his cowboy-attired classmates. His stuttering is accompanied by head jerking and arm waving. As is common, the stuttering increases in tension situations. Jack's birth occurred when his mother was 33. His father had wanted a boy; his mother, a girl. Jack was bottle-fed, weaned to the cup at five months, and in general was an "easy" baby to care for. Toilet training, begun at six months, was not completed until the twenty-fourth month. Jack began using words at one year and was speaking two- and three-word sentences at two years. Stuttering was first noticed by parents and teachers soon after his entrance into the first grade. Jack had pneumonia at age three, German measles at age six, and mumps at age seven years. There have been no serious accidents or operations. Thumb sucking was a problem to his mother when Jack was about three years of age. His mother reported that he would sit for hours sucking on his thumb inserted "almost down to his wrist." After much maternal restraining action, he stopped. Jack's report cards are sprinkled liberally with A's. On the Stanford-Binet, Form L, an I.Q. of 115 was obtained. His attitude toward his teachers is somewhat conforming and dependent. Jack is a shy, controlled boy who strives to please. His behavior suggests a strong need for social approval. He strives to be a model of cleanliness, orderliness, conformity, academic achievement, and propriety. He internalizes his aggressive feelings, allowing them to escape only by the safe means of teasing.

Jack's father is coordinator in a manufacturing concern. He is inclined to be tense and anxious, engaging in much social drinking in order to reduce his tensions. It is necessary for him to be away from the home frequently while he travels to the various branches of the organization. Jack's mother is a good-looking woman who prides herself on her grooming and over-all attractiveness. She was not allowed to go to college because she was a female. Her father, a heavy drinker, perceived females as inferior in status. Jack's mother has strong feelings about her brothers being allowed to go to college. She perceives males as threatening and thwarting. Because of her father's excessive drinking, she overreacts to her husband's social drinking with chronic nagging and strong anxiety. The mother is seen weekly for parent counseling; intermittently, both parents are seen together. At the father's first meeting with the clinician, he commented, "So you're the person my wife has been talking so much about. I had the feeling you'd be so big. She keeps telling me that you say this and you say that." The clinician, in counseling the mother, had not up to that time given any direct advice or suggestions. Such incidents are but confirmations of the fact that our manner of perception influences our attitudes and actions.

Structuring Therapy (Excerpt from First Session)

CL. 1: This is the playroom. You may come here every week to play at this time. You may play here for 50 minutes in any way that you wish. In other words, you may spend your time here in whatever way that you wish, and things we do here we'll keep confidential—this will be *our* group. We'll all meet together at this time each week. (The clinician, who knows the boys from previous individual meetings, introduces the boys to each other. The boys nod and say "Hi" to one another). Here are the toys and the play materials (indicating by a wave of the hand in the general directions of the toys and equipment). This is your time, boys, to use as you want to use it. The only things we don't do is to hit people or to damage any property. I'll let you know when our time is almost over. (Each boy seeks out the familiar materials of paper, pencils, and crayons. Francis begins to draw a cowboy picture. Bruce draws a picture of trees and a lake, while Jack writes this original poem):

> There's a tiny, little gray mouse
> He lives with us at our house
> He likes to eat some yellow cheese
> He runs as quickly as a breeze.
> But, there's a trap waiting for him
> And life for him will be so grim.
> Snip, snap, snip, snap—right on his head.
> Executed—he'll be found dead.

(During this phase of diversified activity, there is silence and complete lack of even nonverbal communication. These pencil, crayon, and paper activities continue for 20 minutes.)

FRANCIS (F.): I'm going to try the finger painting. This cowboy is lousy. I'm a lousy drawer, anyway.

CL.* (F. 1): You feel that you are not good at drawing, so you want to try finger painting, Francis.

* Numbers following clinicians' identification indicate answers made to boy identified; for example, J2 indicates Jack's second statement.

BRUCE (B. 1): I like to draw, and I like to finger paint. I really like drawing better. But I guess I'll try finger painting. (Addressing the clinician) Can I?

CL. (B. 1): You may do whatever you wish, Bruce. You don't have to ask permission. You may do whatever you like.

JACK (J. 1): I wrote a poem—an original poem. It's about a mouse. I finished my poem, so I guess I'll finger paint too.

CL. (J. 1): You finished your poem and now you guess you'll finger paint.

JACK (J. 2): (Jack is very generous in his use of the paint.) This is messy—really messy.

CL. (J. 2): It's really messy.

FRANCIS (F. 2): (Using red paint and smearing it around and around the paper with his hands.) It looks like blood.

CL. (F. 2): Just like blood.

JACK (J. 2): (Crumpling up his paper). This is no good.

CL. (J. 2): You don't like your painting so you crushed it.

BRUCE (B. 2): I love to paint (continuing with his designs).

CL. (B. 2): You really enjoy it.

FRANCIS (F. 3): I'm going to wash up; this is too messy.

JACK (J. 3): Me too. Ugh, messy. (Bruce continues to work on his paper while Francis and Jack wash at the sink. Francis and Jack walk to the puppets, and they look them over. Francis picks up a bird puppet, and Jack selects a chick puppet. Bruce finishes his painting; walks to the sink, washes his hands; and goes to where the two boys are and stands looking at the puppets. Francis and Jack eye the nursing bottles. Francis picks up a bottle, fingers it, fills it with water. He holds the bottle to the mouth of the puppet.)

FRANCIS (F. 4): I'm going to give him a drink.

CL. (F. 4): Give him a drink. (Jack picks up a rubber sword and he hits Francis' puppet, saying, "Take that!" Bruce picks up another sword quickly and says in a loud voice

BRUCE (B. 4): Break it up (swooping down on the puppet with the sword. Speaking, he says quickly to Francis) Do you want my sword? (He quickly gives the sword to Francis. He appears frightened by his brash act of trying to break up Jack's sword fight.)

FRANCIS (F. 5): (addressing Bruce) Do you know how to Indian-wrestle?

JACK (J. 5): That's easy; anyone knows how to do that.

BRUCE (B. 5): Sure, I do.

JACK (J. 6): (Goes to the pounding board.) Hey, let's have a contest. The winner will be the one who gets the most nails pounded into the board with the least number of hits.

FRANCIS (F. 6) and BRUCE (B. 6): (almost in unison): O.K. O.K.

FRANCIS (F. 7) and JACK (J. 7): First!

FRANCIS (F. 8): Let's settle it fair. We'll play fingers. (Francis, Jack, and Bruce engage in the fingers game in order to determine the order of play. Jack comes out first. Francis is second. Bruce says that he wants to be last. The contest proceeds. Bruce wins. After his win, Bruce takes the hammer and pounds furiously on all but four of the nails—one right after the other—about six in all.)

FRANCIS (F. 9): Wow!

JACK (J. 8): That board has really had it.

CL. 5: Bruce really had a workout. (A shining look of success and achievement sweeps across Bruce's face, followed by a trace of a smile.)

The Handling of Limits (Excerpt from Second Session).
Laissez-faire (maximally permissive) approaches are not desirable forms of any play therapy. Disregard of all external directions and restrictions tends to produce confusion in both clinician and children, plus unhandled anxiety. In such settings, aggressive group members become more hostile, while withdrawn members become more encapsulated. If children are to adjust to the communicative demands of society, they must learn to accept restrictions imposed by external sources. Acceptance and tolerance of realistic restrictions without a sense of disorganizing frustration can more easily occur in speech therapy settings which serve as a testing ground prior to acceptance and usage outside of the therapeutic situation.

One of the goals of play therapy is to help the child to become more able to tolerate frustration. The child who is able to accept societal restrictions and limitations has had earlier experience in learning to adjust to frustration. In play therapy, the child's emotional absorption of therapy's

emandatory, restorative elements encourages an inner forti-
tude which gives to the child a higher frustration tolerance
as well as an awareness of his own deviant behavior. A *completely* permissive therapy structure fails to help the child
to appreciate the realistic limits of his world, making it extremely difficult for him to form reasonable goals, to see his
necessary role in life situations, to understand and accept the
realistic boundaries in behavior which are not only socially
acceptable but personally rewarding.

The boys enter the playroom as greetings are exchanged
by all. Francis goes to the puppets and looks them over somewhat carefully. Bruce takes the clay and proceeds to roll it
into long, stringy snakes. There is no immediate verbalization.

J. 1: I don't know what to do.
Cl. 1: Can't make up your mind.
F. 1: You can do what you want.
J. 2: (Irritably) I *know* it! I was hunting up a girl to take to
    the movies on Saturday afternoon.
F. 2: That's all baloney.
J. 3: Baloney, nothing!
F. 3: Girls are crazy.
Cl. 2 (F. 3): Francis doesn't seem to like girls, but Jack does.
F. 4: You can say that again.
J. 4: You should see my girl. Is she a dish!
F. 5: Girls, phooey! (Going to the rubber knives, picking one
    out.) Come on, let's have a fight—left hand behind your
    back. I got you.
J. 5: (Singing *The Blue Danube* as he manipulates his knife.)
    Oh no you don't. Come on, man, fight. Fight, I say.
    (Francis and Jack close in on each other in a wrestle-like
    hold, each striving to make contact on the other's body with
    his knife.)
Cl. 3: (F. 5, J. 5) We can't touch or hit or knife each other or
    do anything that could hurt anyone. I can see that you feel
    like fighting and you may do it with one of the toys, but not
    with each other.
F. 6: Hey, how old are you?

J. 6: Ten years old. (Going to the playhouse and picking up a toy car, putting it in the garage of the play-house that was standing nearby.) Nice model of an old jalopy.

F. 7: Jalopy! Are you crazy? You don't know a car when you see one.

J. 7: (Picking up a rubber knife and going after Francis.)

Cl. 4 (J. 7): Francis made you mad when he called you a dope and you want to pay him back. But we don't fight with each other that way. You can use the toys if you want or talk about it, but we don't hit or hurt anyone.

J. 8: Rich people have that kind of a car. I'm going to have that kind of a car when I grow up.

Bruce (B. 1): My sister has a dollhouse like that.

J. 9: I'd love to live in a house like that. I will too, when I'm working. That's a mansion.

F. 8: Yeah, its a real mansion.

J. 10: Rich bitches live in that kind of a house.

F. 9: Oh, what you said! (Bruce looks up quite aghast.)

J. 11: I said, Rich bitches live in that kind of a house.

Cl. 5 (J. 12): Jack likes to say that because it's considered such a bad word. But he likes to say it.

F. 10: I'm going to draw. (Talking baby talk) I'm going to "dwaw." That's the way my baby brother talks. Boy, is he a pest. I feel like throwing things at that kid brother of mine.

Cl. 6 (F. 10): Your kid brother can be pesty, and he bothers you sometimes. (Bruce goes to the nursing bottle, turning it over in his hands. Jack touches the nipple and starts to release the water on to the floor drop by drop.)

F. 11: Hey, watch out! Look what you're doing. You're getting the floor all wet.

J. 12: I can wet the floor if I feel like it. We can do what we feel like—anything except hit or hurt people. You're lucky too, or I'd beat you up. You're always bossing.

Cl. 7 (J. 12): You know that here you can do what you wish except hurt someone or hurt property. You feel cross when Francis tells you what to do or what not to do.

F. 12: (Going to the toy drum, and beating out rhythms on it) Bongo, bongo, bongo.

J. 13: Just like the natives in the jungles of Africa.

F. 13: This is fun. (Continuing to beat out rhythms on the toy drum.) (Bruce stands watching Francis, as he sucks on the nursing bottle.)

J. 14: Hey, Francis, look at Bruce! (Francis continues to beat the drum, grinning.)

Cl. 8 (J. 14): Bruce knows that he can do what he feels like doing here. (Bruce continues to suck on the nipple and to drink from the bottle.)

J. 15: (Going to the balloon box, selecting a red one, blowing it up, making a knot around its neck, throwing the balloon into the air, keeping it afloat with little hand thrusts.) Hey, kids, let's see who can keep the balloon up in the air. Come on, let's go! (Bruce places his bottle down on a table, and Francis leaves his drum. The three boys engage in keeping the balloon up in the air.)

F. 14: Hey, let's pop it. (Francis pops the balloon with the sharp point of a pencil.)

J. 16: Let's blow up a lot of balloons and pop them. (The boys rush to the balloon box and each boy takes out several.)

B. 2: This is hard to do.

F. 15: We'll be all out of wind. Whew! I'm winded.

J. 17: Blow hard so we'll have a lot of them to pop. It'll sound like firecrackers. (The boys apply themselves to the task of blowing up the balloons, building a stockpile of about a dozen.)

J. 18: That's enough, now. Let's have a balloon fight. We'll throw them at each other, and we can pop them with the pencils. We'll bomb each other. (There is much running around the room, throwing of the balloons, and the repeated sounds of the balloons as they pop, intermingled with the shrieks, shouts, and laughter of the boys.)

B. 3: The last balloon. POP! I GOT IT!

Continuing Release and Acceptance in Developing Group Synthesis (Excerpt from Third Session)

F. 1: (Drinking from a nursing bottle.) I'm a little baby (laughing and speaking in a falsetto voice), a "ittle, bitsy, witsy baby." (Bruce watches for a moment. He goes to the shelf where the nursing bottles are kept. Bruce selects a bottle and fills it with water. He sucks on the nipple, making no comment.)

F. 2: You're doing it, too (directed to Bruce).

B. 1: Yup (continuing with his sucking).

J. 1: Throw some water out of the window.

F. 3: You can't do that. You can do what you want, but you can't hurt anyone. If you throw the water out of the window, someone would get wet. You know that. (Jack picks up a bear puppet and a ball, making the puppet bounce the ball.)

F. 4: Big deal. Anyone can do that.

F. 5: (Putting the bottle down and taking a balloon from the balloon box, blows up the balloon with one breath, causing his face to get very red) I did it with one breath.

B. 2: Your face is all red—you blew it up so fast.

J. 2: (Taking a sharp pencil, and stabbing Francis' balloon, causing it to pop.) Oo-o-o! what I did. I'm a *naughty, naughty* boy (using a mocking voice of rebuke).

F. 6: What did you do that for? Cut it out. I'm warning you. I'm a poor loser. I'm warning you. I really get sore.

Cl. 1 (F. 6): When things don't go your way, you get mad.

F. 7: You can say that again. I get really mad.

Cl. 2 (F. 7): You really get very mad.

B. 3: I get mad, too, when I lose in games. My mother and father get mad with me when I do and that makes me more mad.

Cl. 3 (B. 3): You get mad when you lose and when your mother and father get mad with you you feel even more mad then.

J. 2: I was playing animal rummy once—with my mother. She won and I got so mad that I waved my cards in the air and poked my mother in the eye. I didn't mean to, and I got scared. She told me that I had blinded her in that eye and that she couldn't see out of her eye. She was trying to scare me so that I wouldn't be a sore loser again. I thought that I really blinded her and I started to cry and kiss her. She said, "Now maybe you'll learn not to be such a sorehead." I was glad that I hadn't blinded her, but I was mad because she kidded me all that time. I'll never forget it.

Cl. 4 (J. 2): You really worried when you felt that you had hurt her. When you found out that you hadn't hurt her you felt better, much better, and then you began to feel a little mad because she had fooled you.

F. 8: It's foolish to get sore. It's only a game. But you do get sore even though you know it's only a game.

CL. 5 (F. 8): Even if it's foolish, you can't help feeling that way.

F. 9: I like coming here and I like being here.

CL. 6 (F. 9): You feel good about being here.

B. 4: It's nice here—you can do what you want to do—you're your own boss—here.

CL. 7 (B. 4): It feels good to be your own boss.

J. 3: It's funny here, but I like it.

CL. 8 (J. 3): Funny here.

J. 4: Not really funny—but different—no boss like at home, no boss like at school. You really are your own boss here.

CL. 9 (J. 4): Different from home and school where you're told what to do.

F. 10: (Picks up his nursing bottle and begins to drink) It's good. I'm taking a long, long drink. (Bruce picks up his bottle and begins to drink. The two boys drink from their bottles, sucking on the nipples and making many lip-smacking noises.)

F. 11: (Grinning) I'll save some of this water for next time—for next week. (The three boys laugh uproariously. Bruce bites the nipple off of the bottle and chews on the nipple, holding it between his teeth.)

F. 12: (Picking up a toy telephone, dialing) Hello Bruce, Good-bye Bruce. Hello Jack, Good-bye Jack. (Putting the telephone down and singing *McNamara's Band* at the top of his voice).

B. 5: (Picking up a plush dog, slapping the dog several times, saying mockingly) "Poor doggie, poor, little doggie." (He throws the dog into a corner of the room.)

J. 5: (Picking up a baby puppet and inverting the head of the puppet so that the head is hidden. Holding up the puppet.) Punch baby puppet in the head. Punch it on the head, I said. (Jack puts the baby puppet down and replaces it with the mother puppet. He takes the mother puppet and hits it over the head with a rubber gun.)

B. 6: (Taking the baby puppet and the father puppet, putting one on each hand, engaging them in conversation, saying for the father puppet) Bad, bad girl. You naughty girl. Go sit in the corner (flinging the girl puppet into a corner).

J. 6: (Picking up another baby puppet and touching the tip of Bruce's hair—unbeknown to Bruce, a smile on Jack's face as he walks away.)

Cl. 10 (J. 6): Jack likes to fool people.

F. 13: (Picking up the father puppet which Bruce has put down. He covers his right hand with the puppet, places the puppet's hands over its eyes) That's what some kids do in the movies when the picture is scary. I don't do it, but some kids do. I'm not afraid of anything.

Cl. 11 (F. 13): You feel that you are not afraid of anything.

F. 14: I'm afraid of *some* things, but I'm not afraid of a lot of things. I am afraid of the dark, but I'm not afraid of thunder and lightning. My mother—boy is she afraid of thunder and lightning (laughing). She's really scared of that. I don't like the dark in my bedroom. I like to have a light on when I go to sleep.

Cl. 12 (F. 14): You're not afraid of a *lot* of things, but *some* things you're afraid of.

F. 15: My mother says I'm too big for that stuff, but I don't care.

Cl. 13 (F. 15): Even though she thinks you're too big, you still really feel that way.

J. 7: I don't like the dark really, but I don't have a light on.

Cl. 14 (J. 7): Uh huh.

B. 7: I used to have a night light, but my big sister teased me so much about it that I don't have one now. But I hate the dark. There are creepy shadows in the dark, and you feel so alone—so all by yourself. It's creepy.

Cl. 15 (B. 7): She teased you so that you gave up the light—but you still feel scary about it.

J. 8: It's O.K. after you get to sleep.

Cl. 16 (J. 8): It doesn't bother you if you can't think about it—wonder about it. I see that we have five minutes left.

J. 9: Only five more minutes left.

F. 16: I wish that we were just beginning.

Cl. 17 (F. 16): You'd like to have more time here.

B. 8: Let's go out the door and come in again. We'll pretend. Then we'll have a long time.

Cl. 19: You all wish that you had more time to be here.

F. 17: (Looking down at his slacks) Yipes! My pants are all wet; the water must have leaked out of the bottle. Will I catch it. My mother will kill me.

CL. 20 (F. 17): You're afraid she will get angry at you because of this.

F. 18: Yeah, and I don't want her to know what I do here, either.

CL. 21 (F. 18): You don't want her to know what goes on in here.

B. 9: I don't tell my mother or anyone what we do. When she asks me, all I say is, "We have fun and we play."

CL. 22: (B. 9): You don't want *anyone* to know.

J. 10: (Laughing) It drives my mother crazy when I don't tell her what we do. I just say, "Oh, Francis, Bruce, and I just play." She says, "What do you play?" I say "Just games."

CL. 22 (J. 10): You feel the same way—about not telling them—and then they get mad.

J. 11: Rip-roaring mad! (The three boys laugh.)

CL. 24 (To all the boys): Our time is up now; see you next week, boys.

J. 12: Bye-bye; see you next week.

B. 10: See you next week. Bye.

F. 19: Good-bye. I hope that next week comes fast.

Working Through to Insight (Excerpt from Seventh Session)

FRANCIS (F. 1): Let's play cards.

BRUCE (B. 1): O.K.

JACK (J. 1): O.K. with me. (The boys and the clinician sit around the table.)

F. 2: (Francis deals in a professional manner with an exaggerated swagger that would befit a TV or movie cowboy) Let's play "Old Maid" and then "Animal Rummy." I've got two packs of cards.

J. 2: Ugh! I don't want to play "Old Maid." It reminds me of my teacher. She's not an old maid, but boy does she act like one! She yaks, yaks, yaks—all the time. Never shuts her mouth for a single minute. You can't even think in that room. Never can please her—no matter what. Can't talk to her. She's the last word; she's the law. I hate school this year and I hate her.

CL. (J. 2): She rules the situation—you feel like that about her. . . .

J. 3: She's impossible—just plain impossible. That's what we call her—out in the yard—that's the name we picked for her.

One day something funny happened. She got after me, and I whispered under my breath "impossible"—she heard me and she said, "What's impossible?" The kids were surprised to hear her ask me that. Boy, they were scared that I'd tell her. But of course I didn't. I told her, "My work's hard and I think it's impossible for me to do it." She told me if I'd put my mind on my work instead of fooling around and muttering I could do anything. Everyone wanted to laugh, but we didn't dare. At recess time, boy did we laugh at HER! Mrs. Impossible. She's sick—really sick—sick in her head. Boy is she sick!

CL. 2 (J. 3): It makes you feel good to think that you put something over on her.

B. 2: I don't like my teacher this year. She's so bossy! She won't let anyone move. It's work—work—work—all the time. It's do this; do that page. She doesn't make the work interesting, either. She's such a boss. She won't let you move. You have to stay in your seat. Can't even sharpen your pencil—even if it breaks. Most of the time when you do put up your hand to ask her a question or to ask if you can sharpen your pencil, she'll say, "Put your hand down and get to work."

CL. 3 (B. 2): You feel about the same as Jack does, Bruce.

F. 3: This year my teacher is pretty good. But last year, I went to a different school. What a teacher! She made you stay after school if you dropped one single piece of paper on the floor. She would empty the wastebasket all over the floor, and make you pick up each paper and put each one in the wastebasket by her desk. Some teachers are nice, and some are mean.

CL. 4 (F. 3): Different teachers act in different ways.

B. 3: I match; I'm out.

J. 5: I'm not; I match. (Addressing the clinician) It's either you or Francis.

CL. 5 (to all of the boys): I'm out.

F. 4: I'm the old maid (mockingly) Poor me, I'm the old maid.

J. 6: I don't want to play cards any more.

B. 4: Me, either.

F. 5: (With some irritation in his voice) "O.K. O.K." (The boys get up, and go to the nursing bottles. Each fills the bottle

which he is holding. There is much giggling as the water
empties into the bottles, sprinkling the floor).

F. 6: (Beginning to drink, saying) Down the hatch! (Bruce and
Jack giggle. Each repeats "Down the hatch," as he begins
to drink his bottle.)

J. 7: Let's have a bombing raid. (The boys go to the airplane
box and each takes out several toy airplanes of various sizes.)

F. 7: Bombs away! (Each boy throws an airplane into the air.
When the airplane lands upright the boys call out excitedly,
"Perfect landing!" When the planes overturn they cry,
"That one crashed" or "Oh, boy a crash!" As the airplanes
glide through the air, the boys simulate bombing and crash-
ing with "K, K, K, K, K, Kr, Kr, Kr, Kr, Kr, Kr" at various
levels of intensity. This activity continues for approximately
15 minutes.)

F. 8: Boy, I'm tired!

B. 5: Me, too.

J. 7: Whew, I'm pooped. Got all the steam out of my system.
(Walking to the place where the clay is located.)

B. 6: I'm going to paint.

J. 8: I'm going to make some clay bombs. I'm going to take all
that clay, and make one huge monstrous bomb. It can blow
up anything into pieces. Boom! And everything will
splinter.

F. 9: (Francis sits down, engaging in no activity at all.)

J. 9: You're really pooped, just sitting there doing nothing.

F. 10: I don't have to do anything if I don't want to.

J. 10: I know it! My bomb is getting bigger and bigger. I've
got to get it smooth—round and smooth.

F. 11: Hey, give me some clay.

J. 11: O.K. Here's some (giving Francis a piece the size of a
pea).

F. 12: Thanks a lot! Gee, thanks a lot.

J. 12: Oh, I was only kidding. Here, I'll cut it in half. You can
make a bomb too, if you want. Watch this operation now.
I cut the clay right in half with this ruler. Here! (Bruce
works on his painting, and the other two boys work on their
bombs.)

F. 13: I made a devil bomb. (Throws the bomb on the floor,
causing a thud which he reinforces verbally) K-K-K-K-K-

CH-CH-CH-CH-CH-CH-CH (long whistle) CH-K-K-K-K-K. That bomb made enough noise to wake the dead. (Going over to Jack, chucking him under the chin)

> Roses are red
> Violets are blue
> Oatmeal is mushy
> And—I like you.

J. 12: Here's the world's biggest H-bomb (throwing the bomb on the floor, running for cover under a table). I made it. I made it; the H-bomb didn't hurt me.

F. 14: Hey, let's draw. I'm going to draw. These are nice crayons. (The two boys pick up crayons and drawing paper. Bruce continues to paint.)

J. 10: (After quick drawing motions) Friends, presenting three of the world's greatest masterpieces, "A Cross Red-Haired Mother" drawn by her son. Look at the big fat arms and the big stick. Ouch, ouch, ouch, ouch. I can't sit down sometimes when she gets through with me. (Holding up the other picture) This is what I'd like to do when she hits me (Punching the air).

CL. 6 (J. 10): You feel cross after your mother hits you, and you'd like to let her know how mad you feel, but you don't.

J. 11: I sure do feel cross, but if I say anything, "Ouch," I only get more. So I shut up, but I hate getting hit. I'm too big to get hit. You'd think—well you'd think that I was nothing but a kid, getting spanked for being naughty.

CL. 7 (J. 11): You feel you're too big to be hit.

J. 12: When I get two years older and my mother hits me I'm going to tell her off.

CL. 8 (J. 12): When you're a little older you think you'll tell her how you really feel.

B. 7: Just like my mother. I want to be an artist when I grow up. But mother doesn't want me to. She wants me to go to college. But I don't want to go. I've never wanted to. I want Art School. Mother says that I'll forget all about that. But I won't—I know I won't. Mother says that I will, but I know that I won't.

CL. 9 (B. 7): You want to do one thing and your mother feels different—doesn't see it your way.

F. 15: My mother is always more cross when she's tired. That's when I watch myself or I really get it.

Cl. 10 (F. 15): You're really careful then.

J. 13: That's the way things are—whether we like it or not—we have to obey our parents—because they are our parents. They take care of us, and even if we don't like to do what they tell us to do all the time—we do owe them obedience. It's our duty, and a duty is a duty.

B. 8: Yeah, even in church and Sunday School you learn that (nodding his head up and down slowly while pulling his mouth to the left side of his face). You should obey your parents.

F. 16: When you don't obey your parents you're breaking one of the commandments, "Honor thy father and mother." When you don't obey "WHAM!" You sure get it every which way! Most times, what your father and mother tell you to do is right, but sometimes it seems as though you have to do everything *their* way—sometimes I'm right, too.

Cl. 11 (F. 16): You feel that you should obey your parents and most times you want to—but sometimes you find it hard to obey.

B. 9: (Looking up from his picture) This picture is lousy—really lousy. I love to draw and paint. I want to go to Junior Art School on Saturday mornings, but I can't. My mother won't let me.

Cl. 12 (B. 9): You enjoy painting and drawing very much, but you don't get enough of a chance to do it . . .

J. 14: Parents sure are funny! They want you to do everything their way.

Cl. 13 (J. 14): Parents are hard to understand sometimes.

F. 17: My mother is bossy—really bossy. She bosses everyone— even my father, and he's almost twice as big as she is. He doesn't seem to mind it when she bosses him. Why should I? But I do! Things sure do go better when you go along with her, though.

Cl. 14 (F. 17): You and Jack feel the same way. It's easier to do what your parents want, although you may not really want to do it—all the time.

B. 10: When something means a lot to you, you just can't go along, even if you do keep out of trouble. Now me—I really want to be an artist and go to Art School. I just can't give that up—even for Mother.

Cl. 14 (B. 10): It's all right to go along on the things that don't mean a great deal to you, but you feel that you must stand up for the things that mean so much.

B. 11: Maybe some day—maybe some day Mother will see it my way.

Cl. 14 (B. 11): Maybe some day, you'll get your mother to change her mind.

F. 18: Hey, let's have a target game. (Taking a crayon and drawing a male Indian figure quickly on a piece of gray, bogus * paper.) Hey, you guys, make the bombs. Make a stockpile. I'll prop this guy up here, beside the wastepaper basket. (As he places the paper, Francis extends his right arm.) How, me pale face. You, Red Skin (laughing uproariously). Let's pelt him—really pelt him right in the guts! Punch him in the nose! Belt him in the bread basket! Split his nose—give him a bloody nose. Let's mess him up—but good. O.K. men, ready, aim, fire. (The boys begin their clay assault, throwing clay balls—bombs—at the Indian figure, causing the paper to split in many places. As each clay ball struck, the boys would laugh and call out) Take that, you bum. I'll get you right in the belly! Right in the heart. Wow-eee! Bingo! Yipee! (etc.)

Preparation for Terminating Therapy (Excerpt from Seventeenth Session). As the boys enter the playroom, greetings are exchanged. The boys seek out individual activities. Bruce works with water colors, making random color designs. Francis molds a massive piece of plasticine into a cliff, patting and smoothing the clay with his fingers and thumbs. Jack picks up a red, black, and white beaded, string figure of Mickey Mouse, manipulating its platform while he hums "Yankee Doodle."

Cl. 1: We're coming to the end of our time together. We have only two more periods left.

F. 1: Yeah, just two more after this.

B. 1: I wish we had a million more.

* A 9 x 18″ piece of gray paper which is heavy but easily torn.

CL. 2 (B. 1): You wish we all could be together even longer.

J. 1: (Pulling a crumpled piece of paper from his pocket) Last night I wrote a poem about it (reading his poem).

Very Soon

Very soon we'll have to go,
How I wish it were not so!
The four of us are good friends
But, our time together ends.
Very soon it'll be good-bye.
Too bad "good-bye" can't be "Hi."

CL. 3 (J. 1): Your poem tells us how you feel about the ending.

F. 2: Gee, that's a good poem, Jack. You're good.

J. 2: You like it? Thanks.

B. 2: That's good, Jack.

J. 3: Thanks, Bruce. You know what? (Smiling) I'm going to start stuttering bad again (Laughing). Then I can start coming again. I'm glad my speech is better—not like it was before—but I wish I didn't have to stop coming.

CL. 4 (J. 3): You have mixed feelings about not coming any more. You're glad that you stutter less, but you wish that you didn't have to stop coming here. You wish that today were not so close to the last time, though.

F. 3: Me, too! I love to come and best of all I love to be here. I love doing what I feel like and saying what I feel like saying.

CL. 5 (F. 3): It's a good feeling—to feel free to say what we really think—how we really do feel.

B. 3: I feel comfortable here—like I feel when I stretch out in bed under the warm covers.

CL. 6 (B. 3): Completely relaxed.

B. 4: I have to go to camp this summer. My father and mother are going on a long trip and my sisters will stay with my aunt. I'd rather go to camp than stay with her. At camp, you can do lots of art work and crafts. You can make lots of things. You can make Indian belts and bracelets. I'll make you a bracelet and I'll make belts for both of you.

J. 4: Thanks. I'll be a bloody Indian (initiating a war dance around the room while making an Indian war cry. There is much laughter in response to this burlesque).

F. 4: Gee, thanks, Bruce.

Cl. 6 (B. 4): Bruce will enjoy the camp—and he wants to make something for us.

J. 5: This summer, I'm going to visit my grandmother in Cleveland. I haven't seen her for a long time. I love her. She's nice. Gives me presents, bakes me cookies. I'll stay with her for a month—the whole month of July.

Cl. 7 (J. 5): You feel happy about that.

F. 4: I've got a job this summer, helping my friend Ernie. He runs a big fruit stand. He pays me 75 cents a week. All I have to do is to go to the drugstore every day at 3:00 o'clock and get Ernie a coke or something. He's a nice guy. I'd work for him for nothing.

Cl. 7 (F. 4): So you'll be spending part of your summer with a very friendly person.

F. 5: Hey, look! I got the cliff all made. It's nice and high. It's smooth now. Let's put the soldiers up on the cliff, all around. Let's try to knock them off; we'll shoot at them. We can load the gun on this here gun boat with a pencil. We'll set it up and see who can knock down the most soldiers with one shot. O.K.?

J. 6: We'll each have one turn.

F. 8: I'm going to aim it. M-m-m-m-m—that's the radar, releasing the trigger. I got four. Wow!

J. 7: I'm going to use my own pencil. I've got a whole bunch of them in my pocket. Here goes! I got six of them. Six!

B. 5: (Picking up a red pencil) I'm going to use this one. (Aiming and pulling the trigger) Hey, that was a misfire. I should get another chance. How about it, boys?

J. 8: Sure, that was a dud. Try it again.

B. 6: I'm going to aim it up at the top, and when that guy on the top falls, he'll bring down a whole lot of them. . . .

REFERENCES

Ali, S. "A Note on Social Climates in Group Psychoanalyses," *Int. J. Group Psychother.*, 7: 261–63, 1957.

Axline, V. "Group Therapy as a Means of Self-Discovery for Parents and Children," *J. Group Psychother.*, 8: 152–60, 1955.

———. *Play Therapy.* Boston: Houghton Mifflin Co., 1947.

Backus, O. "Group Structure in Speech Therapy," in *Handbook of Speech Pathology*, ed. L. E. Travis. New York: Appleton-Century-Crofts, Inc., 1957, pp. 1025–64.

BACKUS, O., and BEASLEY, J. *Speech Therapy with Children.* Boston: Houghton Mifflin Co., 1951.

JOHNSON, W. "Stuttering," in *Speech Handicapped School Children,* 2d ed., ed. W. Johnson. New York: Harper & Bros., 1956, pp. 216–17.

KOTKOV, B. "Vicissitudes of Student Group Psychotherapists," *Int. J. Group Psychother.,* 6: 48–52, 1956.

LEOPOLD, H. "Selection of Patients for Group Psychotherapy," *Amer. J. Psychother.,* 11: 634–37, 1957.

ROSENTHAL, L., and GARFINKEL, A. "The Group Psychotherapy Literature, 1956," *Int. J. Group Psychother.,* 7: 196–211, 1957.

SLAVSON, S. R. (ed.). *The Fields of Group Psychotherapy.* New York: International Universities Press, Inc., 1956.

Chapter 10

Projective Therapy

As the dressing of a tree showeth the fruit thereof, so a word out of the heart of man.——Ecclesiasticus XXVII: 7

The basic assumptions which underlie projective therapy are that therapeutic atmospheres and materials can be structured and selected in ways which will help facilitate the child to

1. Release pent-up feelings.
2. Expose his thoughts and attitudes under conditions which are relatively nonthreatening.
3. Unleash his feelings upon nonretaliatory materials or objects which may serve as direct substitutes for persons and situations which have been self-devaluating or hostility-provoking.
4. Project his feelings in the presence of an acceptant, supportive clinician.
5. Recondition his feelings and attitudes in ways which will promote greater objectivity in his perception of self and others.
6. Ultimately develop self-integration.

In short, projective therapy gives the child opportunities to release, re-experience, test, retest—to *be* and *find* himself. Projective therapy employs such processes as creative dramatics, puppetry, psychodrama and sociodrama, modeling and creating with plastic or nonplastic materials, drawing, painting, finger painting, and music therapy.

THE NATURE OF PROJECTIVE THERAPY

The past is prologue in human dynamics. For, how and what an individual feels, what he thinks or does not think, says or does not say, and how he acts or does not act seem to hinge on the nature of his past experiences. The stuttering child, like any other child, reveals something about the character of his past history. The observer of projective therapy with children who stutter watches the young participants draw from their past, fuse it with their present therapy experiences, and evolve for their future a self-system of greater maturity and security. In projective speech therapy, children are "men in the making," both literally and figuratively.

Whether the child verbalizes or not, projective therapy is always rich in expression. The child is always communicating through his use or disuse of projective therapy's expressive media. With projective materials, many opportunities for dynamic communication are possible. We observe the child sitting before a blank piece of paper preparatory to his drawing or painting; reacting to a blob of paint as it rolls down his painting or to a crayon as it breaks under his pressure; responding to the balls of plasticine which refuse to unite in spite of his efforts to mold them into one; ignoring certain puppet figures which are too close to him emotionally. For, projective therapy is a setting in which speech is neither demanded nor asked. The child may express his feelings, conflicts, and ideas through crayon and clay rather than through words. In time, he may come to feel sufficiently secure to express his feelings in speech, also. Projective therapy is an experience which is unique for each child, for it is he who chooses from the available materials, charts the course of therapy activity, and "signals" when he is ready to move on to a more direct expression of his thought and attitudes. For Billy, projective therapy's main value lies in its cathartic opportunities; for Danny, this therapeutic medium may satisfy fantasy or regressive needs; for Marilyn, the total acceptance of the situation may be enough to lead to speech gains; for Peter, the repetitive acting out of a traumatic experience may bring comfort; for Jane, projective therapy may help very little, for she is so withdrawn and repressed that no therapeutic interaction or projection is occurring. As Allen says:

Therapy must occur within the framework of a relationship that is established through the participation of two people. The child, as one of the participants, may and frequently does, find that play activity is the natural means of bringing something of himself to this new experience. The therapist cannot establish a relationship with a child who does nothing, any more than a child can find a connection with the therapist who is passively inactive. There must be a mutual give and take. Everything centers about the child in this particular relationship, and he must be helped to use freely his most natural medium to bring to this new relationship his interests and feelings. So, there is no mystery to the fact that children are provided with an opportunity to play in therapy. Only through such activity can the element of naturalness enter in (Allen, 1942, p. 125).

Whatever the mode or extent of the child's expression, be it meager or monumental, the clinician accepts this behavior. Many times, a stuttering child is one who has been "over-manipulated" with regard to both general and speech behavior. In projective therapy, the manipulated one becomes the manipulator—of paints, clay, paper, puppets, as well as of his feelings and attitudes. He decrees and "rules" the action; he fixes his own expressional modes and directions; he sets his own therapeutic traveling speed. He does this in an atmosphere free of duress or derogation while he ventilates, creates, tests, and projects in action and words. With increasing security comes greater freedom and spontaneity, a warming and thawing of the behavioral and speech rigidities. In this kind of therapy, the action is very much more "child-directed" than clinician-directed (although, of course, the core structure and the therapeutic goal-ideals are incorporated within the clinician's modus operandi).

The directive clinician moving into the realm of dynamic "child-centered" therapy as a new experience will find the projective process a test of his own ability to accept, to be more permissive, to empathize. The clinician who is introduced to this technique may find it easier, for example, to accept the child's choice of activity than to accept the child's barrage of intense, raw feelings. Slackening the tutorial reins in therapy can be discomforting to the clinician new to projective methodology. Clinician apprehension may arise out of fear and anxiety which springs from self-doubts about maintaining the very necessary therapy limits. The clinician may become alarmed when he fails to introduce and reinforce limiting action; for example, when he allows a child to attack him physically or to sprinkle water on him, or when the child spends most of the therapy period traveling back and forth to the water fountain. Such a clinician may become a very uncomfortable person who, under the stimulus of the anxiety which arises out of such experiences, is apt to revert to a directive role which is reinforced by many clinician-prepared materials of a highly specific (nonprojective) nature.

The core goals of projective therapy are identical with the aims of counseling or play therapy: to achieve the fullest *acceptance* of self and others; to experience a sense of *achievement;* to receive an adequate degree of *affection;* to experience the exhilaration which a sense of *belonging* gives; to feel *recognized* as a person of worth; to know the peace and power of *security;* to enjoy the pleasure of unhindered creative exploration and experimentation in verbal and nonverbal *communication.*

The process of projective therapy is basically the same as those of other dynamics-oriented therapies. The clinician establishes a democratic (as compared to an authoritarian or laissez-faire) climate in which the participants choose their own materials and activities. There are ample opportunities for the children to externalize their conflicts; to master their world; to break down rigidities; to develop spontaneity and to reorganize their percepts. The projective therapy situation is one which enables the participants to come to grips with problems of appraisal and discovery of self and others in an atmosphere of permissive interpersonal relationships. As in all therapeutic practice, a very basic principle in projective therapy is that of flexibility of materials and procedures. The needs of each child will dictate how therapy proceeds and what therapeutic direction it will take. With some children, a few of the activities may be used very little, whereas with others, these same activities will be used quite often. Sometimes several activities will be employed with one child or a group of children within a short period of time. However, regardless of the activity, the basic principles of interpersonal dynamics will remain the same. The focus is always upon the child who is occupied with the action and not upon the action itself.

TRANSCRIPTS OF PROJECTIVE SPEECH THERAPY SESSIONS

Bobby, a Five-Year-Old. Bobby's birth was normal. However, the establishment of a formula proved to be most difficult. At 16 months, he was weaned to the cup. His mother reported that toilet training was a problem. She explained that she exerted too much effort on him. "After all, I was only eighteen, and I didn't know what to expect of him. Now, I know I expected too much. Bobby was our guinea pig." The mother reacted to Bobby's constipation problem by administering suppositories every other day for several months, at which time the condition "cleared up." In other developmental tasks, he was reported as falling within normal schedules.

Stuttering was noticed by the parents when Bobby was 48 months old. According to their report, they made no overt reaction to his speech pattern and "probably we did call it 'stammering' when we mentioned it." In the past few months, both parents have been telling Bobby to "say it again," so that they could understand him, but they say that no pressure has been put on him to speak more proficiently. Bobby's stuttering at present consists of repetitions of most initial consonant sounds with an occasional, severe tonic block of a linguadental nature; the latter type occurring primarily on "self" terms (I, me, mine) and authority references (Mommy, Daddy). In addition to the stuttering, Bobby sucks his thumb

"half the day" and also "refuses to eat solid foods," rejecting
anything but liquids, egg nogs, and melted ice cream. At
52 months, Bobby was hospitalized with pneumonia; he received much friendly attention by nurses, who thought he
was cute when he stuttered, engaging him in much conversation in order to hear him speak.

The father, a police officer, "sees very little of the children"
(apparently about one hour per day, usually between 5 and
6 P.M.). Bobby has one sibling, an active, attractive, three-
year-old sister who "has no problems," and with whom Bobby
fights "incessantly." During the pregnancy with her daughter, the mother had to remain in bed a great deal, as had
been the case with Bobby. She had to relinquish much of
the domestic responsibilities to her husband and her three
married sisters. While in their care, Bobby was kept in his
play pen most of the time. The mother places much significance on this period, and she is "trying to make up to him
for those months." A month ago, she placed him in a small
nursery-school setting, to which Bobby reacts ambivalently,
wanting to go one day, resisting attendance the next.

Bobby's Initial Therapy Interview. Bobby taps several
projective media, beginning with art play, shifting to puppetry briefly, and ending with music. Bobby and his mother
were greeted by the clinician and taken to the therapy room
where Bobby was given the choice of having his mother sit
in during the session or having her go to another room (where
she could read some pamphlets and magazines). Bobby
elected to allow his mother to go to the other room. The
clinician announced that this was Bobby's time to do what
he would like and that he could use anything that he wished
to use. He went immediately to the jumbo box of crayons
and put them on the table. He took a piece of drawing
paper and sat down at a table.

B. 1: I'm going to make a library. Here's the door right here—
back here. I'm going to make steps and a gate on the other
side. I use orange. Here's a big door, I'm going to make

right here. (He puts his picture on a chair which is beside him and takes another paper.)

CL. 1: You made a picture of a library and now, you're taking another paper.

B. 2: I'm going to make a fish this time. Here comes a fish—a mouth; there's the big mouth, and eyes and (said with glee and increased loudness), and here's the fish! (Turning over his paper, saying) I'm going to make another fish. I'm going to make the eye first, and then the mouth—a big mouth. See (holding up his picture, putting it on the chair; taking another paper). I'm going to make another fish. There's the big mouth and there's the eye. (There's lots of paper, as much as Bobby wants.)

CL. 3: Bobby can use all the paper that he wants.

B. 4: I'm going to make another fish and this time, I'm going to make two eyes. A *big* fish. See! (holding it up) Boy! It's done.

CL. 4: You made a big fish with two eyes this time.

B. 5: (Putting this paper on the chair; the paper falls down.) Oh, it fell down. Now, you stay there, fish. Do you hear me, fish? Stay there.

CL. 5: You show that you want the paper to stay where you put it by acting cross.

B. 6: That's all! I'm going to paint (going to the easel, taking a brush and using black paint). I'm going to make a sky. It's rainy, a rainy day (making little, black circles for the rain drops. He stands up to paint and then sits down for a while, painting his little circles). It's all done. I'll put it right here to dry. It has to dry off. (Taking another paper, making round scribbles with his yellow paint and putting that paper to dry.) That has to dry too. I'm going to make a house now, with lots and lots of windows, lots and lots and lots of windows. And steps. Here it is, that's all. (Leaving the table and going to the shelf where the hand puppets were.)

CL. 6: You're finished painting, and you're going to look at the puppets.

B. 7: (Taking each puppet and putting each puppet flat on his back) They're all sleeping.

CL. 7: The puppets are having a sleep.

B. 8: (Taking some stand-up farm animals, Bobby takes each animal to the zoo. As the little truck travels along, Bobby makes a continuous "m-m-m-m-m-m" truck sound. He takes each animal to the zoo in this order: pig, goat, cat, dog, duck, rabbit, sheep, goose, donkey, horse, calf, hen, rooster, and the cow. The m-m-m of the truck's engine drones on as each animal makes his journey. Bobby goes to the pencil sharpener which is filled to overflowing with pencil sharpenings. He turns the handle of the pencil sharpener, and as he does so, some of the sharpenings escape. He catches these sharpenings in the back of a toy dump truck. He works to have the sharpenings fall into the dump truck). This is the food for the animals. (The truck returns to the animals.) M-m-m. (He backs the truck near to each animal.) Eat up, pig. (He gives each of the fourteen animals the opportunity to eat from the truck, giving each the verbal command or direction) Eat up—. (After the animals are fed, Bobby takes up some plasticine.) I'm going to make a fish—a big fish, with a big, big mouth. I'm going to cut out my fish. (He cuts his fish into four pieces.) I'm going to make another fish and cut him up.

CL. 8: There are just a few more minutes left, Bobby, five more minutes for you to use.

B. 9: I'm going to hang up my fish pictures on the wall. (Using the Scotch tape, he hangs up his fish pictures on the wall.) See! (With much joy and a reduction of tension in his voice) See! See my pictures hanging up. See them!

CL. 9: You hung up your pictures so that everyone can see what you did. Your own pictures are on the wall. Everyone can see your pictures. Well, our time is up now, Bobby. You may come back next week if you want, and I'll be here.

B. 10: Oh boy! Do I? I like this school better than my other school.

CL. 10: You really liked being here.

B. 11: (Seeing his mother) Come, see my pictures; they are hanging up on the wall. I made them and I hung them up— all by myself.

Commentary. Bobby's first picture was of a library (B1); his nursery school is located in a library. In (B2) spontaneity is evident. He proceeds to draw many fish, all with large mouths. He addresses them aggressively (B4). Upon moving to the puppets (B7), he puts each one to sleep, avoiding any involvement with these human-like objects. Then he indulges in dramatic play with animals at the zoo (B8). His pencil-sharpener activity is a symbolic acting-out of an oral incorporative type, reminding one of his food problems, as he feeds the animals over and over. Toward the end of this session he returns to the fish theme, cutting a clay model into pieces. He finishes by displaying and admiring his creations. He invites his mother to see what he did "all by myself." Bobby reveals much spontaneity and general freedom of expression. This augurs well as far as therapy prognosis is concerned.

Benny, an Eight-Year-Old. Benny's birth and early developmental history were normal. Weaning and toilet training were not forced. His mother said, "Much to my mother's consternation, Benny weaned himself at the advanced age of two and trained himself at four for bladder and bowels." Stuttering was noticed by the parents when Benny was about three and a half years of age. Little notice was taken of this as his parents believed that he would outgrow this behavior. Upon his entrance to the first grade, Benny continued to stutter. The local school system had no speech therapy services available, and he received no professional aid until the family moved to the present community. His stuttering behavior reveals multiple repetitions of the initial sounds of words. His stuttering varies in severity from complete absence to severe nonfluency, as is so common. Intensity of stuttering does not appear to be related to specific objects or situations.

Benny deals with reality by denial or negation. His school life is troublesome; yet, Benny never appears to take note of it. He has repeated grade one, and at present he is repeating the second grade. His mother tutors him in reading and numbers, buying the basic readers for home use, and incurring the school's disapproval for so doing. The school's position is that Benny's familiarity with the contents of the books diminishes his interest at school. Benny's mother's position is that he fails in school; therefore, he needs supplemental help and that this help should be on the work he is doing at school. Thus, a stalemate exists between home and school. In the first grade an I.Q. of 83 was obtained on the Stanford-Binet Scale, Form L. Two years later, with Form M of the Stanford-Binet, an I.Q. of 96 was obtained.

Benny has strabismus. His condition earns him much teasing from his peers. He is called "cock-eyed," "squinty-squint," "Benny Bean Eyes," and "Porky Pig" (the stuttering cartoon character).

Benny is an only child. His mother is a woman of above average intellect. The father is a machinist who works hard to provide for his family. He tends to be submissive in his relationship with his wife, leaving the care and discipline of Benny to her. The family tends to be socially reclusive, with parental interests which center on home and ground improvements.

Both Benny's parents were seen jointly for counseling for three interviews. Because Benny's father works nights, his mother was unable to involve herself in continuous counseling. Reading materials such as Johnson's *An Open Letter to the Mother of a Stuttering Child,* Pennington's *To Parents of a Child Beginning to Stutter,* as well as our own booklet, *Does Your Child Stutter?* were made available to Benny's parents. Both mother and father seemed to derive some benefits from this bibliotherapy.

Benny's Fourth Therapy Session. This entire therapy session was spent using malleable, plastic materials.

Cl. 1: Hello, Benny—good to see you.
B. 1: Hi! Today - - - (letting voice trail off). Let's see, what will I do. Now, will I draw? No, I don't want to draw. Paint? No, I don't feel like painting. Oh, boy! Play-doh and plasticine! When I was sick with the mumps I had some play-doh, but it got hard and my mother threw it away. I had so much fun with it. I just love play-doh. I'm going to make things. I love play-doh, it's smooth when you touch it and cool, too. I like the colors, bright pink, bright blue,

a whitish color, and yellow-orange. You can make rainbow things, use a little bit of pink, some blue, the white kind, and the yellow-orange. I'm going to make rainbow things (working the clay-doh into a blob of intermingled clay colors). I like to make it real soft and gooey. It gets soft and gooey when you roll it back and forth. The heat from my hands does it. It gets nice and soft and gooey. (Taking a ball of pink play-doh, saying with a grin) This makes me think of strawberry—no, not strawberry but raspberry ice cream. (Laughing and extending his hand which holds the pink clay ball in the direction of the clinician) Do you want some nice raspberry ice cream?

CL. 2: You like to kid me that it's ice cream.

B. 2: I think I'll make some dinosaurs. I'm very interested in dinosaurs, and I know a lot about them. Every Saturday my mother and I go to the library. I get books on dinosaurs. Dinosaurs are reptiles. They're cold-blooded animals. Once the whole world had dinosaurs on it. They're extinct now. Dinosaurs were big—bigger than anything (molding a large dinosaur with care and interest as he continues his discourse). The word dinosaurs means "terrible lizards." Some dinosaurs were flesh-eaters. They had teeth and big mouths, little fore arms and big hind legs and a long, long tail. They have small eyes like these (digging out the eyes on his model). Brontosaurus dinosaurs liked to wade in lakes and swamps. I'm going to make some dinosaur eggs now. They're pointed at both ends. They're 8 or 9 inches long. Soon we'll have some more dinosaurs (laughing softly at his joke). Brontosaurus dinosaurs were the largest animals ever! Some big dinosaurs had armor for their own protection. They were big—maybe 15 feet long. Imagine that! But, the dinosaurs weren't smart. Dinosaurs have very small brains. They were stupid—big, stupid lugs. Peter—is a dinosaur. I say to him, "Hey, you big dinosaur, come over here." He laughs when I say that; he thinks it's funny. I hate him—well I don't hate him all the time, but I do hate him when he calls me names. He calls me "Porky Pig" because I stutter and "Benny Bean Eyes" because my eyes need an operation. I do hate him. No, I like him when he's nice and I hate him when he's a wise guy with me. I call him dinosaur. I really mean stupid, but he doesn't know that. He doesn't know much about dinosaurs. So I put it over on him (laughing spiritedly).

CL. 3: It makes you feel good when you get the better of Peter without his knowing it. Get back at him that way.

B. 3: I'm interested in dinosaurs, but Peter isn't. He's a big stupe, and I don't care if he does call me names. Well, I care, but I won't let it bother me. I won't always stutter, and after my operation on my eyes, they'll be O.K.—just as good as anybody.

CL. 4: You're not going to let Peter upset you. You feel that your stuttering will not always be with you, and that your operation will take care of your eye condition. Things will really be a lot better then.

B. 4: (Making more dinosaur eggs.) When I grow up, I'm going to find fossils and go on expeditions. Dinosaurs are extinct now. They couldn't get enough food when the climate changed, so they died. I just love books about dinosaurs. They were the biggest of animals—the biggest ever.

CL. 5: I'm learning a lot about dinosaurs today. You really know a lot about dinosaurs—know a lot about them.

B. 5: Oh, I get books out of the library. Even in the books I can't read, I look at the pictures.

CL. 6: You're really interested in dinosaurs.

B. 6: See (pointing to the dinosaurs and the dinosaur eggs, which he has made). This one is a Brontosaurus, and here are the pointed eggs. Here is a Lambeosaurus. See, he has two blades on the top of his head. Here is the dinosaur that has bony plates—like armor—right down the middle—from his head to his tail. I made a lot of dinosaurs; didn't I? They're fun to make and talk about. (See Fig. 3, Appendix.)

Commentary. Benny's appreciation of therapy's range of activity choice is evident. His past, pleasurable associations with the chosen materials motivate his selection. The smooth, adhesive pliability of the materials satisfies him tactually and affectively. Gratification is evident as he responds to the colors, intermingling them and enumerating the shadings. He associates the effect with ice cream, which he offers to the clinician. Soon he centers his activity on objects aeons removed from his contemporary world, dinosaurs. Self-enhancement accrues as he verbalizes his knowledge of them, almost in lecture form. His facility with the subject makes us wonder about the reported low-average intelligence. He talks of the "small brains" of the dinosaurs, then releases hostility upon his heckling classmate, Peter. The aggression is regarded as a joke. Such humor appears to be a safety valve with Benny. He regards his evaluation of Peter as unacceptable, changing insightfully to a positively toned self-evaluation. He communicates verbally an objectivity concerning his stuttering and visual deficit. We see here in action the inklings of self-acceptance and acceptance of others, too. We see the feelings of capacity, worth, the need for recognition, the comfort-giving character of unthrottled manual and verbal release, and the externalization of socially unacceptable impulses. In short, we see the appraisal, reappraisal, and differentiation of the self.

Dick, a Nine-Year-Old. Dick's birth was normal. His early motor development was accelerated, but his verbal development was delayed. His first word appeared at 16 months and three-word sentences came at 36 months. The mother reported that Dick was shy, even as an infant. "He broke my heart every time that he screamed whenever any strange person visited, especially when my mother and sisters came." Although his mother tried numerous deterrents, Dick sucked his thumb until age seven. He has a mild overbite. The father, a druggist who owns his own pharmacy, engages almost everyone who comes into his store in conversation concerning Dick's stuttering. The mother does likewise in her own everyday situations. These rather constant preoccupations and ruminations probably serve not only as ventilators for parental discomfort but also as apprehensive permeations in the day-by-day family relationships. Both parents emphasize high achievement, concentrating on Dick's future rather than his present situation. Though receiving an I.Q. rating of 116 on the Binet (L), Dick's academic progress has been average. The parents cite the desirability and necessity for better report card grades ("A's" and a few "B's"). Dick's only sibling, six-year-old David, idealizes Dick, wanting to be near him at all times, and tries to duplicate his general manner. Dick considers this a nuisance most of the time.

The stuttering behavior was noticed by parents and teacher upon Dick's entrance into grade one. After several weeks of repetitive speech, complete fluency returned. At the beginning of the current school year, however (grade four), the stuttering returned and persisted. Dick's stuttering is characterized by mild tonic, glottal blocking and gasping before word release. After an initial diagnostic interview with both parents, Dick was assigned to speech therapy and the mother arranged to attend weekly group parent-counseling sessions.

Dick's Seventh Therapy Session.

CL. 1: Hello, Dick. How are you today?

D. 1: O.K. But I have a little cold. I feel O.K., though.

CL. 2: Not too uncomfortable, is that it?

D. 2: It's just a little cold. I'm going to put on a U.S.A. army play. I like the army. My uncle was in the army.

CL. 3: That's what you like to do. (Dick goes to the bag which contains small plastic soldiers, a cannon, jeeps, army trucks, tanks, and airplanes of assorted sizes. With quick movements, he separates the soldiers into "good and bad," i.e., the Americans and the enemy. He counts each soldier as he divides them. He moves the army trucks and jeeps under the cover of a chair to one side. He makes the sound, "br, br, br, br, br, br," as he moves each vehicle to the side. He puts the soldiers into position and sounds the bugle call.)

D. 3: Mmmm . . . Mmmm . . . Mmmm . . . (holding on to an army officer whom he places at the head of the Americans). Attention! Men, we have 12 men who volunteered to go into action, 1 platoon leader, 3 machine gunners, 3 rifle men, 3 action men, and 2 rifle men. Action! Good luck, men! (moving the 12 troops out carefully) Look out men, K-K-K-K-K, take cover, men! He got me (knocking a soldier over) Oh ———— (groan—more gun fire) K-K-K-K-K-

K-K-K-K-K-K. Take care, men. Now, we are only 11.
Mmm. Mmm. An air attack! Take cover, men. Ah, they
are ours, now going out to attack. Advance men! (Sticks
clay balls on underside of airplane fuselage, circles the airplane over the enemy field and bombs enemy by releasing
one bomb at a time, using a quick tap of his index to do so.)
Bombs away—K-K—missed K-K-K—missed K-K-K. K-K-K-K
—missed—K-K-K-K—got one—K-K-K—got two—K-K—. That
will knock them out. Three more men K-K-K-K-K. Airplane
is returning to home base, v, v, v, v, v, v, v————. Replace-
ments will come, (holding airplane aloft, circles the field
back to home base) v, v, v, v, v, v————, v, v. Men, be
careful. We are getting close to the enemy lines now. Take
care men. (Using a babbling sound to denote a foreign
tongue) juki, juki, wiki, juki, wiki, juki, juki, wiki, wiki, juki,
wiki, juki, juki, (moving cannon into position) Aim cannon.
Ready, aim, fire! It got them right in their bellies. K-K-K-
oo-oo—(groaning) K-K-K-oo-K-oo-K-K-K-K-oo-K-K aw—
ouch—K-K-K-K-oo-K-K-K-K-K-K—men, move in with the
machine guns, K-K-K-K-K-K-K-K-K-K-K-K. Drop that
gun; I surrender! Come here! (Goes to enemy and brings
him in, singing.)

"You're in the army now,
You're not behind the plough
You'll never get rich in digging a ditch
You're in the army now."

Move up, machine gunner. K-oo-K-K-K-K-K-K-K-oo-K-K-
K-K. Watch out men. They may be tricky. They want our
ammunition. Go over, men. Knock them out. K-K-K-K-K-K-
oo—ouch—oo (groan)—oo-K-K-K-oo-K-oo-K-K-K-oo-oo-oo-K.
Advance men. Split up! Attack! Good fight, men. Good
fight! Hey men, take cover. Enemy bombers! v v v v v
K-K-K-K-K-K v v v v v v v v v r r r r r (sirens) K-K-K-K-K-
K-K. They're gone. Advance, men! Charge. K-K-K-K-K-
K-K-K. Good fight. Take care of the wounded. Doctors!
Ambulances! But take care; they're tricky and sneaky
(groaning) oo-aw, oo, oo, oo, oo. Be careful; this man is
wounded bad. His guts are spilling out. Go, two by two,
men; spread out. Get them all. Take them to the ambu-

lances—the doctors will take care of them. These men are gone. (Bugler plays taps. Humming.)
> M-m-m
> M-m-m (hums entire "Taps" melody)

CL. 4: Boy, you really did it in that play.

D. 4: I like to put on plays.

CL. 5: You really enjoy yourself when you're making believe like that.

D. 5: The captain was brave and his side—our side won. He knew just what to do.

CL. 6: You enjoyed playing the part of the captain because he was brave and he was smart. It feels good to be brave and smart.

D. 6: Yeh. These are all over the floor.

CL. 7: All over the place.

D. 7: I like to put on plays. Do I have time to put on another one?

CL. 8: Just about, Dick, if you'd like. (Dick walks to the plastic bag where the hand puppets are. He selects fox, dog, and bear puppets. He goes to the toys, stops at the toy bag, selecting a toy drum and a plastic boat.)

D. 8: (Dick takes the parts of the fox puppet, the bear puppet, and the dog puppet, changing his voice with each part. The bear puppet on his right hand beats the drum).
> Fox: Hey, that's my drum.
> Bear: It's not. It's mine. You're a dirty liar.
> Fox: It is not your drum. I'll punch you right in the mouth. Give me my drum, do you hear me? (taking the drum away from the bear).
> Bear: Take your old drum. I have a boat.
> Fox: Hey, that's my boat.
> Bear: You're crazy. (Puts the bear puppet down, slips the dog puppet over his right hand. The dog puppet goes near the fox puppet, growls, and bites the fox.)
> Fox: Ouch! What's the matter with you, you dog, you?
> Dog: Leave my friend the bear alone or I'll bite you into little pieces. Do you hear me?
> (The fox goes away, and he is placed on his back in a sleeping position. Snoring ensues.)
> Dog: Hey, let's put him in the boat, and we'll push him down the river. Then he won't bother us. He'll sail

down the river. Help me and we'll lift him up and put him into the boat. Careful, ready. Now, we'll push him down the river. Ready, push (both puppets push the boat which contains the fox). The circus is in town. Do you want to go?

Bear: I like the circus. What time?

Dog: We'll go tomorrow night. O.K.?

Bear: Tomorrow night. I'll meet you. O.K. I'll meet you at the ticket office.

D. 9: Scene II. The Next Night.

Dog: Hi, here I am—over here.

Bear: Hi, did you get the tickets?

Dog: Yes, I got them. Come on.

Bear: Oh, look at all the animals in the cages. Oh-oh, look at that cage. It's the fox. He's in the cage; let's go. He's where he belongs now—right behind bars in his cage. He won't bother us now. Let's go right inside. We don't want to be late. Oh, look, here comes the fox! He escaped! He's after us! He got out of his cage. He's coming after us. Run, run, as fast as you ever can.

Dog: Run, run, as fast as you can.

Bear: H-h-h-h-h-h-h-h, we got home safe, but we didn't see the circus.

D. 10: The end! Applause!

Cl. 9: (Applauding as directed.)

D. 11: The fox was a creep.

Cl. 10: The fox upset things for the bear and the dog.

D. 12: The bear was a creep, too.

Cl. 11: You don't care for the bear either.

D. 13: No, he's too dopey. He's just a D-O-P-E.

Cl. 12: You don't like him because he is not too bright.

D. 14: I like the dog. He knew how to take care of things.

Cl. 13: The dog is your favorite because he knows just what to do.

D. 15: He knows how to take care of himself.

Cl. 14: You like it when people know how to take care of themselves.

D. 16: I sure do!

Cl. 15: That's important to you.

D. 17: Yeah.

CL. 16: Well, now, our time is up again. That was some time today. Really good. See you Thursday, same time Dick.
D. 18: Right. That's right. So long.

Commentary. Here we see Dick, a shy, withdrawn boy, acting as the aggressive, authoritative, efficient captain who plans, leads, executes plans, and encourages those whom he commands. Oral play and release of hostility permeate the action; he babbles, blurts, hums, sings, shouts, commands, and groans. After the battle, he "atones" for the hostility by making sure that ambulances and doctors will care for those he has hurt and that a respectful "Taps" is sounded. In the puppetry action, the aggression is symbolized more in words. There are many oral releases—snoring, panting, and reference to biting. He castigates the bear puppet for his inadequacies, a possible projection of self-perception in this regard.

ART THERAPY WITH CHILDREN WHO STUTTER

Drawing, art, and painting have been used both diagnostically and therapeutically. Art is a means of expression. For the child who stutters, verbal expression is sometimes blocked. Art can be the child stutterer's entrance to unimpaired, open communication with himself, his clinician, and other members if he is in group therapy. Allen accredits therapeutic consequence to the freedom of expression which is given to the child, affirming:

My conviction is that the therapeutic value of talking lies less in the particular content and more in the freedom to talk. Talking is a sharing medium, a means of communication between related individuals. A child who has gained freedom to talk, whatever the content, has gained a freedom to share himself (Allen, 1942, p. 67).

Projective speech therapy's art activities provide the child stutterer with this freedom to give of himself in both speech and performance. The child is free to communicate through its expressive media of paints, paper, pencil, crayon, pen and ink, as well as through any verbalizations which he may make. In play, the child creates and organizes his experiences in a way which reveals his perception of his world and self—as a part of his world or separated from it. Play is the most telling mode of childhood communication. The child uses a great variety of materials, structured or more indistinct, in a most uniquely personalized way. He projects and expresses his abilities, his ideas, his problems, his feelings—in sum, his total personality. The following are some of projective speech therapy's materials which can be helpful in stimulating self-expression, self-discovery, and self-adequacy in young stuttering people:

ART EXPERIENCES MATERIALS

brushes, various sizes
chalk, white and colored
chalk board
crayons, jumbo size and standard size
cupcake papers
easels for painting
erasers, pencil and chalk
hat boxes, round
ice-cream cartons, round
jelly jars for poster paint
loam in a coffee can
nail polish, bright reds
newsprint, for drawing and easel painting
paint, finger
paint, poster
paint, water colors
paper, colored poster
paper, finger paint

paper, tracing
paper, writing
paper bags
paper fasteners
paste
pencils, colored and lead
pens, ball
pens, Flo-master, in various colors
pipe cleaners
plasticine
play-doh: red, blue, yellow, white
sand in a plastic square dish pan
scissors
shoe boxes
stapler and a box of staples
string, colored
wax paper
yarn, colored

Drawing and Painting. Be it pencil scribbling or an elaborate graphic representation in crayon or poster paint, the child stutterer can express as a Gestalt his ideas and his feelings about himself and others in his world. He can hold his paper at any angle or he can sit in any position he wishes to assume. He is able to make his picture large or small. He may place it in the center or in the corner of his paper. His picture may be reality-bound or phantasy-laden. The child is free to create what he wants, when he wants, and if he wants.

Paul, an eight-year-old stutterer, upon entering the therapy room, sat down and drew his family (see Fig. 4, Appendix).

Significantly he drew each family member as an adequate person, but after he finished with his own picture, he blocked it out with dark, black crayon lines. When he did this, the clinician, rather than jumping in with an interpretation, waited, feeling secure that when Paul was ready to do so, he would bring his feeling out verbally. Two sessions later, Paul made a large, irregularly pointed star which he colored with yellow crayon and cut out with scissors. He went to the shelf where the Scotch tape is kept. He measured off two pieces. Then he walked to the closet door of the therapy room. Paul taped his cutout star to the door, saying, "In here, I'm the star. At home, I never do anything right. At school, I'm just a dumb bunny who gets D's on my report. I never can do anything that is right. Here, I feel I'm O.K. I matter." This release was followed by several therapy sessions of exploration of this theme.

Frankie, a six-year-old, drew a picture of his family while he knelt on the floor. When he finished his picture (see Fig. 5, Appendix), he stretched out on the floor on his back, surveying his picture as he held it up, saying, "I made a picture of my brother and my sister Joan. Bob is four. He's the roughest. He starts fighting with me a lot. My mother hits me sometimes. She's 31. My father hits me sometimes, too. Bob starts the fight, and I finish it. Will you write the names under the pictures?" (Getting up and coming to the clinician, saying) "This is Bob and Mummy and Joan and Daddy and me." Frankie's pictures of his family are interesting for their emphasis upon orality. Each figure has sharp teeth and a magnified mouth, suggesting oral aggression and sadism. This emphasis upon the oral area is not at all unusual in the drawings of children who stutter. A random selection from the case folders of children and young adolescents who stutter demonstrates that for many children and adolescents, the world is orally centered and orally confined. For them, the oral zone assumes prominence and importance. Alschuler and Halliwick (1943) enlighten us on such occurrences, stating that young children exaggerate, usually by size or number, those parts—eyes, mouth, thumb, hat, etc.—

which from their own experiences have become particularly meaningful to them. Certainly, the pictures in the Appendix, Fig. 6, bear out this thesis.

When speech is blocked by stuttering and when direct, parental-imposed correction of nonfluent speech is given to the child, frustration can develop. In concurrence with the earlier writings of Dollard and his coworkers (1939), the concomitant of frustration very often is aggression. Stuttering can be the breeding ground for frustration and aggression, in addition to being their consequence. Art media can be used as ventilators for aggression when the person who stutters depicts pictorially aggressive and punitive themes. In the Appendix, Fig. 7, we see aggression and hostility given expression through bombing and fire scenes. These were drawn many times by heavy line pressures and colored in the red of aggression and hostility.

Tommy, an eight-year-old stutterer, was the victim of rejection by both the maternal and paternal grandparents who favor Tommy's older brother, an adventitiously deafened 12-year-old. Tommy utilizes the mechanism of regression—babbling in an immature manner which his mother characterizes as Tommy's "goofy" behavior. Tommy's mother is inconsistent in her handling of him, sometimes trying to fill his void by being warm and affectionate in her relationships with him, but just as often being quick to punish him. On occasion, she has punished him for misdemeanors in which he had no part. Tommy counters the rejection by his peers in his classroom with aggressive behavior. He physically attacks his age-mates. Tommy is a problem to his teacher, who describes him as possessing a very short span of attention and inclining toward noise making. Fig. 8 (Appendix) is a picture which Tommy painted during his second therapy session. The hate and aggression which pours out of Tommy spills out of his picture with its gunfire, bombings, and explosions. Fig. 8 also includes a picture which he painted during his next to the last therapy session. The security and the adequacy of personality and speech which Tommy found for himself in his 18 months of therapy, are reflected in the serenity which he expressed in this picture in which blue birds fly, an airplane cruises, and the sun shines.

Beverly, an eight-year-old girl, presents the problem of "secondary" stuttering characterized by blocking which she releases by a clearing of her throat. Beverly, at the age of three, was corrected frequently by the parents for her inaccurate articulation. The parents noticed that after they had begun their corrections, stuttering became evident. Consciously, Beverly's parents know that correction redoubles the very stuttering which they are trying to eliminate, but their unconscious motivations do not allow them to accept without correction Beverly's variant speech. The mother reported that Beverly is always polite and obedient. She indeed appears compliant in relation to the demands pressed upon her by perfectionistic parents. She is a tense little girl whose palmar sweating attests to her anxiety. Beverly internalizes and represses her feelings, having no vent for them with the exception of her stuttering speech. When Beverly entered therapy, she lacked spontaneity and affect, playing in a controlled and spiritless fashion with the materials in the playroom. During her first therapy session, Beverly drew a picture of a person (Fig. 9a, Appendix) which consisted only of a head, quite indicative of a girl who was repressing her emotional responses and responding on an intellectual level. The mouth is a single line with one side depressed downward and the other side extended upward. The eyes stare out dolefully. The absence of the body attests to her feelings of inadequacy. Though Beverly used an economy of line, her picture achieves a quiet but penetrating pathos.

In Beverly's eighth session, she showed herself to be more volitional and unfettered. She sat at a table and scribbled with crayons and pencils, drawing a figure which sprouted the rudiments of a body, two legs, arms, hair, and ears (Fig. 9b, Appendix). She scribbled over this figure with red, brown, and green crayons. Beverly asked the clinician how to spell "Miss Ugly." The clinician spelled out these words, and Beverly lettered them on her paper.

During her fifteenth session, Beverly drew a picture (Fig. 9c, Appendix) in which she manifested the emerging, more integrated self which she was discovering in therapy. Her figure, house, and tree are planted solidly on the ground. Oral aggression shows itself in the big mouth which is filled by many teeth in the female figure. The human figure lacks definite sexual identification, having the hair of a female and the clothing of either sex. It is drawn in black crayon.

As therapy neared its termination Beverly drew another house, tree, person picture (Fig. 9d, Appendix). Adequacy is reflected in the realistic proportions of the human figure of a little brunette girl who is dressed in a matching lavendar dress, socks, and hair bow. Stuttering is no longer a problem for Beverly and her parents. The smiling lips of the figure show that Beverly's world is no longer orally dominated. Beverly's drawing of a person appears as adequate and integrated as Beverly herself.

Painting. Here is an appealing medium for the child of three or the adult of three score and beyond. There is a feeling of freedom as one moves a wet brush over a paper while he sees his thoughts and feelings come into being in form and color. Mixing colors and changing the primary red, yellow, and blue into the secondary orange, green, and purple can provide the child with a feeling of magical mastery befitting the most accomplished prestidigitator. The child can experiment subjectively, making blobs of isolated or intermingled colors as did *Charlie,* a five-year-old, whose communication was word-locked by the consonantal repetitions of "primary" stuttering. Charlie announced, "I'm going to paint," and he proceeded to make a bubble of blue paint on his paper. Next he painted a yellow spot of paint over his blue, changing the color patch to a green tone. Brown paint appealed to Charlie and he gave his paint spot a coat of brown which was followed in turn by red, purple, and black, fluently announcing, "I'm all done; where am I going to put that?"

Jimmy, a 7½-year-old boy with severe secondary stuttering, walks to the painting easel with the wolf puppet on his right hand. Jimmy continues to hold the wolf puppet in his right hand as he picks up the large paint brush, announcing, "Wolfie is going to paint a polka dot, paint picture, red, orange, yellow, green, blue, violet, black, and brown, spatter, spatter all around, spatter, spatter on the ground." Humming a nameless little tune, Jimmy continues to spatter the paint in polka-dot fashion. With a feeling of satisfaction registered by the soft, relaxed look on his face, and with the wolf puppet on his right hand, Jimmy removes the paper from the easel and places it on the floor to dry. "Now, I'm going to make some nice green grass (laughing as he says this); I'll have to mow the lawn. Now, I'm going to make a tree, a big tree. You can't erase paint. Once you paint a thing it's there, unless you paint over it like this (blotting out the tree picture). Now, I'm going to make a teensy weensy tree, see how teensy it is, a little, teensy, weensy, baby tree." Ripping off this paper and putting it on the floor to dry, Jimmy, still with the puppet on his hand, says, "I'm going to make a skinny 'Jimmy,'" calling out each letter as he makes each, thin and tall. "Now, I'm going to make a fat 'Jimmy' underneath it." Once again, calling out the letters in his name and taking this paper off the pad of paper which is stapled on the easel and putting his paper on the floor to dry, Jimmy says, "Now I am going to make my name as good as I can." Jimmy looks at his completed papers with a feeling of achievement as he says, "Look at all of the papers *I* did!" Smiling broadly, Jimmy adds, "I should say 'Wolfie did.'" Turning to the puppet on his hand and addressing it, Jimmy says, "You did good work, Wolfie."

Finger Painting. Finger painting as an educational, diagnostic, and therapeutic means has been reviewed extensively from its introductory use by Ruth Shaw to its more diversified uses by many other workers (see References at the end of the chapter).* Through finger painting, the child stutterer can gain expressive and personal freedom as he experiences

* For an account of finger painting to music, for example, see Alexander's protocol on pages 365–66.

its various incentives. Finger painting provides: visual appeal as the child responds to its colors; motor-tactual appeal as the child rubs and smears his hands around on the paper; and messing appeal as the child indulges in the gelatinous mass without reproof. Finger-painting experiences can enhance close child-clinician interaction, as the clinician, on request, supplies more paint; opens hard-to-get-off jar tops; helps with pushing up the long sleeves of shirt, sweater, or jacket; gives assistance with hand washing and the removal of stubborn paint patches from arms, necks, and faces; accepts, encourages, and praises the child's attempts and productions; verbalizes along with the child or just listens appreciatively as the youngster vocalizes or verbalizes. It is a medium which can open the door for the child to discuss his parents and their reactions to the process or its effects: for example, he may comment on his anticipation of parental, censorious reactions to a paint spot on an article of his clothing. With one omnipotent rub of his hand, the child can wipe out his creative products if he wishes, or he can give his finger-painting products an acceptance by allowing them to dry.

Raymond, a fifth-grade pupil, whose educational and speech adjustments were impaired by a militant teacher, looked over his paint-smeared hands, saying as he bowed mockingly low, "Wouldn't I like to meet Brown now? (Mrs. Brown, his teacher.) I'd go right up to her and I'd say, 'How do you do, Mrs. Brown? Shake hands.'"

Stuart, a compulsively neat, seven-year-old gives a typical reaction to the finger-painting experience, saying: "It feels funny—goo—goo—gooey. Look how nice it comes when I run my hand flat. (Laughter) Hey, this is fun. Hey, let me get some brown. Look how nice it's coming, nice and thick. Ugh, gucky. I don't like that color. Nyuh. I'm going to put some orange in it. It's nice and smooth—smooth as ice cream. Look. (Running his finger tips around on the paper.) It looks like noodles. If you don't want it one way, you can change it, just rub it all with your hands. Look, I'm using my arms. (Laughing.) Now, my elbows." (More laughter.)

Stephen, a 12-year-old stuttering boy, gives us an idea of how even older youngsters lose themselves in the freeing, expression-stimulating experience that is finger painting:

"Around, around, around, around, faster, faster, faster, I go as I go around in big circles and little circles. Look, mine is gray now. I'm going to make a rainbow, here I go (using his five fingers to span his paper). Look at mine now. Oh, this is fun. Look at this scribbly snake (using his two hands.) Now there are ten snakes. Look at my hands— paint all over. Who cares? (Laughing) I'm going to write my name (singing up the scale) S-t-e-p-h-e-n. I'm going to make somebody's head. That's Karl. He hits girls and he kicks them. My teacher shakes him. Guess what color I like? (Adding blue paint.) I love blue. Here I go, all ready. This is mud, plain mud. Now, I need red. Red blood, bloody, bloody. Look at my hands. That's how *real* men do it. (Wiggling his hands and fingers.) The red monster, the deadly sea monster. Now I'm going to make the foamy sea waves. It feels so good when my hand moves along on the paper, scallop waves" (filling his paper with free floating, uninhibited horizontal waves).

Mud Play. Mud play and mud painting are closely akin to finger painting. Playing and painting with mud can enable the child to relive in a pleasurable reconditioning situation the activities which are here devoid of the pain of social disapproval, the anal pleasures of the earliest years. A coffee can filled with sifted loam and topped with a hole-punched cover can serve as a shaker as well as a container. Heavy-duty wax paper cut into generous pieces can serve as the paper on which to "mud paint." A water sprinkler can moisten the loam so that fingers and hands can swirl around in the "old, brown, swishy goo" to use Marlene's own descriptive phrase.

Marlene is a seven-year-old whose stuttering is manifested by many word repetitions. She is an orderly, overly conscientious little girl (a seven-year-old prototype of the adult "anal character") who discovered mud painting during her third therapy session. Marlene was exploring the contents of the play-room shelves when she found the can of loam. To her inquiry concerning the can's contents the clinician replied, "It's mud pie dirt—you may use it if you want to, Marlene. We use it with this water on this paper" (pointing to the water sprinkler and to the wax paper). And use it, Marlene did—for five weeks of therapy—once she overcame, by herself, her initial resistance which showed itself in her use of only one finger, the utterance of many "ugh" sounds as well as the emitting of little startled screams as she felt and saw the grainy and brown substance on her hand.

Plasticine and Play-Doh. Plasticine and Play-doh are formative plastic materials which are attractive to children. These yielding substances provide kinesthetic satisfactions for a child as he molds, rolls, softens, and kneads. Their malleability supplies creative satisfactions as the child formulates the amorphous clay into shape and form, providing him with a feeling of authorship. (The report on Benny is a case in point.) A survey of our case records of child stutterers shows that clay became many things to many children who projected onto these unformed, unstructured materials. Long ropes of plasticine became boas, cobras, snakes, and serpents. Plasticine and clay were formed into sausages, frankfurters, bologna, pizza, pies, pancakes, ice cream, roast turkey, mashed potatoes, and candy. Figures, both human and fanciful, are used in the roles of people, snowmen, witches, wizards, ghouls, and vampires. Animals, from the common to the prehistoric, abound: cats, dogs, rabbits, seals, sharks, starfish, hawks, and vultures, beetles, grasshoppers, flies, fleas, and bumblebees. In short, clay can turn into anything in the hands of a child.

Most school systems stock plasticine. This can be considered a schoolroom staple. Play-doh is a material that would have to be procured on special order in most school systems. However, "flour and salt" dough is a molding medium that can be made in the speech therapy room. In preparing it, mix the flour and salt together by hand; add liquid slowly, a small amount at a time; then knead with fingers and shape into a ball.

Richie, a ten-year-old with severe secondary stuttering and sibling rivalry toward his nine-year-old sister, made a small female figure out of pink Play-doh. He smashed it between his two hands, saying, "Judy really gripes me." This action and this statement were followed by an out-pouring abreaction concerning his distorted perceptions of his role in his family constellation.

Helen-Marie, a five-year-old, overprotected, only child who stuttered severely, concentrated upon the action of making a long plasticine rope about 3½ feet in length. She got up from the table and started to jump rope with her clay rope. After one jump, her clay jump rope broke, and Helen-Marie broke into laughter.

Gene, a six-year-old first grader whose primary stuttering occurred with great frequency and intensity, rubbed a piece of Play-doh between his hands and laughingly chanted, "A rub-a-dub-dub, three men in a tub, the butcher, the baker, the candlestick maker, all jumped out of a hot potato," speaking this rhyme with a fluency which reflected the accepting, free-therapy conditions.

Walt, an 11-year-old sixth grader whose stuttering interfered with almost every communicative attempt, molded with extreme care a round clay "bomb" into which he inserted a pipe cleaner. He threw the bomb against the wall with force, saying, "They make me sick." This action induced a distillation of troubling feelings.

Sand Modeling. Modeling with sand has a kinship with clay modeling. Sand and sand boxes may be found in some speech clinics; they are usually not found in the public school setting, however. A square, plastic dish filled with beach sand may be stored and managed easily in the public school. Sand is a molding medium that offers the child expressional opportunities in which he can be passive or aggressive. It is a less-threatening molding medium to the neat, orderly child with obsessive-compulsive characteristics than are the media of finger paint, clay, mud, or plasticine.

Larry is an eight-year-old second grade pupil. He has superior intellectual ability, although his academic standing borders on low-average achievement. He has deep phobic reactions to speaking and stuttering. He is a shy, reticent boy who lacks affect and appears wooden in his reactions. Larry's mother has said that he makes her both angry and anxious because she sees in him a replica of herself. She wants him to be more outgoing and more extrovertive, for this is the personality which is her self-ideal. This lack of support which Larry receives from his mother shows itself in Larry's total behavior.

Larry's Fourth Therapy Session. Larry went to the plastic dish pan which contained the sand. He sat before the pan and ran his fingers through the sand, drawing little rings in it, and letting the sand run through his fingers for a few minutes.

CL. 1: You like to work your fingers in the sand.

L. 1: You can make things with sand. I make sand houses down at the beach. I like sand.

CL. 2: You like to make sand houses. If you want to, you can make things in this sand. You can wet the sand, and you can use the water in this bottle. If you need more water, we can go to the sink and get more. You can wet the sand in the pan. We can put this board on the table (a piece of heavy cardboard). You can make your house in the pan or on the cardboard—whichever way you want.

L. 2: (Pouring some water out of the bottle onto the sand.) The water is all gone.

CL. 3: Uh huh.

L. 3: (Going to the sink and filling the bottle, coming back to the table where the sand is, pouring out the water.) I need more water.

CL. 4: You used that all up.

L. 4: (Getting the water, sitting down and pouring out the water, picking up the sand in his hand.) The sand is wet. It won't run through my fingers.

CL. 5: Not any more—it's wet now.

L. 5: You can pat it together now. I'm going to make a big, round house (piling up the sand with his hands).

CL. 6: Round and big.

L. 6: Now I'm going to make it smooth. I'll have to pat it all around. I'll have to be careful so I won't knock it down.

CL. 7: You're going to smooth it carefully.

L. 7: No bumps—nice and smooth.

CL. 8: Nice and smooth!

L. 8: (Working carefully, patting the sand house on all its sides.) Now, I have to make windows. I'll draw them with my finger. Windows upstairs and downstairs! So we can see everything.

CL. 9: Windows all over!

L. 9: (Working quietly on the windows.) Windows on the top floor and windows on the first floor. Now, I have to make the front door.

CL. 10: Windows upstairs and downstairs.

L. 10: There, the house is finished. I'll have to clean the yard. I'll pat it down hard.

CL. 11: You're working on the yard now.

L. 11: I'm making a winding walk up to the door (working away).

CL. 12: Right up to your door.

L. 12: There, it's all done (surveying his work). I'll put this pencil on top for a flag.

CL. 13: All finished and there it is.

L. 13: Don't you think that it's a very good house?

CL. 14: You want to know if I like your house.

L. 14: I want to know if you like the good house I made.

CL. 15: Because you feel that you made a good house—a very good house.

L. 15: It's a very nice sand house.

CL. 16: You're proud of your very nice sand house.

L. 16: It's the best sand house I ever made.

CL. 17: A *fine* house.

L: 17: I'm going to make sand houses every time I come. I love to make sand houses (Appendix, Fig. 10).

CREATIVE PROJECTS: DIORAMAS, MASKS, AND MOBILES

In these art activities, which lend themselves very well to projective speech therapy, it is important for the clinician never to assume the teacher role, i.e., the director or the selector of the art activities. Completed activities (for example, a diorama, a mask on a stick, and a mobile, plus the necessary materials needed to make each item) can be displayed with the other play materials. In this way a child is free to indicate his interest in an activity if he *feels an interest*. The clinician can mention that the materials to make the article are located beside the item in which the child has indicated his interest. In this way, the child is free to go his way as he wishes. The making of a diorama, a mask on a stick, or a mobile may serve these valuable ends:

1. It can contribute to the child's sense of achievement.
2. It can provide the child with a feeling of success.
3. It can supply opportunities for the child to work and talk under emotionally favorable circumstances.
4. It can give the child avocational interests which he can carry on in his after-therapy hours.
5. It can give the child a freedom of choice in activities on which he can project his feelings, attitudes, and experiences.
6. It can enlarge interpersonal experiential opportunities between child and his clinician and among the clinician, the child, and the group members.

The Diorama. A child can make a diorama, peopling it with his own cutout drawings that depict any theme which has significance for him. In content, the dioramas made by child stutterers can be wishful, realistic, rich in phantasy, and representative of conflict areas which were covertly or overtly expressed. As the child draws, cuts, pastes, or staples his background and foreground figures within the walls of his diorama, he is expressing something of himself and his relationships with those who are important in his milieu. In order to make a diorama, a child needs a shoe box from which the long side of the box has been removed, crayons, construction paper on which to draw his figures, scissors to cut his drawings, stapler and staples or paste with which to fasten his cutout figures in an upright position within his box. The outside of the shoe box can be decorated with paint, construction paper, or aluminum foil.

Peggy, a seven-year-old of average intelligence and achievement, whose stuttering was severe, made her diorama of a little girl who was crying, standing all alone near a tree in the rain and puddles—a projection of her own isolation within the family constellation which consists of a parentally highly valued, intellectually and socially gifted ten-year-old sister, her father, and her mother (see Fig. 11, Appendix).

Martin, an eight-year-old third-grade pupil, whose stuttering symptom was indeed oppressive, made a diorama in which he placed some trees, two tigers, one bigger than the other, and a small curled-up white bunny which huddled in the lower right-hand corner. He was projecting feelings of helplessness experienced as he witnesses the bitter quarrels which ensue between his mother and father, who are both orally and physically aggressive in relation to each other and to Martin (see Fig. 11, Appendix).

Masks on a Stick. In order to make a mask on a stick, the child needs a paper bag, newsprint paper (for stuffing the mask), crayons or paint to decorate the mask, an empty wax paper or paper towel roll, and string to tie the paper bag mask on the roll. The children draw whatever face they wish with crayons or paints. When the face is finished, newsprint paper is crushed and stuffed into the paper bag in order to make a full mask. The stuffed paper-bag mask is placed in the cardboard roll, and the bag is held tightly and firmly with string. The edge of the bag can be fringed or scalloped. Then the child has a mask which he can hold and which he can use in made-up, creative plays.

Mike, Lloyd, and *Anne,* nine-year-olds who stuttered, put on a play with their just-finished masks on a stick (Appendix, Fig. 12). They crouched behind a table, saying:

ANNE: (Holding a blonde, blue-eyed girl mask) Let's go for a walk down the road.

LLOYD: (Holding a boy mask) O.K. Let's go.

ANNE: I see something purple over in the field. See? Is it a purple flower?

LLOYD: I see it! Let's go get it.

ANNE: It's not a flower—it moves.

LLOYD: Don't stand here talking. Let's go. Come on, slow poke.

ANNE: (With irritation in her voice) Oh, keep still! I'm no slow poke. Come on, let's go.

MIKE: (Holding a clown mask) Well, what are you looking at? Haven't you ever seen a clown before? Don't stare so hard or you'll both pop your eyes.

ANNE: It's a clown. (Whispering) He's a cross clown. I thought clowns were funny. He's not funny; he's mean.

MIKE: Mean! Who's mean? Speak up, little girl. Speak up. You kids make me sick. Don't you think clowns get sick and tired of being funny all the time? You kids are all alike!

ANNE: I didn't say anything!

LLOYD: Do you live at a circus? Where is the circus? Why aren't you at the circus now?

MIKE: You ask too many questions—didn't your mother ever tell you that's not polite?

ANNE: I'm scared. Let's go home.

LLOYD: O.K. Let's go. We have to go now, Mr. Clown. Goodbye.

ANNE: Good-bye.

MIKE: Why did you come in the first place? You and your questions. GOOD-BYE!!!

Through mask making, these children expressed themselves nonverbally and verbally, creating their masks and using their creations to communicate through speech their feelings and thoughts.

Making Mobiles. Mobiles have an attraction for children. They like the fluttering stirs of the mobiles as they oscillate in the air. Mobiles can elicit creativity, projection, catharsis, and abreaction as the child composes his mobile and converses about his creation. Children can draw human figures, animal figures, a combination of both, as well as designs for their mobiles. They can use cutout magazine pictures of parental figures, sibling figures, both big and little, infants, and pets. For children who do not choose to draw their figures, the clinician can have a stockpile of magazine cutouts. Mobiles have their figures tied by pieces of string which are cut in various lengths so that each part of the mobile does not touch the other, upsetting its balance. Strings are tied onto a coat hanger.

The following is a summary of a verbatim record of two boy stutterers, *Gil* and *Keith*, both age nine, as they worked at mobile making, a self-selected, self-initiated activity, each making his own mobile in his own way (see Fig. 13, Appendix). Gil announced that he was going to work on the floor and Keith echoed this plan. Gil commented on his lack of ability in art, saying: "I'm not too good in art, but here I just draw the way I want to, and I think about drawing. It doesn't matter how I draw, the fun is doing the drawing, not how it looks after I draw it." As the boys worked, there was considerable laughter when they drew the mother and father figures. Gil, after he looked at Keith's drawing of the father, said, "If your father ever saw that, he'd kill you. You know how fathers are." To which Keith rejoined, "I know, I know, you don't have to tell me! All fathers are good for is to get mad. Even when you're good, they still yak and yell at you." The boys worked at drawing their figures. When Gil took up the task of drawing his father, he proclaimed: "Here's daddy-long-legs. You're nothing but a daddy-long-legs. Now I'm making me. I'm almost as tall as my father—almost." Keith, looking in the direction of Gil who was working on drawing his sisters, said, "You have a lot of peewees in your family. Two peewee girls." (Keith is an only child.) Gil picked this up, saying, "Two itsy-bitsy peewees, double trouble. I should have cut them out with double paper—they're both pesty—they get me into trouble if I touch them—they take my things and mess them up. But I can't do a thing about it!" When the mobiles were tied, the boys waved them back and forth, singing in loud voices, "The Man on the Flying Trapeze." After the singing stopped, the boys began to blow with their breath onto the figures, making the cutouts move. Gil, directing a steady stream of air on the father figure, said, "Dance, poppy, dance. 1, 2, 3 dance." Keith hung his mobile onto the venetian blind which covered the upper portion of the window. As the figures moved from the air which came through the open window, Keith said authoritatively, "Stop that, daddy. Do *you* hear me?" Gil hung his mobile on the venetian blind also, and he picked up a music box. He turned the handle of the music box while he addressed his mobile figures. "Dance, I say, dance. Now, you do what I tell you!" On this autocratic note, the boys left the mobiles and went to the finger paints.

Both the placement of the family figures on the coat hangers and the ways in which the figures were drawn hold considerable interest. Keith's father is placed at the far right of the hanger. His mother is located in close proximity to the father. Keith, himself, appears at the extreme opposite side. Near Keith one finds Keith's dog. A nine-inch space separates Keith from his parents. Keith drew his parents with enormous oral zones. He gave his mother an orally aggressive, huge mouth which he circled in sharp, irregular teeth. (In reality, Keith's mother is deserving of this orally aggressive characteristic; she tends to be orally punitive in her discipline and punishment of Keith.) Though Keith's figure and that of his mother are clothed, Keith, with his black crayon, placed a navel near the midsection of each body region, denoting rebellion against society, particularly his mother. The figures of both Keith and his mother are most inadequate except in the head and oral areas, while the hands and legs are mere sticks.

Gil's placement of his family constellation is of interest in that his parental figures are placed closely together at one end of the hanger. His younger sibs, age five and six, are placed together in the other far corner. Gil is placed alone in the middle, denoting, perhaps, the isolation which a solitary junior male feels because of the cohesiveness which exists between his father and his mother as well as between his two sisters. Gil's drawing of each figure is characterized by sameness: rigidity with the arms extended away from each body, denoting an exteriorization of his aggressive needs.

What did the mobile-making experience mean to these boys? They were able to take off cultural, communicative, and emotional padlocks, ridding themselves of conflicted feelings both verbally and nonverbally. They spoke under conditions which were pleasurable, nonthreatening, and accepting. All this has come to pass within a relationship with a clinician whom the boys like, understand, and respect and who likes, understands, and respects them—conditions which are both therapeutically necessary and therapeutically productive.

ROLE-PLAYING THERAPY

Thomas Brown's words, "Not picked from the leaves of any author, but bred amongst the weeds and tares of mine own brain," are descriptive of productive role-playing procedures. Though role-playing processes are basically very similar, the following differentiations can be made: *Psychodrama* usually concerns itself with the individual involvement of a person with others (such as the hostility of a stuttering child toward a peer group which is making him a scapegoat); *sociodrama* ordinarily is concerned with conflicts of societal or special subgroups (such as attitudes of rejection of nonhandicapped toward certain handicapped groups). Essentially, however, the two processes are quite similar in rationale, method, and aims. *Creative dramatics* has been described as follows by two leading proponents of the art:

Creative dramatics is the term given to the form of the drama which exists for the child participant. It is *playing with purposeful group planning and significant evaluating,* and it affects each individual who actively participates in this experience. Staging and costume are of little concern, for it is the process rather than the product which is the region of emphasis in this activity. The process is the end in itself from the standpoint of child growth and development; however, to the children who are creating it, the play is vitally important. The teacher guides rather than directs the children through the process of creative playing. Creative dramatics . . . *is aimed toward the development of the whole child, socially, emotionally, intellectually, physically, and spiritually* (Lease and Siks, 1952, p. 2).

Finally, *puppetry* may be considered as one form of creative dramatics as far as its therapeutic utilization is concerned, although there are some distinguishing features.

In these projective media, the child is an author without an editor—an actor without a director. There is never any clinician dredging for dramatic depth, nor is there clinician drill for dramatic interpretation. In therapeutic role playing, the child, once again, can *be*, think, act, feel freely and completely. The benign and free psychological relationship between the child and his clinician allows the child myriad emotional, motor, and verbal explorations.

Role-playing procedures are dependent upon speech more than any other media in projective speech therapy. The child stutterer, with his oral equivocations, engages in creative dramatics, puppetry, and psychodrama with speech that may be unacceptable to his fluency standard as well as to the fluency standards of persons who are important to him. As the child expresses himself verbally and emotionally in his role playing, his stuttering speech is received without attempts at modification, just as his original play lines are accepted without attempts at change. The focus is on feeling rather than on fluency. The stuttering child speaks under communicative conditions which can give him a comfortable feeling and speaking milieu. Role-playing opportunities can help the child to become more empathic, too. As he clothes his own personality in the personality of another being, he develops insight and understanding, and in so doing, he enhances his own personality. He recreates and relives the past experiences of his perceptual field through projection as he casts himself in the inventive situations for which the role calls. These experiences can help the child stutterer to become more spontaneous as he responds affectively, motorically, and verbally with his *total* personality, reducing *total* behavior which is flat, controlled, and lacking in both personal and speech autonomy.

Psychodrama. Psychodrama * or its modifications can hold effective therapy worth, not only with stuttering persons of almost any age but also with the parents of young stutterers. Psychodrama was developed by J. L. Moreno as a special method which allows emotionally involved persons to act out roles, situations, and fantasies in their experience. Although of Freudian background, Moreno believed that most psychotherapeutic situations were inadequate because the person in therapy is seen alone and the interaction between the person and the therapist was through words alone. Moreno wanted more realistic conditions to exist. He wanted the persons to be able to act out their feelings *spontaneously* in a social setting (the kind of life situation out of which much of the difficulty arose). Psychodrama was his solution.

In psychodrama, the person is given no limitations. He may act out spontaneously and freely whatever he wishes—actual situations or imagined ones. Sometimes trained persons act along with the person to set the process in motion. Perhaps the person finds himself acting out his fears, dislikes, or desires; perhaps he takes the part of other persons who are meaningful in his life. Usually there is an audience (the other members in group therapy, for example). The person can act the part of another group member. Many times the members alternate roles or they may all act out a situation together. Myriad variations are possible. The clinician may analyze the action or suggest a discussion of what took place. In this way, many insights can develop as the participant works through the reasons for the interpretations which he made in his role, the avoidance of certain types of roles or actions, as well as the specific types of "scenes" which are anxiety-provoking for him. In such ways, he can reformulate his self-image. Clinician understanding, the varying responses of the group to his releases, and his

* The reader is referred to References at the end of the chapter, which contain the representative works by Moreno, the leading proponent of psychodramatic technique. Other works by other less orthodox practitioners are included.

persistent and increasing awareness and attempts to understand self contribute to his reformulation of self. All this is based on unhampered motor and verbal catharsis which is self-initiated in a thoroughly acceptant "social" atmosphere. If spontaneity is to develop within the person, it should do so in this ideal setting (of course there are those who are not able to bring themselves to participate in the process; when this does occur, this behavior has important clinical significance for the clinician).

The problem situations which follow were submitted by preadolescent and adolescent stutterers for use in role-playing situations which were designed to offer opportunities for *self- and group exploration, experimentation,* and *problem solving.* A perusal of this list will bring to mind that most of the items listed may be categorized as illustrating a self-defensive process. It is interesting to so identify these items:

1. A pupil gets "called down" by the teacher. He is cross. When he gets home, he gets angry at his little brother. Just then, his mother comes in.
2. A child is mad because his mother scolds him. She sends him to his room. The child takes his piggy bank and smashes it.
3. Billy picks on Tommy, who is fat. Billy teases and ridicules him.
4. A child is afraid of dogs (tigers, lions, snakes, etc.).
5. A play about:
   a. A child who is the smartest pupil in the room.
   b. A man who is the richest man in the world.
   c. A person who is the most famous in the world.
   d. A girl who is a beautiful movie star.
   e. A boy who is the best athlete.
6. A girl is scolded by her mother for using bright-red nail polish. After that she doesn't use any nail polish at all.
7. Two boys are being scolded by a teacher. One of the boys says, "Well, he kicked me first."
8. A boy isn't invited to join the gang's club. He says, "I wouldn't want to join anything with that bunch, anyhow."
9. A child does not like his little sister, but he plays with her and acts as though he loved her more than anyone.

10. A child has a temper tantrum, and his mother comes in.
11. A seven-year-old child is watching TV, sucking his thumb. His father sees him.
12. A child stayed out to play. He didn't make it to the bathroom.
13. A child won't go to bed without his old Teddy Bear. His mother thinks that he is too old to have it. She hides it.
14. A child stays home all the time. The gang comes and asks him why he never comes out.

The three psychodramatic protocols which are about to be reproduced demonstrate spontaneous psychodrama (No. I), the monologue (No. II), and role reversal in which the members of a parent counseling group participate (No. III). These three protocols show the use of psychodrama with a wide age range: child stutterers, an adolescent stutterer, and the parents of stuttering children.

I. *Psychodrama with a Group of Nine-Year-Old Boys.* In this spontaneous psychodrama, the boy stutterers (Alvin, age 8½; Hal, age 8½; and Addison, age 9) assumed their roles on an unassigned basis. The group-selected subject of the psychodrama to be acted out was "Being Afraid."

ALVIN: Hal, are you ever afraid?
HAL: Lots and lots of times.
ADDISON: Me, too.
ALVIN: What are you afraid of?
HAL: I'm afraid that I won't get promoted. I'm no good in reading, and I just hate school to pieces.
ADDISON: I'm not afraid of not getting promoted. I'm afraid of not getting a good report card. I got all C's last time. My mother and father were mad when I didn't get a good report card. They want me to get all A's and B's and I'm afraid that I won't. Report cards come out at the end of January.
ALVIN: I'm afraid of the dark. I'm afraid without my night light on. I don't move in my bed, I'm so scared. I'm all stiff. I just stay in bed and listen. I keep my eyes wide open so that I can see everything. My father calls me a sissy, and he gets mad with me. He thinks I'm too big for a light. My mother lets me have the light, but when my father gets mad, she picks on me too.

HAL: I hate to have people mad at me. I feel all crumpled up inside. Why are you afraid of the dark? Everything is the same as it is when the light is on. The dark don't change things. Why be afraid of the dark?

ADDISON: What you're afraid of isn't real. The dark can't hurt you. Getting a bad report card or getting kept back—they can hurt you. The dark can't hurt you, Alvin. What we're afraid of is real, but what you're afraid of isn't real.

ALVIN: The dark is, too, real.

ADDISON: Yeah, the dark is real. You can see the dark. But what you're afraid of isn't the dark; it's what you think of that scares you. The dark makes you think of scary things.

ALVIN: It's scary—creepy—so still except for little creaks. I think of scary things.

HAL: The dark can't hurt you. Creaks can't hurt you. You're not alone in the house, nothing can hurt you.

ALVIN: Well, I'm afraid, and I can't help it. But, when the light goes off and the room gets dark, it looks scary and shadowy. Even the furniture looks black. I'll keep telling myself—not to be afraid and who knows maybe I won't be scared, maybe.

ADDISON: Maybe.

HAL: I'll be the father and you go to bed in the dark—without a light. O.K.? You be the mother.

ADDISON: (In a falsetto voice) I'm the mother.

MOTHER: Alvin, it's time to go to bed. Get washed now. Right this minute.

ALVIN: All right, in a minute.

MOTHER: Not in a minute—right now.

ALVIN: O.K.

FATHER: Now, remember, son, don't use that baby night light. You're a big boy now and act like one. Good night, son.

ALVIN: (Walking away) Good night, daddy.

FATHER: Remember what I said—no light.

ALVIN: Good night, mother.

MOTHER: Good night, dear, and don't forget, make us proud of you. Remember what daddy said.

ALVIN: O.K. (Going through the motions of washing, undressing, and getting into pajamas, turning off the light, getting into bed.) Oh, it's so dark. I'm scared, what was that? Oh, that's just a leaf blowing against my window. What's that

light? Oh, that's just a car going down the road. The dark
won't hurt me. The dark won't hurt anybody. I think I'll
take my flashlight to bed with me. Then I won't have to have
a light on. I'll keep my flash light right by my side. Then
when I'm scared I can put it on—and I can put it off and
make the room dark again. That's what I'll do and I won't
be afraid—(closing eyes, making snoring sounds).

Commentary. Hal's self-indequacy feelings are expressed.
Addison's fear centers around his inability to meet parental
standards. Alvin's anxiety is not rooted in reality; his is nonspecific, unconsciously motived anxiety which he displaced
onto fear of the dark. All the boys ventilate their feelings
of lack of parental understanding and acceptance of them
as they are. Hal and Addison, whose fears are reality factors, fail to understand Alvin's nonspecific anxiety. The boys'
protestations over the lack of reality features in Alvin's
anxiety cause him to become somewhat defensive. The action centers around Alvin's anxiety as Alvin verbalizes and
reassures himself about his fear of the dark, identifying with
Hal and Addison who maintain that fear of the dark is a fear
without reality. As Alvin enacts his anxiety during the course
of this spontaneous psychodrama, perhaps he is on his way
to desensitizing his anxiety in his own way. In individual
therapy, Alvin can explore this—if he chooses to do so.

II. *Psychodrama with a 15-Year-Old Girl.* This is a monologue in which a 15-year-old girl stutterer selected this life
situation and enacted all the roles. The subject of this monologue is fear of stuttering and answering in school. This
took place in a group setting in which each of three group
members enacted a monologue.

CECELIA: I hate Mr. Charles' class. I wish his period never came.
   If he would only be more understanding; he'd know that
   everyone hates to be called on in that order. I just hate to
   sit there and wait and wait until he gets to me. If only he
   didn't call on us that way. If we could only volunteer. But,
   no. That foolish way that he does it. We all know when our

turn will be. We spend too much time worrying about our turn that we miss out. If he would only skip around instead of calling on us in the order that we sit. I'm so scared by the time that he is two or three seats away from me that I freeze. My lips stick together, and I can't get a word out. The way he calls on us is hard on everyone—even when they don't stutter. Everyone is just scared stiff. I wish we'd get a committee and present a petition to him—maybe that would show him how we all feel. If I were on that committee, I'd go right up to him before class and say, "Mr. Charles, I represent the pupils in Home Room 321. We request that you consider our signed petition. We wish that you wouldn't call on us the way you do—that you'd let us volunteer—we promise that we'll contribute just as much—even more. Everybody likes to be able to volunteer. Nobody likes the way that you call on us in the order that we sit. We get uncomfortable. Could we volunteer, Mr. Charles, instead of being called on?"

MR. CHARLES: Are you finished now, Cecilia? You go back and tell Room 321 that I am the teacher in this room and, as long as I am the teacher, I'll do things my way, the way that I think is best, without help. Tell them that when they get to be the teacher that they can do things their way. Any questions? Now, get back to your seat; you've taken enough of my time already.

CECILIA: (Giving a withering look, walking away, sitting down in a chair.) Oh, that Mr. Charles! He's terrible. You just can't change teachers. I'll have to get used to his way; he won't change. No, I won't without trying. I think I really will speak to him about it tomorrow. Not fresh—the way I did here, but just polite. I'll tell him about my stuttering and about how nervous it makes me when I have to wait and wait to be called on. I'll do it. What have I got to lose? All he can say is "No."

Commentary. Cecelia experiences affective release as she ruminates about her feelings concerning her teacher who makes continual use of a controlling, nondemocratic question-and-answer method in his teaching. In this classroom, Cecilia finds herself involved in an avoidance conflict; both goals repel her, i.e., answering a question with stuttering speech in compliance with the teacher-imposed conditions that increase her anticipatory anxiety response of stuttering, and taking action about these conditions, discussing her problem with the teacher, risking his ire and more personal derogation. She deals with this conflict by fantasy as she enacts her role as a chairman of a class committee. She perceives Mr. Charles as a nondemocratic, authority figure and she assigns him this role in the psychodrama. Cecelia ends her psychodrama in a way which shows some insight development as she decides on a course which leads her to positive action to do something about her conflict.

III. *Psychodrama with Parents: Role Reversal.* This is a protocol of the use of psychodrama with parents of children who stutter, using the reversal of role technique. This parent counseling group was comprised of three husbands and their wives, plus one mother whose husband was unable to attend. Clinical experience in the use of psychodrama with parents in a parent-counseling group has demonstrated that before psychodramatic action is introduced, the parents should know well the group members and the clinician. For, with parents of children who stutter, no warming-up period, however successful, can take the place of a period of group interaction over a period of time. With parents particularly, the role-reversal technique is therapeutically advantageous, enabling more empathic feelings to be experienced as parent becomes child. Also, with parents, the post-psychodramatic discussion is most helpful in insight development.

This psychodrama takes place in the home of Mr. and Mrs. X., before dinner. Mr. and Mrs. X. have two children: Cary, a boy stutterer of seven, played by Mr. X.; and Jacqueline, age eight, played by Mrs. Y. Mrs. X. is preparing dinner. Mr. X. has not arrived home yet. The children are watching TV. The audience is comprised of other group members: Mr. and Mrs. Z., Mr. Y., Mrs. A., and the clinician.

MRS. X.: Will you two tune down that TV? You'd think war were declared.

CARY: O.K., but it's not loud.

Mrs. X.: Never mind talking about it, just do it. Do you hear me, Cary?

Jacqueline: Mummy, mummy! Cary turned the audio all off. I can't hear a thing. He thinks he's smart. I want to hear my program, Mummy. (Crying) Mummy, make him turn it on, Mummy!

Mrs. X.: Cary, turn that TV on. Do *you hear me?* If I hear one sound out of either of you, one sound, I'll turn that TV off and it will stay off for a week and you'll march right up to your rooms. Now, be quiet and let me do my work. Your father will be here very shortly.

Cary: Hey, cut that out, Jackie. I don't want to see that dopey program. It stinks! Don't change the channel.

Jacqueline: Leave that alone! It does not stink. You stink. It's not stupid. You're stupid. Leave it alone, do you understand?

Mrs. X.: What's that trouble? What did I tell you? All right! I wasn't talking to hear myself talk. I have more to do than referee that TV set. I'm coming right in as soon as I can leave this chicken. I'll turn off that set and march both of you right upstairs.

Cary: Now, see what you did; you big creep.

Jacqueline: *I* did! You mean, *you* did.

Mrs. X.: Cary! Jacqueline! (Stomping over to the two children, snapping off the TV.) Now, both of you go right up to your rooms and shut your doors. I don't want to hear one word from either of you. Let's have a little peace and quiet around here. I have enough to do without you two adding to it. Just wait until your father gets home. I'm worn out—you two just wear me out. My nerves feel as if they will snap. You're like a cat and a dog when you get together. I don't know what makes you that way. The way you two fight, you'd think I never taught you any manners. I refuse to have that smart-aleck behavior from either of you. I just won't accept it. I don't care if you have to spend every afternoon in your rooms. If you act like a cat and a dog, I'll treat you like they treat cats and dogs. I'll just separate you. Now, get up there. My head is splitting.

This scene is played once again with a reversal of each role. This time Mrs. X. plays the role of Cary, Mrs. Y. plays the mother, and Mr. X. plays Jacqueline. Following this second session of acting out, the group has a discussion, a small portion of which follows:

MRS. A.: All that fighting—I'm worn out, just from listening.

MR. X.: You know, dear, you really were quite a fishwife in that.

MRS. X.: Well, dear, sometimes I have to be a fishwife. By the time you arrive home, Cary and Jacqueline have knocked themselves *out*, along with me. That constant bickering! By the time you, my lord and master, arrive, we're really battle-scarred. So you don't hear it all.

MR. X.: You know, when Cary and Jacqueline fight, we should be more calm. What we do is add our fuel to their fire.

MRS. Y.: Well, it's hard to do everything. I found that if I get everything ready for dinner in the morning, when I have the house to myself, I do lots better. Then, I'm not so rushed, and I don't get so excited. Just before dinner, I watch TV with David and Anne. In that way, I'm more calm. It's cut down my being unpleasant with David and I, for one, certainly know what being unpleasant does to his speech. It lets me share TV watching with the children, too. Also, if the 5 o'clock movie isn't something that I want them to see, I am right there, and I introduce something else, like playing monopoly or cards. I cut down a lot of tension that way—tension in me and tension in David. His speech certainly shows it. This has really worked *for me*.

MRS. X.: You know when I was playing Cary I really hated to have all that cross-fire of talk directed at me. Just think, if I feel that way when it's only acting, how my poor darlings, especially Cary, the poor dear, must feel when I really get going.

MRS. Z.: Well, I know that when I keep after Fred all of the time, his speech shows it. We try to cut the correction and criticism to the bone. It's hard; isn't it honey? (addressing her husband). But we've learned from experience what unpleasantness does to Fred. He just goes to pieces. And so does his speech. You have to make a decision, give up criticism, or have a son who can hardly get a word out without stuttering.

MR. Z.: Hard! It was damned hard. But it's worth it, and after a while it can become a part of you so that you save your corrections for the big things. There was a time when our house was a correctional institution. It's better now, and we're all happier for it.

Commentary. The clinician was freed from any authoritarian role as the parents and clinician interacted as actors and discussants. Spontaneity characterized the psychodrama, the role reversal, and the post-psychodramatic discussion. As the parents enacted, listened in, and discussed their feelings, they received release and insight awareness.

As the authoritarian mother, Mrs. X. released in every way. Cary and Jacqueline appear to displace their hostility toward their mother onto each other as they bicker. The parental comments regarding the oral aggression indicate that they are listening with highly sensitized ears that find the orally aggressive outflow to be something that they react to negatively. Mrs. X.'s comment shows that role reversal can awaken understanding of the personality of the person whose role one is playing. Three of the parents (Mrs. Y., Mr. Z., and Mrs. Z.) are emphatic in their viewpoints that stuttering reflects an increased anxiety level, reinforcing their position more than once.

Creative Dramatics. Creative dramatics have been used in many settings. For the child stutterer, creative dramatics can be used to advantage by the speech clinician during his speech-therapy sessions and by the classroom teacher who wants to help the pupil who stutters, especially during the language arts program. In creative dramatics, the child stutterer can lose himself—the self which lacks confidence and speech adequacy; and find himself—the more adequate self which he has the capability of becoming. In creative dramatics the child stutterer makes a *total* response of self to the self of another personality (the role that he is playing), providing he is working with an accepting, nonrestricting clinician or teacher.

In creative dramatics, the child can play-act a poem, a song, a story, his own experiences, or the experiences of someone whom he knows. When poetry, songs, and stories are used, they must have a strong emotional impact that can stir the child affectively so that his response to the role that he is playing is real, deep, and meaningful. Stories can be those which the children know and love, or they can be stories which are new and which the clinician and the child read together and later play out together. When books and stories are used as source materials for creative dramatics, we have them available so that the choice of book or story rests with the child. This is most important because, in creative dramatics, the clinician does become more directive than he is in play therapy, for example. The clinician may say, "Would you like to play a story that you know or a new story that we can read together before we play it?" In spite of this clinician lead, the climate must always be such that a child is free to say, "I don't want to do that," if that is his true feeling. In creative dramatics the clinician provides the frame, leaving the child free to build the inner structure as he wishes. Slade's book (1954) is rewarding reading for the clinician who thinks in terms of child needs and expressional needs. A listing of some books and stories which we have used therapeutically in creative dramatics with child stutterers can be found at the end of the chapter.

Creative Dramatics with an 11-Year-Old Boy. An 11-year-old boy stutterer, the only son in a family of six girls, picked up the book, "Too Many Sisters," saying, "Boy, he's just like me. He has only four of them, lucky stiff, *but me,* I got six of them." Thumbing through the book, reading as he went through its pages, making some biting comments as he went along, "The little ones are O.K.; it's the big ones—they are bossy. Boy, I'd like to put a sign up on my room, 'Keep out,' but that wouldn't stop *them.* Mike's sisters help him, but that will be the day, when my sisters help me!" His clinician asked, "How would you like to play out this story, Clark?" Clark replied with a "Boy, this is going to be good!" Clark took all the parts, using a different voice for each role that he played.

CLARK AS MIKE: (Holding his head with his hands, raising his
    eyes skyward) Oh, so many of them! They crawl all over
    the place—girls, girls, how I hate them.
    (Raising his voice) Come on, we want you to be in our play.
    You be the rich uncle!
    I will not (decisively). I don't want to be anybody's old
    rich uncle. Now, go away. Get out of here! (Walking to
    the other side of the room.) I'm getting out of here—away
    from those pests. Girls, pests, pesty girls.
    Hi, guys! What are you doing. Gee, look at that shack.
    What a swell club house that would make, and there'll be
    no girls allowed. Let's put up a sign, "No girls allowed."
    Girls are pesty, plain pesty!
    (Bending down) Let's build a snow fort. O.K. Hey, who
    are those guys? What do you think you're doing. This is
    our club house.
    It is not.
    It is too.
    It is not.
    It is too, we got here first. Hey, cut that out. O.K. you asked
    for it. (Bending over, making snow balls, and throwing
    them.)
    (Raising voice) We came to help, you look as if you need it.
    We need help.
    "oo—ouch oo—oo."
    We won. You helped us.
    We won. Let's go home.
    oo—
    What's the matter.
    I turned on my ankle.
    (Raising voice for sister part) You need first aid.
    Here.
    Oh, a stretcher. That's really good.
    Put down that sign. Girls can be O.K. sometimes—some-
    times.

At this point, the clinician may wish to suggest that the
child discuss the scene, act it out again under slightly changed
conditions, or even, under certain circumstances, act the
scene out in pantomime.

Creative Dramatics with Three First-Graders. Creative dramatics can be a therapeutic experience for one child as he role-plays every part that is called for in his play drama, or for a group of children, filling affiliative and related needs of three, four, or five children as they interact in their roles. Three first-grade child stutterers, two boys and one girl, play-acted "David and His Silver Dollar," a story which they chose for the clinician to read and for subsequent play acting. Edward, whose stuttering is compounded by a food allergy problem, plays David. Harold play-acts two parts, that of David's father and Ralph, who works for David's grandmother. Marjorie, a smiling towhead, role-plays David's mother, his grandmother, and the girl who sells the puppy.

FATHER (Harold): Happy birthday, David. Here is your present. Here is a silver dollar for you. Spend it on something you want the most of anything in the world.

DAVID (Edward): Thank you, daddy. I wonder what I'll buy.

MOTHER (Marjorie): I'm going down town. Do you want to come with me?

DAVID: Yes.

MOTHER: You can spend your silver dollar. Hurry up now. Well, here we are. Do you want to eat? Are you hungry? Do you want to eat?

DAVID: Yes. Let's go to the Chinese restaurant.

MOTHER: All right. Let's go.

DAVID: I want a glass of milk and a peanut butter sandwich and a piece of chocolate cake.

MOTHER: All right, but eat it all.

DAVID: This is good! The chocolate cake is so good. It's as good as grandmother's cake.

MOTHER: Have you finished? Let's go.

DAVID: I want to go to the toy store.

MOTHER: I'll wait for you here.

DAVID: (Walking away from his mother.) No, I don't want that (pointing in the air). No! No! I don't want that or that or that. I'll save my dollar.

MOTHER: What did you buy?

DAVID: Nothing—not today.

MOTHER: David! David, we're going to grandmother's house.

DAVID: I'm going to take my silver dollar.

MOTHER: Now, don't go away, and don't lose your silver dollar. (David and mother walk close together, side by side, around the room with mother play-acting driving the car and David's making a "br, br, br, br" sound for the car motor.)

GRANDMOTHER: Hello. Hello. Hello, Davy boy. What have you got in your hand?

DAVID: My silver dollar. Daddy gave it to me for my birthday.

RALPH: Hi, Davy, I'm going to town. Do you want to come Davy? Ask your mother.

DAVID: Can I go to town with Ralph?

MOTHER: All right, Davy, but be careful.

DAVID: I have a silver dollar and maybe I'll buy something down town (looking around) No! No! No—nothing here that I want to buy.

RALPH: We have to go home now, Davy. Did you spend your silver dollar?

DAVID: No, not yet.

RALPH: I have to stop here. You go and play.

DAVID: Oh, look at the cute, little puppies. I like the little one. I know what I want to spend my silver dollar on. Could I buy that little puppy for a silver dollar?

GIRL (Marjorie): I think so. Ask your mother.

DAVID: (Running across the room) Mother, mother, can I buy a puppy with my silver dollar?

MOTHER: All right, Davy. Grandmother will ride over with us and we can buy the puppy.

DAVID: I'm going to buy a little puppy with my silver dollar. That's what I want more than anything else.

DAVID: Here's my dollar.

GIRL: Here's your puppy.

MOTHER: What are you going to name your puppy?

DAVID: I know. I'll call him Dollar because I bought him with my silver dollar. Hello, Dollar!

Creative drama can help to give the child a self-autonomy. If the child uses a story or a book as the basis for his creative drama, he may adhere to its story line strictly or loosely. If he plays out a personal experience, he may be authentic and realistic or extravagant and illusory. In creative drama, the child has the freedom to express himself *in his own way* in many languages: the language of emotion, the language of gesture, the language of the body, the language of inflection, and the language of silence.

Puppetry. Hand puppets, stick puppets, potato puppets, paper-bag puppets, and marionettes placed on a shelf or a table in the therapy room are all that are needed to excite the imagination of the child in speech therapy. Puppets and marionettes, for a child, are "such stuff as dreams are made on."

The withdrawn child may respond to the puppet nonverbally, fingering the puppet gingerly. The acting-out child may respond both verbally and nonverbally, causing the puppet to "act out" as well as to expel words of aggression. The mere presence and availability of puppets and marionettes are usually enough to spark spontaneously a puppet play which may last for 1 or 20 minutes. Rarely does a speech-play therapy session go by without the occurrence of at least one or more puppet plays.

With puppets and marionettes, the child takes over, and he carries the therapy ball. Puppetry usually demands speech from the child, and it is speech which the child gives freely and spontaneously. In order for speech to have therapeutic significance, it must be volitional on the part of the child. With the shy, noncommunicative child who is not ready for free, elective speech, string marionettes can be used to break the verbal ice. The child can manipulate the marionette strings, causing the various body parts to move at the command of his will and touch, giving him complete mastery without a dependency upon that usual mastery modality— *speech*. Puppetry can facilitate the important therapeutic relationship (for it is this "very nice" clinician to whom these fascinating puppets belong and it is this "very nice" clinician who lets *me* play with his miniature puppet persons and puppet animals). Puppets facilitate therapy by enabling the child to abreact and pour forth his feelings either as pure or disguised projection. They give the child the safety of disguise, if he needs it, and the clinician does not pounce on each and every cue which is to be found in the child's puppet activity with an interpretation. Rather, the clinician reacts to the child as he does in speech play therapy, offering acceptance, support, respect, and understanding whenever possible.

Commercial puppets are available, or the children can make their own puppets. They can be human or animal figures. Puppets which call forth a stereotyped imagery from the viewer (for example, Donald Duck) are not productive for projective purposes. As in creative dramatics, puppet plays can come out of the child's own experiences or they can come out of a story in a book.

A Second-Grade Girl's Puppet Play. Anna, a seven-year-old second-grade girl who stuttered, entered the therapy room and announced, "The teacher read us 'Henny-Penny' today; I like it. I'm going to draw Henny-Penny and the animals. Then I'll cut them out and put them on sticks and I'll have stick puppets. We made a stick puppet last week. They're fun. That's what I'm going to do." She sat down and drew the Henny-Penny characters, drawing, coloring, cutting them out, and pasting each animal onto a tongue depressor. Addressing the clinician, Anna said, "Now, you sit over there, and I'll put on a play about Henny-Penny for you. I hope I can remember all their names. Let's see now—Henny-Penny; that's easy, and Turkey-Lurkey, Cocky-Locky, Ducky-Daddles, Goosey-Poosey, Foxy-Woxy." (Holding the Henny-Penny stick puppet in her right fist) "Ouch, my head! What was that? Something hit me on the head! I'd better tell the king. The sky is falling." (Making the stick puppet march along on the table, with a clicking sound) "Hello, Henny-Penny, where are you going? I'm going to tell the king the sky is falling. Can I come? O.K." (Picking up Cocky-Locky puppet and holding it with the Henny-Penny puppet, and making them march along on the table.) (Picking up Ducky-Daddles.) "Where are you going, Henny-Penny and Cocky-Locky? To tell the king that the sky is falling. Can I come? All right! Come on." (Picking up Goosey-

Poosey) "Where are you going Henny-Penny, Cocky-Locky, Ducky-Daddles? To tell the king that the sky is falling. Can I come? All right." (Picking up Turkey-Lurkey) "Where are you going Henny-Penny, Cocky-Locky, Ducky-Daddles, Goosey-Poosey? To tell the king that the sky is falling. Can I come? All right." (Picking up Foxy-Woxy) "Where are you going Henny-Penny, Cocky-Locky, Ducky-Daddles, Goosey-Poosey, Turkey-Lurkey? To tell the king that the sky is falling. This is not the way to the king. I know the way. Do you want me to show you the right way? Oh, yes. Come, follow me. This is the short way to the king's. I will go first and you come after me. O.K.?" (Putting Turkey-Lurkey near the fox, "Mmm," throwing Turkey-Lurkey over her left shoulder. Each animal was put close to Foxy-Woxy's mouth, a "Mmm" was emitted, and each animal was thrown over Anna's left shoulder. Holding Cocky-Locky and saying) "Don't come Henny-Penny." (Henny-Penny was rushed to the other side of the table safely) "Oh, I got away. Am I lucky! I didn't get caught. I'm staying home."

Anna smiled a smile of pleasure and satisfaction. Her feelings of success and achievement (both personal and speech) were evident when one viewed her facial and postural expressions. Her vocal inflection reflected the meanings of her original dialogue, i.e., concern over the sky's falling, curiosity when the animals inquired about Henny-Penny's destination, authority when consent was given to the animals to accompany Henny-Penny; cunning when the fox gave the wrong directions; avarice and finality when the fox attacked the animals; and pure, sweet relief when Henny-Penny reflected on her good fortune in being alive—all this without clinician direction and clinician control.

A Fourth-Grade Boy's Puppet Play. Eric, a nine-year-old fourth-grade pupil with a history of dislike for school and a resultant poor achievement record, picked up two boy hand puppets and a witch string marionette during the course of his therapy session. He sat down behind a table, causing the puppets to interact in a puppet play in which he projected his feelings and attitudes towards school in general and teachers in particular.

Holding up a boy hand puppet, as an announcer, Eric said, "This is a play called 'Trouble.' Scene I. At the Railroad Station. The characters are a good little boy and a mean teacher."

WITCH PUPPET: (Making the marionette jump up and down with impatience) Hurry up! Get my bag! Hurry up. Get it! You're too slow. Hurry up, there! Hurry, hurry, hurry!

BOY: I wonder who that old, crabby lady is. I wouldn't want her for a teacher.

ANNOUNCER: Scene II. At school, the First Day of School.

BOY: I wonder who the teacher will be. I hope she's nice.

TEACHER (witch): Good morning, boys and girls. I am your new teacher. My name is Miss Knuckles.

BOY: Oh, no! It's that old crabby lady who was at the railroad station. Oh, no! She's an old crab. I'd like to put ants in her desk. I wish it was the last day of school instead of the first day—a whole year—a whole year of her—oh——.

TEACHER: Now, I want to see how much you know. How much are 3 + 3? 4 + 4? 5 + 5? 2 + 2? 1 + 1? No! No! No! You're wrong. No, that's not right. No! What's the matter with you? If you can't do this easy arithmetic you must be stupid—plain stupid. I'll have to put you back in the baby room. This is terrible work—just terrible! You should be ashamed of yourself! I'm ashamed of you. I'm ashamed of having a class that is so stupid. Terrible!

BOY: (Whispering) Oh, shut up! This is the worst day in the world—the first day of school. I thought last year's teacher was bad—but this one—what a pain!

TEACHER: Well, you don't know arithmetic! So I'll test your spelling. Spell "cat," "crocodile," "hippopotamus." Well, I don't know why I think that you could spell that word, you can't even spell "cat." I am ashamed of you.

BOY: (Mockingly) Yeah, it's terrible!

TEACHER: Now, we'll do social studies. Who were the Pilgrims? You don't know! This is terrible. I'm going to tell the principal about how stupid you are, and he'll have a talk with you, one at a time, in his office. I never had such a class! Now, stop that noise! I don't want babies in my room.

What's that noise? Who did that? Quiet class! Quiet! Now, be quiet! (Slamming the marionette up and down for emphasis) Now, I said, *Quiet!*

BOY: Why don't *you* be *quiet;* you're the one who is making all the noise.

TEACHER: Now, do your writing. Time's up. Let me look these papers over; this one is not finished. They are terrible, just terrible. I never saw such papers.

BOY: What a teacher! She doesn't teach you anything—always crabbing. She doesn't give you a chance. She just talks and crabs—

ANNOUNCER: Now, a word from our sponsor—

Eric's title for his puppet play is indicative of what his school history has been to him and to his parents. It is interesting that Eric selected the witch marionette to play the teacher. Eric has frustrated every teacher whom he has had because his intellect is high average; yet, he plods along at a most mediocre achievement pace. His teachers have been aversive in their handling of Eric's lack of achievement with their use of negative reinforcement followed by more negative reinforcement. Eric's selection of the surname "Knuckles" (something which knocks) is revealing. His entire puppet play shows his perception of teachers as nonaccepting, punitive, and aversive in their pupil-teacher relationships. Eric exteriorizes his perceptions in the nonthreatening perceptual therapy field. Eric ended his catharsis by means of a commercial which removed the reality factors which he wove into his play, absolving him of any guilt reactions, by placing his play in the realm of make-believe.

MUSIC THERAPY

Because speech handicaps are complex, clinicians use many approaches in treatment. Psychiatry, semantics, educational and clinical psychology, and physical therapy—all these fields have been investigated in the search for improved ways of helping the speech-handicapped (Murphy, 1955). Recently, speech clinicians have surveyed still another field, music (Kaplan, 1955; Murphy and FitzSimons, 1958; Palmer,

1952, 1953). Although music has been used as therapy since ancient times, it is only lately that workers have tried to learn what help music can offer to those who are under emotional stress (Light, 1946). However, research on the subject is still meager.

Despite the paucity of objective study, many music therapists are enthusiastic about the power of music. It contributes to socialization, they maintain. It is an aid to relaxation; helps release anxiety; stimulates free association; and helps summon the powers of concentration (Gutheil, 1952; Schullian, 1948). Though there is little objective evidence to support these allegations, some experimentation and much practical experience have convinced many in medical and allied fields that music can be a worthy aid in altering the moods of the emotionally disturbed (Greene, 1947). Physical therapists are turning more and more to music therapy (Brown, 1956); clinicians and teachers have used it to help the hearing-handicapped (Uden, 1949), the blind (Sabin, 1954), the mentally retarded (Weir, 1953), and others (Schorsch, 1950). The success that workers have experienced in using music to treat such disabilities hardly justifies the use of music therapy for persons with speech disorders. However, because speech and music, especially vocal music, have many qualities in common—pitch, rhythm, inflection, volume—the technique has merited exploration.

Speech therapy which is combined with music therapy as a help for children who have various speech problems, including stuttering, can be one more procedure which is available in the therapeutic warehouse. In an earlier writing, the authors reported on the use of music therapy with emotionally involved speech cases (Murphy and FitzSimons, 1958). The clinicians (students under supervision in most cases) followed the principles of client-centered play therapy as defined by Axline (1947), creating a warm, permissive atmosphere, allowing the children to express all feelings, supporting and respecting the behavior of each child. Each clinician made it clear to the children that they were free to do as they wished—to choose activities, to set the tempo, while at the same time he set limits on time and other considerations. Songfests played a valuable part. For accompaniment, an autoharp (a compact, zither-like instrument that is easy to play) was used by the children. Each child contributed in his own way. Most of the children gained in a sense of achievement as they lengthened the list of songs which they could sing. The assumption was that speech tends to improve if children enjoy hearing and making sounds, especially speech sounds (Mowrer, 1952). The children were encouraged to make up their own songs, which were then shared with the group. For some of the children, larger, freer movement was called for, and plenty of opportunity was given to march, dance, and participate in the rhythm band. Activities were developed for experience in auditory discrimination and enjoyment as well as for the physical release of tensions. The practice was to have several clinicians rate the speech-voice behavior of all participating children prior to and following the speech-music therapy sessions. In the majority of cases, improvement was noted in intelligibility, inflection, fluency, and spontaneity.

Under wise guidance, music therapy can enhance a child's speech skills as well as his general perception of self. Its group processes can give the child a feeling of belonging; its songs, games, and rhythms can help him release and relax; its effect as the child learns each new song and game is an increase in self-esteem and self-confidence. The reader interested in more information about this particular therapeutic approach may wish to inspect a bibliography on the music therapy literature (Green, *et al.*, 1952); a list of songs which have been found to be particularly helpful may be found in an earlier writing by the present authors (1958).

Finger Painting to Music. Finger painting by the child stutterer in response to music can offer him tension release, opportunities for regression, mood mutation, affective enhancement, and verbal as well as nonverbal communication under the benefaction of a positive child-clinician relationship. Alexander, an 11-year-old stutterer with an overly stringent conscience, is exhausted by feelings of guilt and inferiority which arise after frequent temper tantrums, Alexander's coping device for parentally imposed frustrations. Alexander selected the RCA Victor record, E-79, 45-5033 B, *March of the Dwarfs* by Grieg, as the record to which he wanted to finger-paint. An excerpt from Alexander's therapy protocol follows:

A combination of red and blue finger paints, which were fused into a depressive purple, covered Alexander's paper. He began his finger painting in the right-hand corner of his paper, using his first two fingers decisively while he made primitive, circular movements which climbed in spirals to the rhythm of the music. While he finger-painted, he said, "A guy is trying to sneak up on someone. When he gets him, he's going to give him an awful beating." Every time the music's tempo increased, Alexander responded with circular movements which became more and more accelerated. Alexander continued his verbalization, saying, "The guy is still trying to sneak up on that guy and get him. He's looking every way, but he still can't get him." Alexander made horizontal lines that ended in circular movements when he said, "He's still trying to get that guy. He's trying a new crazy way to get the guy." As he said, "new way to get the guy," Alexander changed his method of finger painting from finger movements to pressure strokes with the side of his hand. Alexander commented, "He's sneaking around, trying to get that guy." He made more primitive, circular movements, saying, "he almost had him, but he lost him," indicating this with a quick, sliding motion of his hand.

Alexander projected aggression as he listened to the descriptive music, and as he worked at finger painting. His theme is based in aggression which is expressed by ruminations concerning a physical attack. The action in finger painting, the listening to the music, and the verbalizations which flow in response to this activity and audition provide Alexander with a substitution for overt aggression while still supplying him with a release outlet which can reduce his aggressive motivations.

MULTIPLE PROJECTIVE SPEECH THERAPY

Let's Play Hide and Seek. (FitzSimons and Murphy, 1959.) This is a series of projective speech therapy experiences which were designed for use with children who have articulation problems and for hard of hearing children who need practice in speech (lip) reading. However, clinical use in both the university and the public school speech-therapy settings has demonstrated its value for children who stutter, as well. This section is based to some extent on the manual which accompanies *Let's Play Hide and Seek.* Concepts which have evolved out of learning theory and experiments are basic in *Let's Play Hide and Seek.* The theoretical positions of Mowrer (1952), Dollard and Miller (1950), and McCarthy (1954) in relation to verbal learning, learning in general, and emotional-social needs show their influence in *Let's Play Hide and Seek.* The therapeutic learning experiences in it meet some of the requirements which Skinner (1957) sets forth as necessary to efficient learning: the absence of negative consequences for the child if and when he does not reach a desired learning goal; immediate reinforcement to the child's every response; a planned series of learning experiences which build skill; the availability of automatic and natural reinforcement. The therapeutic relationship between the child and the clinician while they work in either individual or group therapy on *Let's Play Hide and Seek* creates intrinsic motivation within each child, avoiding the tedium of extrinsic motivation.

Let's Play Hide and Seek consists of ten picture cards which are contained in a plastic composition-covered, large stand-up easel. These picture cards allow for the projection and discharge of feelings. One child may project feelings which center on sibling rivalry when he talks about the merry-go-round picture, while another child may perceive this same card as a happy family fun time. Another child may perceive the supermarket card moralistically as he over-reacts to the shopping expedition of the bear family. Another child may identify with the junior bear figures, while still another may see only fun and humor in a bear family that shops in a supermarket.

Hidden throughout each of the ten pictures are little pictures (of words which begin with the same initial sound). These little hidden pictures are woven into the large drawing so that the child who plays *Let's Play Hide and Seek* has to really seek before he finds. The clinician gives the child or children a riddle; (there are 10 to 20 riddles for each large picture). The child guesses the answer to the riddle, and he is started on his search for the little hidden picture; for example, the riddle's answer. *Guess What!* (FitzSimons and Murphy, 1959), the child's workbook which accompanies *Let's Play Hide and Seek,* contains more riddles for the child to read and guess as well as space for him to draw or to paint pictures of the riddle answers. The reading vocabulary of these riddles is controlled so that it never exceeds a first-grade reading level. (With the nonreading child of five or six years of age, the clinician can read the riddles aloud.) Perforated pages in *Guess What!* allow the child to take home the pages that he completes as he progresses in his workbook. In this way the child can share the riddles and his drawings with his family and his out-of-therapy friends, enjoying a feeling of adequacy as he displays his riddle-solving ability while testing theirs.

Hide and Seek's activities hold many projective values. The large pictures offer cathartic release to the child as he comments about them. As the child puzzles over the answers to the riddles, projection can play its part. This riddle elicited a projection:

> "Sometimes I'm happy.
> Sometimes I'm sad.
> Sometimes I'm pretty.
> Sometimes I'm mad."

The answer (and hidden picture to find) was an "f" word; for example, "a face," but an overprotected, seven-year-old boy stutterer said, "Oh, I know that, my mother! Oh, no! That's not right; 'Mother' doesn't begin with 'f.'"

Feelings of adequacy or inadequacy are projected as the child perplexes over a riddle's answer or as he hunts for a hidden picture which remains illusive for him. *Hide and Seek* gives the child opportunities for motor expression as he projects his thoughts and feelings into his free drawings in his workbook. A 9-year-old stuttering girl, who was drawing a Jack-in-the-box in answer to a riddle, drew her picture of a box without a "Jack," saying, "That's the way my Jack-in-the-box is now. My little brother broke mine; He gets into my things all of the time. I get mad. When I get mad with him, I get it."

Terminus Point. Speech play therapy, speech counseling, and projective speech therapy emphasize the attitudes, feelings, and perceptions which make up the "me" of the person who stutters—the "self-as-object"; as well as the "I" who thinks, recalls, and perceives—the "self-as-process." Such therapy lets the person who stutters come to terms with the "me" and the "I"; to be more acceptant of the "me" and the "I"; and to be a more autonomous, more productive *total* self, possessing an inner security which recalls these lines of Victor Hugo:

> Be like the bird who
> Halting in his flight
> On limb too slight
> Feels it give way beneath him,
> Yet sings
> Knowing he hath wings.

REFERENCES

ALLEN, FREDERICK H. *Psychotherapy with Children.* New York: W. W. Norton & Co., Inc., 1942.

ALSCHULER, R. H., and HALLIWICK, L. A. "Easel Painting as an Index of Personality in Pre-School Children," *Amer. J. Orthopsychiat.*, 13: 616–25, 1943.

AXLINE, VIRGINIA. *Play Therapy.* Boston: Houghton Mifflin Co., 1947.

BROWN, M. E. "Motor Games for Crippled Children and Adults," *Amer. J. Nursing*, 56: 44–48, 1956.

DOLLARD, JOHN, and MILLER, NEAL E. *Personality and Psychotherapy.* New York: McGraw-Hill Book Co., Inc., 1950.

DOLLARD, JOHN; DOOB, LEONARD W.; MILLER, NEAL E.; MOWRER, O. H.; and SEARS, ROBERT R. *Frustration and Aggression.* New Haven, Conn.: Yale Univ. Press, 1939.

FITZSIMONS, RUTH, and MURPHY, ALBERT T. *Guess What!* Magnolia, Mass.: Expression Co., Publishers, 1959.

———. *Let's Play Hide and Seek.* Magnolia, Mass.: Expression Co., Publishers, 1959.

———. *Manual: Let's Play Hide and Seek.* Magnolia, Mass.: Expression Co., Publishers, 1959.

GREENE, RAY, *et al. Bibliography on Music Therapy.* Chicago: National Association for Music Therapy, 1952.

GREENE, RAY. "Music in Veterans' Hospitals," *Music Educators J.,* 36: 22, 1947.

GUTHEIL, EMIL, *et al. Music and Your Emotions.* New York: Liveright Publishing Corp., 1952.

KAPLAN, MAX. "Music Therapy in the Speech Program," *Except. Children,* 22: 112–17, 1955.

LEASE, RUTH, and SIKS, GERALDINE B. *Creative Dramatics in Home, School, and Community.* New York: Harper & Bros., 1952.

LIGHT, SIDNEY. *Music in Medicine.* Boston: New England Conservatory of Music, 1946.

McCARTHY, DOROTHEA. "Language Disorders and Parent-Child Relationships," *J. Speech Hearing Disorders,* 19: 514–23, 1954.

MOWRER, O. H. *Learning Theory and Personality Dynamics.* New York: The Ronald Press Co., 1953, pp. 573–616, 688–726.

———. "Speech Development in the Young Child: 1. The Autism Theory of Speech Development and Some Clinical Applications," *J. Speech Hearing Disorders,* 27: 263–68, 1952.

MURPHY, ALBERT T. "Counseling Students with Speech and Hearing Problems," *Personnel and Guidance J.,* 33: 260–64, 1955.

MURPHY, ALBERT T., and FITZSIMONS, RUTH. "Music Therapy for the Speech-Handicapped," *Elem. School Journal,* 59: 39–45, 1958.

PALMER, MARTIN F. "Musical Stimuli in Cerebral Palsy, Aphasia, and Similar Conditions," *Bull. Nat. Assn. Mus. Ther.,* 2: 7–8, 1953.

———. "Viewpoints on Music Therapy," *Music J.,* 10: 21, 1952.

PODOLSKY, EDWARD. *Music Therapy.* New York: Philosophical Lib., Inc., 1954.

SABIN, ROBERT. "Lighthouse School Music for Blind Students," *Musical America,* 72: 300, 1954.

SCHORSCH, M. J. "Music Therapy for the Handicapped Child," *Education,* 70: 434, 1950.

SCHULLIAN, DOROTHY, and SCHOEN, MAX. *Music and Medicine.* New York: Abelard-Schuman, Ltd., 1948.

SKINNER, B. F. *Verbal Behavior*. New York: Appleton-Century-Crofts, Inc., 1957.

SLADE, PETER. *Child Drama*. London: Univ. of London Press, Ltd., 1954.

UDEN, A. V. "Music and Dancing for the Deaf," *Volta Rev.*, 51: 386, 1949.

WEIR, LOUISE E. "Music Therapy for Retarded and Autistic Children," *Bull. Nat. Assn. Mus. Ther.*, 2: 6, 1953.

ADDITIONAL SUGGESTED READINGS

On Projective Psychology

ABT, LAWRENCE E., and BELLAK, LEOPOLD. *Projective Psychology*. New York: Alfred A. Knopf, Inc., 1952.

ANDERSON, HAROLD. "Human Behavior and Personality Growth," in *An Introduction to Projective Techniques*, eds. H. H. Anderson and E. L. Anderson. Englewood Cliffs, N. J.: Prentice-Hall, Inc., 1951.

BELL, JOHN ELDERKEN. *Projective Techniques*. New York: Longmans, Green & Co., Inc., 1948.

BLAKE, R. R., and RAMSEY, G. V. (eds.). *Perception: An Approach to Personality*. New York: The Ronald Press Co., 1951.

FRANK, L. K. *Projective Methods*. Springfield, Ill.: Charles C Thomas, Publisher, 1948.

FREUD, S. *The Basic Writings of Sigmund Freud*, ed. A. A. Brill. New York: Random House, Inc., 1938.

MURPHY, LOIS BARCLAY. *Personality in Young Children*. New York: Basic Books, Inc., 1956.

RAPAPORT, D. *Diagnostic Psychological Testing*. 2 vols. Chicago: Year Bk. Pubs., Inc., 1946.

———. "Principles Underlying Projective Techniques," *Charact. and Person.*, 10: 213–19, 1942.

SYMONDS, PERCIVAL, and KRUGMAN, NORRIS. "Projective Methods in the Study of Personality," *Rev. Educational Research*, 14: 1, 81-98, 1944.

WHITE, ROBERT W. "Interpretation of Imaginative Productions," in J. McV. Hunt, *Personality and the Behavior Disorders*, Vol. II. New York: The Ronald Press Co., 1944.

WOLFF, WERNER. *The Personality of the Pre-school Child*. New York: Grune & Stratton, Inc., 1946.

On Art Therapy

ALSCHULER, R. H., and HALLIWICK, L. A. "Easel Painting as an Index of Personality in Pre-school Children," *Amer. J. Orthopsychiat.*, 13: 616–25, 1943.

ALSCHULER, R. H., and HATTWICK, L. B. W. *Painting and Personality.* Chicago: Univ. of Chicago Press, 1947.

CALIGOR, LEOPOLD. *A New Approach to Figure Drawing: Based upon an Interrelated Series of Drawings.* Springfield, Ill.: Charles C. Thomas, Publisher, 1957.

GUNZBURG, H. C. "Projection in Drawings: A Case Study, *Brit. J. Med. Psychol.*, **28**: 72–81, 1955.

MACHOVER, KAREN. "Human Figure Drawings of Children," *J. Proj. Tech.*, **17**: 85–91, 1953.

———. *Personality Projection in the Drawing of the Human Figure.* Springfield, Ill.: Charles C. Thomas, Publisher, 1949.

NAUMBURG, MARGARET. "A Study of Art Expression of a Behavior Problem Boy as an Aid in Diagnosis and Therapy," *Nervous Child,* **3**: 277–319, 1944.

NAPOLI, P. J. "Interpretative Aspects of Finger Painting," *J. of Psychology,* **23**: 92–132, 1947.

OBROOK, I. "The Therapeutic Value of Fingerpainting," *Crippled Child.*, **13**: 172, 1935.

SCHMIDLE-WAEHNER, TRUDE. "Interpretation of Spontaneous Drawings and Paintings," *Genet. Psychol. Monog.*, **33**: 1–70, 1946.

SHAW, RUTH F. *Finger Painting.* Boston: Little, Brown & Co., 1934.

STEVENS, K. H. "Fingerpainting for Little Deaf Children," *Volta Rev.,* **48**: 454–57, 1946.

STONE, L. J. *Finger Painting, Children's Use of Plastic Materials.* (Guide to the Film.) New York: New York Univ. Film Library, 1944.

On Role-Playing and Psychodrama

BLAKE, R. R. "Experimental Psychodrama with Children," *Group Psychother.*, **8**: 347–50, 1955.

BRUK, M. "An Example of the Use of Psychodrama in the Relieving of an Acute Symptom in a Psychiatric Children's Clinic," *Group Psychother.*, **6**: 216–21, 1954.

HAAS, ROBERT BARTLETT (ed.). *Psychodrama and Sociodrama in American Education.* New York: Beacon House, Inc., 1949.

HAHN, ELISE. "Role-playing, Creative Dramatics and Play Therapy in 'Speech Correction.'" *Speech Teacher,* **4**: 233–38, 1955.

KLINE, N. S. "Psychodrama for Mental Hospitals." VI. *J. Clin. Psychopath.*, **9**: 96-107, 1948.

LAVALLI, ALICE, and LEVINE, MARY. "Social and Guidance Needs of Mentally Handicapped Adolescents as Revealed Through Sociodramas," *Amer. J. Mental Defic.*, **58**: 544–52, 1954.

LEMERT, E. M., and VAN RIPER, C. "The Use of Psychodrama in the Treatment of Speech Defects," *Sociometry,* **7**: 190–95, 1944.

LIPPITT, R. "Role-playing," *Amer. J. Nurs.*, **53**: 693–96, 1953.

MORENO, J. L. *Introduction to Psychodrama* (film). New York: Beacon, Therapeutic Film Production, Inc., 1951.

———. *Psychodrama,* Vol. I. New York: Beacon House, Inc., 1946.

———. "Psychodrama and Group Psychotherapy," *Sociometry,* **9:** 249–53, 1946.

———. "Theory of Spontaneity and Creativity," *Sociometry,* **18:** 361–74, 1956.

PARKER, SEYMOUR. "Role Theory and the Treatment of Anti-social Acting-out Disorders," *Brit. J. Delinq.,* **7:** 285–300, 1957.

SARBIN, THEODORE R. "Spontaneity Training of the Feebleminded," *Sociometry,* **8:** 389–93, 1945.

SCOTT, L. B., and THOMPSON, J. J. *Speech Ways.* St. Louis, Mo.: Webster Publishing Co., 1955.

STOKVIS, B. "Group Psychotherapy of Enuretic Children by Psychodrama and Sociodrama." *Am. J. Psychother.,* **8:** 265–75, 1954.

TURNER, R. H. "Role-taking, Role Standpoint, and Reference-Group Behavior," *Amer. J. Sociol.,* **61:** 316–28, 1956.

WOLPE, ZELDA S. "Play Therapy, Psychodrama, and Parent Counseling," in *Handbook of Speech Pathology,* ed. L. E. Travis. New York: Appleton-Century-Crofts, Inc., 1957, pp. 991–1024.

On Creative Dramatics

GILLIES, E. P. "Therapy Dramatics for the Public Schoolroom," *Nervous Child.,* **7:** 328–36, 1948.

HAHN, ELSIE. "Role-Playing, Creative Dramatics, and Play Therapy in 'Speech Correction.'" *Speech Teacher,* **4:** 233-38, 1955.

HARTLEY, RUTH E.; FRANK, LAWRENCE K.; and GOLDENSON, ROBERT M. *Understanding Children's Play.* New York: Columbia Univ. Press, 1952.

OGILVIE, MARDEL. *Speech in the Elementary School.* New York: McGraw-Hill Book Co., Inc., 1954.

PRONOVOST, WILBERT. *The Teaching of Speaking and Listening.* New York: Longmans, Green & Co., Inc., 1959.

SIKS, GERALDINE BRAIN. *Creative Dramatics: An Art for Children.* New York: Harper & Bros., 1958.

TRAVIS, LEE EDWARD, and SUTHERLAND, LAVERNE DEEL. "Psychotherapy in Speech Correction," in *Handbook of Speech Pathology,* ed. L. E. Travis. New York: Appleton-Century-Crofts, Inc., 1957, pp. 805–31.

Source Materials for Creative Dramatics

ALDRICH, MARY M. *Too Many Pets.* New York: The Macmillan Co., 1952.

ARBUTHNOT, MARY HILL. *The Arbuthnot Anthology.* Chicago: Scott, Foresman & Co., 1953.

AYME, MARCEL. *The Wonderful Farm*. New York: Harper & Bros., 1951.

BEIM, JERROLD. *Andy and the School Bus*. New York: William Morrow & Co., Inc., 1947.

——. *Jay's Big Job*. New York: William Morrow & Co., Inc., 1957.

——. *Too Many Sisters*. New York: William Morrow & Co., Inc., 1956.

BELL, THELMA HARRINGTON. *Mountain Boy*. New York: The Viking Press, Inc., 1947.

——. *Yaller-Eye*. New York: The Viking Press, Inc., 1951.

BROWN, MARGARET WISE. *The Runaway Bunny*. New York: Harper & Bros., 1942.

COLLODI, CARLO. *The Adventures of Pinocchio*. New York: The Macmillan Co., 1951.

CONGER, MARION. *Day at the Zoo*. New York: Simon & Schuster, Inc., 1958.

CROWLEY, MAUDE. *Azor*. New York: Oxford Univ. Press, Inc., 1951.

DuBois, WILLIAM PENE. *Bear Party*. New York: The Viking Press, Inc., 1951.

ESTES, ELEANOR. *Ginger Pye*. New York: Harcourt, Brace & Co., Inc., 1951.

——. *The Hundred Dresses*. New York: Harcourt, Brace & Co., Inc., 1944.

EVERS, HELEN, and EVERS, ALF. *Copy-Kitten*. Chicago: Rand McNally & Co., 1937.

FENNER, PHYLLIS. *Yankee Doodle: Stories of the Brave and the Free*. New York: Alfred A. Knopf, Inc., 1951.

FLACK, MARJORIE. *Ask Mr. Bear*. New York: The Macmillan Co., 1932.

——. *Wait for William*. Boston: Houghton, Mifflin Co., 1935.

——. *Walter, the Lazy Mouse*. New York: Doubleday & Co., Inc., 1937.

GAG, WANDA. *Nothing at All*. New York: Coward-McCann, Inc., 1941.

HAYES, FLORENCE. *Hosh-Ki, the Navajo*. New York: Random House, Inc., 1943.

HAYWOOD, CAROLYN. *Eddie and the Fire Engine*. William Morrow & Co., Inc., 1949.

HIGGINS, LOYTA. *Let's Save Money*. New York: Simon & Schuster, Inc., 1958.

JACOBS, JOSEPH. *The Fables of Aesop*. New York: The Macmillan Co., 1950.

JONES, E. O. *Little Red Riding Hood*. New York: Simon & Schuster, Inc., 1958.

MARTIGNONI, MARGARET E. *The Illustrated Treasury of Children's Literature.* New York: Grosset & Dunlap, Inc., 1955.

MASON, MIRIAM. *The Middle Sister.* New York: The Macmillan Co., 1947.

O'HARA, MARY. *My Friend Flicka.* Philadelphia: J. B. Lippincott Co., 1941.

RAWLINGS, MARJORIE KINNAN. *The Yearling.* New York: Charles Scribner's Sons, 1939.

REYNOLDS, QUENTIN. *The Wright Brothers.* New York: Random House, Inc., 1950.

SCOTT, SALLY. *Blinky's Fire.* New York: Harcourt, Brace & Co., Inc., 1952.

SEREDY, KATE. *Gypsy.* New York: The Viking Press, Inc., 1951.

SQUIRES, ELIZABETH B. *David's Silver Dollar.* New York: The Platt & Munk Co., Inc., 1950.

TERHUNE, ALBERT PAYSON. *Lad: A Dog.* New York: E. P. Dutton & Co., Inc., 1947.

TUNIS, JOHN R. *All-American.* New York: Harcourt, Brace & Co., Inc., 1942.

VERRAL, CHARLES S. *Play Ball.* New York: Simon & Schuster, Inc., 1958.

WARD, LYND. *The Biggest Bear.* Boston: Houghton Mifflin Co., 1952.

WOOLEY, CATHERINE. *David's Railroad.* New York: William Morrow & Co., Inc., 1949.

YATES, ELIZABETH. *A Place for Peter.* New York: Coward-McCann, Inc., 1952.

On Puppetry

BATCHELDER, M. *The Puppet Theatre Handbook.* New York: Harper & Bros., 1947.

BATCHELDER, M., and COMER, V. *Puppets and Plays, A Creative Approach.* New York: Harper & Bros., 1956.

HAWKEY, L. "The Use of Puppets in Child Psychotherapy," *Brit. J. Med. Psychol.,* **24:** 206–14, 1951.

JAGENDORF, MORITZ A. *The First Book of Puppets.* New York: Franklin Watts, Inc., 1952.

JENKINS, R. L., and BECKH, ERICA. "Finger Puppets and Mask Making as Media for Work with Children," *Amer. J. Orthopsychiat.,* **XII:** 294–300, April, 1942.

LANCHESTER, WALDO. *Hand Puppets and String Puppets.* Peoria, Ill.: Charles A. Bennett Co., Inc., 1949.

OGILVIE, MARDEL. *Speech in the Classroom.* New York: McGraw-Hill Book Co., Inc., 1954, pp. 45–67.

PELS, GERTRUDE. *Easy Puppets*. New York: The Thomas Y. Crowell Co., 1951.

RICHMOND, ARTHUR. *Remo Bufano's Book of Puppetry*. New York: The Macmillan Co., 1950.

SCOTT, LOUISE B. "Puppetry," *Amer. Childh.*, **42:** 13–15, 1956.

WOLTMANN, A. G. "Puppetry as a Means of Psychotherapy," in *Encyclopedia of Child Guidance*. New York: Philosophical Lib., Inc., 1943.

———. "Puppetry in Therapy," in *An Introduction to Projective Techniques*, eds. H. H. Anderson and G. L. Anderson. Englewood Cliffs, N. J.: Prentice-Hall, Inc., 1951.

———. "The Use of Puppets in Understanding Children," *Ment. Hyg.*, **24:** 445–58, 1940.

Chapter 11

Client-Centered Counseling

Give everyone thy ear, but few thy voice.——Shakespeare

Client-centered therapy is a relatively new approach to counseling persons with emotional problems. The leading advocate of this form of counseling is Carl R. Rogers, whose book *Counseling and Psychotherapy*, published in 1942, was the pioneer work in this field. Rogers' approach to therapy was based on a theory of personality representing "a synthesis of phenomenology . . ., of holistic and organismic theory, . . . of Sullivan's interpersonal theory, and of self-theory . . ." (Hall and Lindzey, 1957, p. 478). Interestingly, Rogers included a complete counseling record of his therapeutic sessions with an adult stutterer. His case of Herbert Bryan is a classic, showing the therapeutic progressions of a stutterer from a neurotic adult to a more integrated self. Since 1942, scores of clinical and experimental publications have been produced, amplifying (Snyder, 1947, 1954; Seeman, 1949, 1957; Seeman and Raskin, 1953), supporting (Rogers and Dymond, 1954), and criticizing the client-centered approach (Smith, 1950; Thorne, 1944).

A sequel to *Counseling and Psychotherapy* is the later *Client-Centered Therapy* (1951), a title which reflects the change in nomenclature from "nondirective," a term which produced what nondirective counselors felt were many misinterpretations as to the true nature of the process. The popularity of the client-centered system has increased, it has been said (Hall and Lindzey, 1957, p. 476), because (1) it is

377

an approach which has its origins in psychology (as compared to other well-known psychotherapeutic practices whose geneses have been in the field of medicine), (2) because it is easier to learn, (3) because it requires no knowledge of personality diagnostics to use it, and (4) because the treatment period is briefer than other forms of psychotherapy. The present authors would say that no disagreement can be made with the first reason given; sharp disagreement could be made to the second; agreement must occur at point three in relation to client-centered counseling as currently practiced (wherein diagnosis in the usual sense is considered unnecessary); and, finally, agreement is possible with point four, providing the severity of the disorder is taken into account as a variable.

THE NATURE OF CLIENT-CENTERED COUNSELING

Basic Assumptions. Client-centered counselors claim that the psychological cause of behavior emanates from the individual's mode of perceiving and that the client is the *only* one who has the potentiality of knowing fully the dynamics of his perceptions and his behavior. For behavior to change, perception change must be *experienced*. Mere exposure to intellectual knowledge is no substitute. Thus, simply telling a stuttering person that he stutters with authority figures because he stuttered with his father would not, in itself, produce basic personality changes. He would need to have reached this connection on the basis of his *own* working through of conflict areas in order for full acceptance to occur. Dynamic relationships must be experienced inwardly. The person in counseling cannot be told what the conflict pattern is and be expected to mature because of the telling. Forces which will eventually alter perception, and which lead to reorganization of the self through perceptual relearning, reside primarily *within the client*. The therapeutic process, then, is basically one of seeing misperceptions; making perceptions more realistic; and seeing perceptual relationships more meaningfully. The stuttering individual, like all persons, tends to react to objects and situations as *he* perceives or experiences them. This perceptual field is his "reality," as compared to the "objective" reality. It is self-reality which motivates the person's behavior.

The core of client-centered philosophy lies in a clinically derived hypothesis which states that ". . . the individual has a sufficient capacity to deal constructively with all those aspects of his life which can potentially come into conscious awareness" (Rogers, 1951, p. 247). The counselor accepts the person as an individual who has the capacity to direct himself; as one who can work through to the solution of his own problems. This basic hypothesis must not be shifted.

"If the counselor feels . . . that the client may not have the capacity for reorganizing himself, and if he shifts to the hypothesis that the counselor must bear a considerable responsibility for this reorganization, he confuses the client and defeats himself. . . . This confused eclecticism, which has been prevalent in psychotherapy, has blocked scientific progress . . . it is only by acting *consistently* upon a well-directed hypothesis that its elements of truth and untruth can become known" (Rogers, 1951, p. 24). Stuttering individuals, from this viewpoint, are to be regarded as individuals who have a basic capacity to improve, a "growth impulse" which, in appropriate settings, will trigger and enlarge into more mature behavior, including speech behavior.

Rogers put it this way: "One of the most revolutionary concepts to grow out of our clinical experience is the growing recognition that the innermost core of man's nature, the deepest layers of his personality, the base of his 'animal nature,' is positive in character—is basically socialized, forward-moving, rational, and realistic" (Rogers, 1954, p. 56). It can be seen that, in a client-centered setting, responsibility is placed upon the stuttering person, and that therapy proceeds at a pace "chosen" by him. In addition, a completely free expression of feelings is encouraged by the clinician through his attitude of *full acceptance* of the stutterer's verbalizations (or lack of them). The clinician accepts without judgment, without qualifications, whatever comes into the stutterer's mind; it is an acceptance that is experienced deeply within the counselor and by the person who stutters.

In addition the clinician tries to *recognize* and *reflect* the attitude patterns of the person who stutters. This technique has a deceptive simplicity. The clinician attempts to identify the feelings being experienced by the client. He then reflects or mirrors the feelings the client has been expressing; but in so doing, he tries to *clarify* the feelings for him, tries to help him perceive these more meaningfully than he has been able to do alone. Here is an example of simple reflection:

CLIENT: I should be able to go to that dance—if I had the nerve. Funny thing, here I am on the football team—that takes guts you know—and I should be able to use some of it to have fun. But here I am scared stiff I'll stutter.

CL.: You feel that your football field abilities should help you socially.

CLIENT: Yeah, and not only that. . . .

This kind of feeling recognition helps the person to continue ventilating his feelings, and it does not make him at all defensive. On the contrary; theoretically, he feels understood and free to move on, therapeutically, into broader and deeper realms of attitudes. *Clarification* reflections are designed to convey in a clearer and often briefer manner the attitudes being expressed by the client, again without arousing defensiveness. This is an example:

CLIENT: I go to a party and most of the kids ignore me—it's always been like that. In school the teachers don't call on me cuz they're afraid I'll stutter and I really want to talk. Everybody else does things and has fun—they're OK—me—this stuttering—what did I do to deserve this? They don't suffer like I do.

CL.: You really feel that you haven't had any of the luck.

Here is another example of clarification:

CLIENT: I get so bottled up and it keeps building up that I finally wind up not going to the party. I act as though I don't give a damn. But down deep I know I do. I'm just kidding everybody—myself mostly.

CL.: The situation gets so uncomfortable you want to escape from it—get defensive.
CLIENT: Yeah, but I kid myself.
CL.: When you're in such situations you feel maybe it's best to give up the ghost and admit defeat.
CLIENT: Yeah, I'd like to, but I have so many things to consider —everybody's counting on me you know—makes me want to go off by myself.
CL.: You feel the others think you should be a very capable person—and this very thought makes you uncomfortable.
CLIENT: That is so right.

"It is as such recognition and clarification of feeling frees the client from all need for defense, since it never in any way attacks the ego, that expression becomes freer, that deeper attitudes are brought forth, and insights are developed. The justification for the development of these nondirective attitudes, and the skills which implement them, lies in the results which they bring" (Rogers, 1944, p. 340).

One of Rogers' major propositions is that "the total perceptual field gradually becomes differentiated as the self" (Rogers, 1951, p. 497). The *self*, according to Rogers, is one's awareness of his being and doing, the conception of the "self-as-object" (i.e., the person's feelings and attitudes about himself, his self-regard or self-perception), and it is produced primarily on the basis of evaluational reactions with others. The self-structure is, then, "the organized picture, existing in awareness either as figure (i.e., clear consciousness) or ground (i.e., hazy consciousness or unconscious), of the self and the self-in-relationship (to the environment), together with the positive or negative values which are associated with those qualities and relationships, as they are perceived as existing in the past, present, or future" (Rogers, 1951, p. 501). Values are added to the self-perception, not only as a consequence of actual experience with his surroundings but also because the person adopts (introjects) attitudes of others, making them part of his own set of values. But such introjections may run counter to his actual feelings and attitudes, thus setting up internal conflicts, and creating discomfort. Clinicians try to help the client modify or resolve such conflicts by fully *accepting* his value systems; though *not necessarily approving them.* (Similarly, parents offset the development of distorted value systems by using such procedures with their offspring.) In addition the person who stutters perceives in a way which is most congruent with his self-image. That is, he may perceive experiences so as to incorporate them into the existing self-picture; he may avoid perceiving certain experiences if they appear to have no connection to the structure of self; or he may misperceive (perceive distortedly) experiences which are inconsistent with the self-picture (see Chapter 5, especially pp. 115–16 and 135, and Chapter 6, especially pp. 143 and 181).

The reader may notice the similarity between this view of self and materials which have been available for more than two decades in the fields of Gestalt and projective psychology, both of which have attributed great importance to the process of *selective perception* or *selective attention.*

There can be little doubt that one of the chief functions of perception . . . is that of making it possible for the organism to protect itself against situations and circumstances which are harmful and painful to it and which do not contribute to its welfare and survival. Perceptual acts establish the grounds for the individual's exercising foresight with respect to potentially harmful situations and circumstances. For this reason, among others, each separate act of perception necessarily involves a judgment of some kind or other by the individual with respect to the consequences that a given course of behavior may involve for him (Abt and Bellak, 1950, pp. 52–53).

Evidence is available which supports the idea that perception functions as a kind of ego protector (McGinnies, 1949). This process of "perceptual defense" has been described in this viewpoint:

. . . perceptual processes function in such a manner that they permit the individual to maintain a state or level of anxiety for which he has, through learning, acquired an adequate amount of tolerance . . . apparently one of the functions of perception is to permit . . . defense mechanisms to operate so that the individual is able to maintain a fairly constant level of anxiety.

. . . as the stimulus field becomes progressively more and more unstructured—a process that forces the individual to rely increasingly upon internal or subjective factors in perception, there is a tendency for his anxiety level to increase markedly (Abt and Bellak, 1950, pp. 53–54).

Perceptual recognition experimentation has often supported such views, but for a full review and references to the supportive and critical literature relating to such perceptual hypotheses and processes, the reader is referred to Hilgard's treatment (Hilgard, 1956). What projective psychologists may refer to as an increasing perceptual sensitivity or discrimination, and the present authors call an "increase in the realm of self-consciousness," Rogers would describe as an increasing awareness of experience, "the experiencing of self." In such a process the client comes to feel free, in the security of the therapy relationship, to examine different kinds of experience, often alien to his self-concept, which he ordinarily would be unable to experience. It is, as Rogers said, as though the client were saying, "I am thus and so, but I experience this feeling which is very inconsistent with what I am" (Rogers, 1954, p. 46). According to self-theory, a client would come to count increasingly upon the experience of his own impressions in structuring a solid foundation of behavior, and decreasingly upon the attitudes and value systems expressed by others but felt to be alien to his own sensory and visceral experience. But how does the client-centered counselor help to bring about such growth? The present authors, setting this challenge in question form, would put it this way: "How can we make that which is unconscious, conscious—how can we extend the realm of consciousness of the client who stutters?" A psychoanalyst may ask, "How can I strengthen his ego and release in a sublimated fashion the forces of the id?" A client-centered clinician would ask, "How can I best help this individual to achieve the harmonious integration of self and organismic reality?" And the client-centered workers would answer their own question by saying that, under certain conditions, client-centered therapy will produce the solution. Let us consider these "conditions."

The Role of the Client-Centered Counselor. As has been said, the counselor is completely acceptant of everything the client says; thus, the client finds himself in a situation which is entirely nonthreatening. This "warm, accepting attitude" encourages the client to experience deeper feelings and attitudes and to gradually become more aware of them. The counselor *accepts*, *reflects*, and *clarifies* the feelings being expressed by the client, and in this way is continuously supportive, conveying support on a feeling level rather than on a purely verbal level which evaluates positively or commends behavior. Underlying these counselor attitudes and functions is the deeply basic belief held by the counselor that the client himself has the capacity to reach the most developmental human solution to his problems, that the client has within him a *positive growth force*. The counselor's aim is to provide understanding of the way the client appears to himself at a given moment. The assumption is that the client can do the rest. The counselor has no preoccupations with diagnoses or professional evaluations. Neither does he try to formulate prognoses nor in any way attempt to explicitly guide the stuttering person. The counselor must relinquish the concern with himself and what he must do, for such concern dilutes his attention and the respect he feels for the other person. His task is to perceive what the client is perceiving and to accept this with deep respect, for only in this fashion can the troubled person come to accept the same feelings about himself. In short, the counselor must assume the "internal frame of reference" (Rogers, 1951, p. 29) of the stuttering individual, perceive as he perceives, avoid all external frames of reference, and communicate this acceptant understanding to the individual.

We know that if the therapist holds within himself attitudes of deep respect and full acceptance for this client as he is, and similar attitudes towards the client's potentialities for dealing with himself and his situations; if these attitudes are suffused with a sufficient warmth which transforms them into the most profound type of liking or affection for the core of the person; and if a level of communication is reached so that the client can begin to perceive that the therapist understands the feelings he is experiencing and accepts him at the full depth of that understanding, then we may be sure that the process is already initiated (Rogers, 1954, p. 44).

A statement which is brief but great with emotion shows the meaning that the client-centered relationship had for a 25-year-old woman who stuttered. She said, "Isn't it a sad thing when we can't say what we think because someone might misinterpret it or that we don't tell an incident because someone won't see the truth in it? It is so much more simple to accept it, but they won't—particularly when, whatever it is, it isn't favorable. One of the reasons I appreciate it here so much is that I don't have to be careful of what I say. You always manage to take it just the way I intended it."

Client-centered therapy provides the person who stutters with a feeling-experience which differs decidedly from any in his past or present. An adult who perceived his imperfect, inarticulate speech to be an intolerable maledict expressed himself as follows:

"When you ask me how things are, I feel that you really want to know—that how I feel is important. It's so different from the way it is with the others. Some of them will ask in an off-hand way—just the way they discuss the weather. But the others—and they are the ones I really hate—they ask not because they care about me or mine. They ask so that people will like them or so that people will think that they are understanding. But they don't give one tinker's dam about how I am. Understanding—they deal only in false understanding—understanding that is counterfeit to both of us."

Counselors who question, interpret, and suggest would be considered by client-centered counselors as having a limited confidence in the capacity of the person who stutters to comprehend and grapple successfully with his problems. On the other hand, if the client asks a question having a straight-forward response which can be answered without implying any evaluation and without giving any advice, the counselor does have the option of "leaving the client's frame of reference momentarily and answering it" (Rogers, 1951, p. 206). Counselor questioning and probing are thought to arouse the perceptual defenses of the client, and it is believed that questions may uncover attitudes which the client is fearful of revealing even to himself, and thus are to be avoided. For similar reasons, evaluative responses are taboo, for they constitute a passing of judgment on the client, and even though some evaluations may be positive, they are said to arouse the client's fears that other attitudes may be judged—negatively, and for this reason he is apt to curtail his verbalizations.

Johnson made an interesting point concerning the consequences of what he terms "evaluate labeling," stating:

Maladjustments occur because of this, in that we tend to make and express highly similar evaluations of extremely different situations. This is to be seen with unusual clearness in what I have called *evaluative labeling*. This term is designed to emphasize our common tendency to evaluate individuals and situations according to the names we apply to them. After all, this is a way of saying that the way in which we classify something determines in a large measure the way in which we react to it (Johnson, 1946, p. 261).

In the client-centered therapy relationship, the person who stutters is removed from any such jurisdictional atmosphere, and he is free to divulge his feelings to a counselor who conceives and interpenetrates affectively without any judgment or interpretation. A male adult stutterer ventilated his feelings and showed his strivings to become a better integrated self in the following way:

"I felt weighted down. The hurt feelings that I carry around, ache and bear down—deep inside of me. I always try to hide my feelings. I always say and do what is expected of me. And do you know? I have a sixth sense; I can feel what the other person expects and wants of me. I know what he thinks about me—what he judges me to be. Then I don't do what I want to do. I can never be myself. I hide my feelings; I try to ignore them. But, they are not to be ignored. They pain and sting me inside. They show in my face—even when I'm on guard. And that is such a strain. I can't keep it up. I hate to be found lacking by other people. But I can't help it. I can't help what they think about me— how they feel that I am. It's too much of a strain—always being what someone else wants you to be. I just can't keep up that strain any longer. And what's more, I don't want to keep it up. Let people think what they will about me. I want to be what I am—not what other people think I should or shouldn't be. I want to just be what I am, and to hell with what other people think I should be."

On the matter of interpretations, the client-centered assumption is that the more adroit the interpretation, the greater the defensiveness it elicits. All such directive methods, then, are thought to place the client on his guard, and for these reasons are not used by client-centered workers.

Structuring Therapy. At the initial meeting with the client, the atmosphere of therapy is cast. The counselor may explain what the relationship between counselor and client will be by merely saying something such as: "This time is yours. You can use it as you wish—talk about whatever you'd like. I don't have any assumptions to make about your problem, no answers to it. But perhaps we can achieve some good by talking and thinking these things out together and seeing what kinds of solutions can be reached. Would you like to go ahead?" This is, of course, not at all what the person usually expects. He expects and wants advice, procedures, assurance, definite answers to his questions; he may even ask for "assignments" or "drills" and the like. The structuring process will have to be repeated many times during the early phases of counseling. In time, in the absence of criticism and judgment and in the presence of a therapeutic atmosphere of permissiveness, warm acceptance, and clarifying responsiveness, the person will feel freer to explore hitherto threatening thoughts and feelings.

The Matter of Diagnosis. To Rogers, psychodiagnostics are unnecessary for effective counseling to occur, and in fact they may be detrimental to the counseling process (Rogers, 1951, p. 219). He believes that diagnostic procedures place the counselor in a "God-like role which seems untenable" to him. It is undemocratic, and it increases the strength of the person's dependency strivings. "The best vantage point for

understanding behavior is from the internal frame of reference of the individual himself" (Rogers, 1951, p. 494). "The
psychologist with his methods of identifying and measuring
stimulus properties and his tests for assessing personality
cannot know the person's phenomenal field as completely as
the person himself is capable of knowing it. Of course, the
person may never develop this self-knowledge although he
has the potentiality for doing so" (Hall and Lindzey, 1957,
p. 479). As Snyder, a well-known client-centered counselor
has explained:

If the client requests them (tests), they may be made available. This
change in approach from the traditional case history and testing
method lies theoretically in the belief that one of two situations is
likely to prevail: (a) the client may be emotionally unprepared to
utilize information about himself, especially in those instances in which
an emotional difficulty, rather than lack of factual information, requires
resolution; (b) the client may consciously or unconsciously use the
psychological test situation as a means of forcing a dependent relationship upon the counselor, thereby making it impossible for the client
to avoid accepting the responsibility for solving the problem (Snyder,
1954, p. 535).

Such a view reveals the almost complete confidence which
client-centered counselors place in the self-reports of clients.
In other words, clients' attitudes and feelings, as expressed
in the client-centered atmosphere, tell us far more about them
than do descriptions and inferences based on testing procedures. Rogers is well aware, however, that a person may
be cognizant of the motivants of his behavior but be unable
to verbalize them coherently, and also that a person may be
unaware of his experiences and thus unable to report them.
In addition the individual may be aware and also able to
verbalize his experience, but may be unwilling to. Nevertheless, it is these self-reports which are, to Rogers, the ideal
clinical material. Self-reports reveal the depths of the stuttering person's nonintegrative and self-defensive behavior as
he, himself, feels it and lives it. Client-centered counseling
with its self-evaluation and self-perception can be likened
to a psychological filter through which the person who stut-

ters filtrates and refines his perceptions and misperceptions about self and others, ultimately evolving a more integrated and less defensive self.

A 15-year-old adolescent who stutters severely was trying to clarify his blemished relationship to his mother:

"If my mother is jealous, and I know that she is—I think I may have substituted my aunt for my mother. I am reaching now, but I want to understand what is happening—what has happened—and if I say it, it helps."

A 21-year-old engineering student, aggrieved by severe stuttering, voiced the significance that the client-centered relationship had for him:

"I have always been a dependent person—submissive, never aggressive—ever since I can remember—'that good John—,' always doing what was expected of me—never what I really wanted to do. When I first came here, I wanted to be told just what to do to help me to get over my stuttering. In fact, at first I felt that you were failing me when you did not (laughing), even would not tell me what I should or should not do. It was the first time in my life that I was really responsible for myself. It bothered me—for if my therapy failed—it was my fault—not yours. But, after a while, the fact that you believed that I could help myself became good for me. I began to think. It is my problem. It does concern me, so perhaps I should assume the responsibility (laughing). In the beginning, because I like you and I feel that you like me—I found myself using a lot of autosuggestion, talking myself into it. Now I feel that it is the most important thing that ever happened. I feel that I really do have the capability to help myself. I am the one concerned, and I am the one who must be concerned."

The Goals and Course of Client-Centered Counseling. The primary aim of therapy is to have the individual develop *insight*. This is the point where the tributaries of counselor acceptance, reflection, and support, plus client release, perceptual reconditioning, increased recognition, and self-acceptance merge to form a stream (a trickle or a torrent) of emotional understanding or insight concerning the web of interpersonal relationships. The successful therapeutic traffic-pattern of a client who stutters may be outlined briefly in the following manner:

1. Advice-seeking, dependent, intellectual, (nonaffectual); attention focused on the stuttering symptom; generally inhibited.
2. Discussion of immediate problems; anxious; defensive; low self-estimates. Attribution of blame to environmental forces.
3. Increasing release of negative feelings (hostility, hopelessness); some increase in anxiety; assumes some responsibility for therapy; ambivalent—becomes more aware of self-contradictions; attention shifting from outside to inside of self.
4. Begins connecting attitudes with causes; increase in motoric and verbal spontaneity; stuttering decreases in therapy; greater acceptance of feelings.
5. Shifting from emotionalized overgeneralizations to more discrimination and differentiating behavior; more positively toned self-references. Diminution in anxiety and in stuttering symptom in and out of therapy setting.
6. Little or no anxiety; greater spontaneity; goal-directed planning action in light of new insights; feeling of personal adequacy and greater independency; realistic perception of self and others; stuttering continues to decrease, becomes minimal or nonexistent.

Throughout, the permeating desire and goal in client-centered counseling is to achieve increasing amounts of insight concerning the affective bonds between outer behavior and inner feelings. Increased insight accompanies or, more accurately, is part and parcel of increased awareness of self, greater self-acceptance and self-realization. Discussing insight, Rogers has stated:

When the client is freed from all need of being in any way defensive, spontaneous insight comes bubbling into consciousness. When the client is talking through his problems in an atmosphere in which all his attitudes are genuinely understood and accepted, and in which there is nothing to arouse his desire to protect himself, insight develops.
Some workers will feel disappointed in the simplicity of this conclu-

sion. They will feel that they have always dealt with clients in an accepting fashion. The fact is, however, that most of the procedures actually used in counseling contacts are such as to make clients defensive. . . . It is not enough for the worker to have an accepting attitude, though this is important. The techniques used must also be such that defensiveness will not be aroused (Rogers, 1944, pp. 338–39).

Some clinicians regard insight as the ability to symbolize (verbalize objectively) ideas formerly unavailable to consciousness due to reduced awareness or repression (Shaw, 1946). Client-centered clinicians would feel that client-centered counseling gives the person many opportunities to verbalize and thus to symbolize more efficiently the previously unavailable ideas. However, completely successful symbolization may not always occur. Elsewhere, Rogers gives us an indication of his intensely personal investment in working with humans in trouble, when he says:

As therapy goes on, the therapist's feeling of acceptance and respect for the client tends to change to something approaching awe as he sees the valiant and deep struggle of the person to be himself. There is, I think, within the therapist, a profound experience of the underlying commonality—should we say brotherhood—of man. As a result he feels toward the client a warm, positive, affectional reaction. This poses a problem for the client, who often . . . finds it difficult to accept the positive feelings of another (Rogers, 1954, p. 50).

TRANSCRIPTS OF CLIENT-CENTERED COUNSELING

If the speech clinician believes that the stuttering behavior is predominantly psychogenically motivated, his concern must be primarily with the pattern of motivations rather than with the end product of these dynamics, the stuttering. He will structure therapy which is focused, not on the stuttering but on the person who stutters. One form of such therapy is client-centered counseling. Although there are several articles in the literature which mention the use of nondirective therapy with stuttering individuals, they tend to be fleeting references (Clark, 1948), brief, subjective discussions of the procedure (K. Thorne, 1947), or inconclusive in terms of value of the technique with those who stutter (Schultz, 1947). One of the present authors (Murphy, 1955), has discussed client-centered procedures in speech therapy and presented ten capsule case histories of young adults with communication disorders who were seen in a clinical setting which incorporated client-centered philosophy. Although some questions were posed regarding the feasibility of adhering strictly to client-centered counseling principles and methods in a setting in which a variety of speech and hearing disorders is treated, the discussion revealed a belief in the value of the methods for many persons with psychologically purposive speech symptoms.

Counseling with a Young Stuttering Adult. Steven is a 16-year-old boy, a junior in high school, of a lower middle-class community. He has been referred to the speech clinician by the guidance department because of a mild stuttering problem. He is a tall, good-looking fellow, neatly groomed, with a Binet I.Q. of 124. Although he has received no professional help for the problem in the past, he is not at all sure, at least consciously, that he needs any now, and at the outset of the first meeting appears reluctant to enter counseling.

Steven's First Session

CL. 1: Well, we have this time to talk over the situation and it will be your period every week. By talking over together the kinds of things that may be bothering you we may help improve things in general. The only way I can really get a good idea—really appreciate the situation—is by seeing your point of view—so I'd like to get that from you. You might say I'm a blank movie screen and you're going to put the picture on it. So it's a situation where we work together—talk together—and sometimes it's very hard work—talking about things that bother us, make us uncomfortable—not easy to do, but it's the way we find very helpful a lot of the time. Now of course, everything we say here is confidential. By talking and thinking together we may make things more comfortable. Perhaps you could let me know the situation as you see it and as you feel about it.

STEVEN 1: Well—how do I begin (laughs) I mean—uh—I don't know—I've got my problems like everyone else—I don't know if I'm different really. It's just that I have this trouble sometimes y'know and—sometimes I don't (pause). I was wondering just what we'd be doing as these meetings—exactly.

CL. 2: Yes, well as I said, I think if we can talk things out and think about it together—how you feel about it—the things that may be bothering you—or things you may be wondering about, we may come up with something helpful.

S. 2: Uh—I have a little trouble talking sometimes and—I've had this trouble—oh for quite a while. Since I was a kid. My mother said since I was about six or seven, but I don't remember it at all. Then—I remember in the fifth grade or so some kids laughed at me at the school and I thought they were jerks, but that's the first time I can think of. Jerks.

CL. 3: You felt that way about them.

S. 3: Yes, they were laughing—well, cause I was having a little difficulty—talking in the group. I've never forgotten that though, I'll say that.

CL. 4: Really stayed in your memory.

S. 4: Yes, cuz I guess I was sore—but I didn't do anything then about it—I mean I acted like I didn't hear them really—but I was sore.

CL. 5: You felt angry about it.

S. 5: Yeh—after all, I think anybody would, don't you?

CL. 6: You feel this was a natural thing to do—reacting like you did.

S. 6: Yes, cuz after all, how often does a person just laugh at you? It's a lousy—queer feeling.

CL. 7: Umhmm.

S. 7: And another time—last year—we were at the beach . . . a summer cottage. Some buddies of mine—we were at the dance pavilion y' know—and I had met this girl—who I thought was—well—very attractive—and I had trouble with her—so I left.

CL. 8: Trouble with her?

S. 8: Yes—I was talking to her and—uh—all of a sudden—I got clutched—really clutched good y' know and—I just couldn't talk to her. I don't know why—I just couldn't and—God it was—not very nice.

CL. 9: You really felt uncomfortable.

S. 9: Oh, boy—it was awful—so I started talking and talking about anything—real queer—and the whole thing was a mess. I got out of there fast.

Cl. 10: The situation was so tough you got away from it.

S. 10: Yeh, I sure did. But heck, that doesn't always happen—on the contrary I—well—I don't exactly suffer from a lack of girls—at parties and dances y' know.

Here (Cl1) the speech counselor has set the initial structure of the situation and the client moves in somewhat hesitatingly (S1). We get an idea of his expectation that the clinician will take control of the action. The clinician restructures the situation (S2). The client reacts by discussing the onset of the stuttering, and the remainder of this session turns out to be a chronology of specific events. It is primarily recall without relating affective commonalities, a not unusual beginning. The clinician continually accepts what is said, reflecting so as to concentrate and refocus the verbalizations on the feelings experienced in the various recollected incidents and in the emotions being felt as Steven recounts the incidences.

Second and Third Sessions. Steven continues talking about specific unpleasant incidents in his life which stand out in his mind. However, he finds it quite difficult to express real feelings about any of them. He talks of being basically an antisocial person who studies hard and thinks he will be successful some day, but he's not sure of what field this may be in. He spends a good deal of time reiterating that his difficulty is actually nothing any more serious than other kinds of problems all other people have. He thinks he may be under too much pressure from relatives who expect a lot of him. By the end of the third hour he has not yet stated that he "stutters." He refers to the problem as "the trouble," "the difficulty," "the little situation," "it," and other synonymous descriptions. In general, his behavior appears to be quite defensive, and he still wants the clinician to take the responsibility for initiating and maintaining therapy. However, through constant acceptance, support, and some clarification, the clinician helps Steven to gradually peel off some of the intellectual layers which have been clouding his and the clinician's perception of basic feelings and attitudes. We see the difference in level of language usage and the breakthrough of feeling content in the following lengthier account.

Sixth Session *

S. 1: Is there anything in particular that you want me to talk about?

CL. 1: Whatever you'd like.

S. 2: I'd like to say that lately I haven't been having as much trouble. That's all I want to say.

CL. 2: Uh hm.

S. 3: But the trouble is I always have that fear that I'm going to have some trouble—at just the wrong moment, you know?

CL. 3: The fear is still there.

S. 4: Yeh, cause I'm always expecting it—any moment—so that's just as bad anyway, you know what I mean? And as a result —of the fear—just because you have the fear—does that mean that you can't possibly have any trouble—even though you don't seem to be having as *much* trouble? There always is that amount of trouble that comes every time when you usually don't want it, like now, see (is stuttering)? It's all the time you always have this strange sound in your voice like you're straining to get the words out—and it doesn't sound very nice, I don't think. And I hate a voice like that. And besides, it makes people nervous—having such a darn time trying to get the words out—it's not very—not very relaxing to the person—some people you can just listen to for hours and hours and you just never mind it—they have all this information and everything—not that I don't have all this information—I'll lose my speech and everything like that —that's what the trouble is—always trying too hard to get the words out and I always seem to have the trouble. Sometimes, I'm talking about nothing—just the way I happen to be feeling or something like that—and I don't care what anybody

* The authors wish to acknowledge the assistance of Jane Scory, speech clinician, Meeting Street School, Providence, Rhode Island, who, as a graduate student at Boston University, helped to collect and organize some of the material presented in this session.

thinks of me—and I don't care about anything in particular—
and I'm not especially thinking about myself and my impression upon anybody—then it just happens that—this doesn't
make any sense—I forgot where I was. Anyways—now what
was I saying?

CL. 4: You were saying that if you're afraid you'll have trouble—
that having the fear can be just as bad as really having the
trouble. And, the way you feel about yourself when you
have the trouble—and how you think people feel about it.

S. 5: I see you're slightly mixed up there. I think I changed my
subject. Sometimes all these things pour out—because most
of the time I'm speaking I'm always thinking so hard about
what I'm saying—word for word—and how I say it—and
therefore when I'm finished saying it—I have a pretty good
idea of what I was talking about—*but* if I just don't give any
darn to what I'm saying and the way I'm saying it, it just
comes out and I say, "what did I say?"—like that.

CL. 5: It just pours out and—

S. 6: Well, like Saturday night I went to a dance—and I'm not
exactly a wallflower—although sometimes I feel like I am—
but I usually know who I'm going out with—and who's going
out with me. I'm usually not in want of anyone to dance
with—so—well, anyway, for some reason I just didn't care
that night about what I was going to say or anything. Every
once in a while I just get that feeling—and I say a lot of
things—things I might not mean—and I might tell a lot of
harmless lies about the way I feel—everything like that—
I tell people I feel that way cuz it sounds—it just comes out—
I don't even think. For instance, now here's something—for
instance—well, first I must tell you that I'm a very peculiar
person—I'm not like anyone else I know—and I feel slightly
crazy or something like that—do you think so?

CL. 6: You've been wondering about this.

S. 7: Sometimes I wonder. Just happens—I don't know—it would
take an awful lot of explaining to do for you to understand
exactly what I mean—but—well, uh—anyways, uh, it's very
hard to explain.

CL. 7: It's really very difficult for you to talk about it.

S. 8: Well, let me see—oh, I just want to come out with this and
don't think of what anyone's saying—like it was something

that was very important I guess—I guess—it better be—uh—
I don't know how to go about this—well, anyway.

CL. 8: You're wondering if you should say this—or whether you
can say it—because it's so very difficult to talk about this.
Perhaps you're wondering how I'll react—this makes it very
difficult for you.

S. 9: I don't know in what direction I should explain this—but,
uh—anyways, I have a girl friend—I don't know if that will
make any difference in my explanation—but—well, let me
think—anyways, uh—what I mean is, uh—what I'm trying to
say is, uh—uh—uh, what was the question?

CL. 9: This may even be one of the most difficult things you've
ever had to say—to tell how you really feel about these things
—most people would find this very hard to do—it's really very
hard to say how we very deeply feel.

S. 10: I say a lot of funny things—funny things—for instance,
I might say—oh, let's get back to my girl friend—it might be
easier to explain. Anyways, uh—hum, some reasons—some—
I am very, very sensitive lots of times and every time I just
happen to be in such a mood—oh, lots of times I feel so *stupid*
compared to her, you know? And—actually, I don't think
I am but I seem that way. Anyways, this might be—uh—
oh, gosh!

CL. 10: (In a relaxed manner, smiles slightly.)

S. 11: For some reason, I don't know but I just start talking and
I talk about all the ways—for instance I might tell her that
I have—I'm a very unique person—and I might have two
completely different sides to me you know? And I just go on
and on and I tell her all these—oh—all these—if I could only
think of what I was saying—not in that mood—I just don't
know why but—oh, like for instance, I can be perfect on the
piano—have a completely different personality and I—just like
that. I just talk and talk and talk and talk—uh—and I can't
think of what I talk about—it's all about—uh, do you have an
idea of what I'm saying right now?

CL. 11: You really feel confused right now and you're wondering if you make any sense to me. You're trying very hard
to get this out and it's taking some time. But these things
do take time—they come along all right.

S. 12: I *want* to get at what I want to say and that's exactly what

I'm trying to do—I've got nothing to hide—it's just—oh—it's just not something you can explain that easily—extemporaneously or something like that (laughs). As a matter of fact I'm a wonderful actor, straight-faced and everything—just things like—and I—oh (like a groan). I can't even explain it to myself.

CL. 12: (One minute pause.)

S. 13: I *don't* know why I do things like that—it's like I'm imagining myself doing something like that—like one time—I just like to—love to fib you might say and I don't know why—just comes out of me—like once—sometimes I'd like to plan these things like—might take me a week to do it. One case—what it was—I saw a perfect chance to do something—to say something—to make up a story you see—something about I was writing this script for this motion picture—I was loaded with details—how they were making a movie out of it—and I lead up to it—and I tell her about how they've already made it and putting the finishing—oh, touches on it and I was going to see the first release of it that week you know—I knew there was a dance on the week end, like and I'll tell her all about it and of course, she not believing me even though I'm giving a perfect performance—it's *fantastic* you know—I tell her that during the showing pieces of film got jammed—a few hundred feet—and how I wrote the script —and I got the piece of torn film and of course she didn't believe me and at the end of it I asked her if she believed it— and well—you know—and I guess she says something like she didn't think so—and I admit as how I guess it is a little bit too fantastic you know—and all of a sudden very candidly I say, do you want to see the pieces of film and she starts to laugh—but I take it out and I show it to her—and it is actually *exactly* as I described it—the pictures, the images all squeezed down—200 feet of it—and so that was really *effective*—things like that—and—uh—of course I did not tell her how I got it though—from a friend—it was very effective—I don't think she knows yet how I got it—things like that—all those crazy things—and she never knows if I'm telling the truth or not— and that's bad but—can't help it.

CL. 13: Something makes you go ahead to—

S. 14: I love to confuse people—some temptation—get them bewildered—is that normal?

CL. 14: You're wondering about this behavior of yours—really wondering.

S. 15: Sometimes I don't have the purpose to bewilder them but I go along anyway. And my urges to become an unsavory character or a snob or something—but I just say that—it's not true. I tell people this.

CL. 15: You try to create this impression for yourself.

S. 16: I just have the urge to talk sometimes and I just blab blab blab blab blab. Sometimes I wonder if that's right but that seems very unusual. I don't know anyone else who does it the way I do it.

CL. 16: This is unique behavior—and you're wondering about this difference.

S. 17: It's not the way I really feel, mind you. It's a lie, all a lie—it's terrible of me but nevertheless I do it every once in a while.

CL. 17: You feel like this and you can't help it.

S. 18: If I don't have anything to say and I want to say something—I say *anything*. Always make it sound realistic.

CL. 18: Yuh.

S. 19: Another thing is this—often when I want to tell somebody something that is the truth—those are the times—it's really something I want to tell them—lots of times those are just the kinds of things I can't get out—so it's not hard for me to lie—and one way to tell if it's a lie or not is to see if I'm having trouble talking.

CL. 19: The more trouble you have talking, the more you're keeping something in, you mean.

S. 20: How much more time do we have?

CL. 20: Seven minutes. Would you like to go on?

S. 21: Well, if you'll notice, I never say—uh, uh, that I'm a stutterer—and I never even mention it, even when I'm talking about that—*that* I have never admitted to *anybody*—or even myself that I was a stutterer—cuz I'm not (laughs). I don't know why. Is that normal?

CL. 21: This too—this not calling yourself a stutterer—you've wondered about this too.

S. 22: I don't think I'm exactly a stutterer—I don't see how I could be but—just something that worked out that way. I don't want to have that label attached and I don't like the word. Is that normal?

CL. 22: Even the word itself—you just don't like it.

S. 23: I *hate* the word—I just loathe it and I wish there were some other kind of word you could use—or, most of all, let's just not have a word for it—that's better. It's just trouble, that's what it is.

CL. 23: You'd rather not even mention it because it is so distasteful to you—in terms of all it means to you.

S. 24: I don't like to say even that I have difficulty talking—but at least it's not as bad as saying I am a stutterer. I hate it—hate that word. I'm just different, that's all—and maybe I'm not—I like to say it—cuz lots of time I just don't have any trouble at all. It's just one of those things that's very annoying. And another thing—do you know that I spend at least two-thirds of my time, my waking hours, just thinking? . . .

The sixth session reveals fairly well that Steven has moved into the region of basic feelings and attitudes, away from the realm of intellectual description of past events to such crucial dynamics as his way of perceiving others and self, his sensitivity to the reactions of others, and his deep doubt concerning just how different he really is from other people. He shares his phantasy life with the counselor and verbalizes his inner promptings concerning his self-adequacy doubts. Increasingly, as his verbalizations concern conflict areas, the anxiety and doubts well up to a point where he becomes quite disorganized and at times incoherent, while his stuttering symptom increases. When he finally breaks through his own state of conflict and says what he is really thinking and feeling, the anxiety begins to decrease and the stuttering lessens in severity, although, at this point, the thought processes and language structure remain somewhat disorganized.

This young man had had twenty-eight 50-minute sessions of therapy before going away to work at a summer camp. During the final two sessions, he expressed the following feelings:

1. "I realize I'm a fairly intelligent guy and I should be able to do all right without posing.

2. "I'm far less tense than I was—not as tied up about what kind of impression I'm making on people.

3. "People are really O.K. Most of them can appreciate me for what I am.
4. "So finally I'm getting to do what I want, not what some other persons think I should do.
5. "I was pretty doubtful about all this (therapy) at first, but it's given me a new look at the world. But I still wouldn't tell anybody I came here. Still, I'm happy I came.
6. "I can see him (father) more as another guy, too—a guy who isn't perfect—just like I'm not.
7. "Being more relaxed—this 'What-the-heck' attitude as you called it—has made my speech more relaxed—that's the main reason I'm not having much trouble now . . ."

Steven came back, as prearranged, for a conference the following September. One or two additional sessions were held, mostly of an informal nature, during which no stuttering was observed. He appeared to be a more comfortable, realistic, self-acceptant person. It is true that he had a lot in his favor; intelligence, motivation, preconscious understanding, moderate emotional involvement and stuttering symptom, plus more independency and pliability than many stutterers.

CRITICISMS OF CLIENT-CENTERED COUNSELING

Before considering some of the objections which can be made to the Rogerian approach, let us read the following passage:

You need not and in fact cannot teach an acorn to grow into an oak tree, but when given a chance, its intrinsic potentialities will develop. Similarly, the human individual, given a chance, tends to develop his particular human potentialities. He will develop then the unique life forces of his own real self; the clarity and depth of his own feelings, thoughts, wishes, interests; the ability to tap his own resources, the strength of his own will power; the special capacities or gifts he may have; the faculty to express himself, and to relate himself to others with his spontaneous feelings. All this will in time enable him to find his set of values and his aims in life. In short, he will grow, substantially undiverted, toward *self-realization* (Horney, 1950, p. 17).

This sounds like a client-centered counselor, doesn't it? But no, these words were written by Karen Horney, a leading psychoanalyst. The point is that forms of dynamic therapy are more alike than different, and it is unfortunate that the few differences have been pounced upon so fiercely at times. In productive counseling with psychogenically motivated speech cases, regardless of what name we give or "school" we attribute to the approach, there are without question certain essentials basic to all. Sensitive, unprejudiced, permissive, warm, feeling-oriented, empathic clinicians do not "attend one school"; they are found everywhere, just as their opposites may be found anywhere. From this point of view, client-centered counseling is more similar than dissimilar to other dynamic therapies. Nevertheless, it is appropriate to mention some of the criticisms which have been directed to the technique, if only for the purpose of avoiding a one-sided presentation.

One of the most outspoken critics of Rogerian theory has been F. C. Thorne (1944, 1948), whose reactions have been made predominantly to the *methodology* of the approach. He cites the following points of vulnerability in the client-centered method:

1. The failure to recognize the importance of valid diagnosis, particularly in research studies, makes it impossible to properly assess the claims and results put forth by adherents.
2. The lack of identification of pertinent diagnostic factors makes it impossible to utilize standardized research designs having equated variables.
3. The failure to control or account for the effects of other treatment elements, such as catharsis and suggestion.
4. The failure to correlate phenomenological material expressed by the client or inferred by the therapist with measurements of objective behavior.
5. The failure to compare the efficacy of client-centered counseling with other therapeutic approaches.

The second criticism concerns the degree to which the process is truly "nondirective." We have seen that the counselor "directs" the client's attention to his feelings, not by request or demand, but by example, as in these two counselor responses made by Rogers in sessions: "You feel the feeling you're experiencing isn't quite what the culture objected to." "You feel that here, at the basis of it as you experience it, is a feeling of real tears for yourself" (Rogers, 1954).

Yet, it does seem difficult to believe that a counselor can completely hold back or otherwise refrain from injecting some directive behavior into the therapy situation, if not on a verbal level then surely on a nonverbal one. The inflection pattern can vary considerably for the simple response, "Uh huh," as can the loudness of the voice and the rate of speaking from one instance to another. The facial expression, the uplifting of an eyebrow, the gross body movements of the counselor certainly tend to influence whether or not the client will choose to "go on" at that point. Even the *silence* of the counselor "reminds" the client that he is expected (directed) to carry the responsibility of the working through process (Greenspoon, 1955). The choice the counselor makes of which statements he'll react to certainly leads the process along certain pathways. A well-known psychologist, Rollo May, in a footnote to one of his writings, comments on the matter of directivism in a way that deserves the following full quotation:

It seems to me clarifying and healthy that the directive implications of any relationship be admitted openly. These directive influences, for example, inhere in the reputation and position of the therapist (which certainly influence the person's choice of him as a therapist); they exist in the unspoken attitudes of the therapist in the session itself, and in countless subtle ways in addition to the outward beliefs and value judgments of the therapist. I believe it essential that the therapist frankly admit these directive influences to himself, and sometimes (though not necessarily always) to the other person. This may not only have a clarifying effect, but it also gives the only basis for moving beyond the actually directive elements in the situation to a greater objectivity . . . the autonomy of the person is best protected by a frank realization on both sides that no human relationship is entirely nondirective. . . . Rogers has performed an invaluable service in his indefatigable attacks on the kinds of psychology and psychiatry which in effect try to make over the client into the image of the therapist's particular school. But such a philosophy of therapy is shared by therapists using different techniques. All good therapy . . . is nondirective in the sense that the primary concern is the need, values, and potentialities of the person who comes for help (May, 1954, p. 27).

A third criticism involves the ancient argument concerning conscious and unconscious processes. To Rogers, the self-reports are the data *par excellence* in conveying information about the client. The person, for all practical purposes, is what he reports himself to be; that is, he is his own best psychologist. Unconscious determinants are hardly considered, an anomalous situation in view of the voluminous evidence supporting the belief that behavior often is propelled by motivations of which the individual is unaware and that it is these deeper wellsprings of human behavior which form the core of defensive reactions. Client-centered clinicians are slowly conceding that defensive systems tend to seriously warp the person's perception of self, an accession which some believe tends to undermine the core of client-centered philosophy, viz., the Rogerian self-theory.

The fourth and final area of disagreement is related to the third, inasmuch as unconscious processes are intimately involved. It concerns the matter of *transference*, the focal point of resistance and the hub around which psychoanalytic therapy has revolved. Very simply, transference is a projection onto the counselor of feelings the individual experienced toward his parents. Thus the counselor is perceived and reacted to as though he were an important, early figure, mainly parental, but also others important in the early emotional life of the person. The existence of transference implies that the client's attitudes are out of date, inappropriate for the present situation. In the course of treatment, the client or patient not only wants to be loved, accepted, and dependent as he wished with his early important adults, but he will also express his hostilities and independency strivings via projection onto the clinician. The transference thus may be positive, negative, ambivalent, superficial, or intense, depending on the degree and type of involvement with the therapist.

Analysts *interpret* these dynamics to the patient so as to provide insight. Here, then, is a process during which the patient relives earlier conflicts in the presence of the clinician, exposing himself to emotional conflicts similar or identical to the old childhood ones. But the clinician does not react as the parents, teachers, and others did; there is no reproach, aggression, or retaliation. Nor does he gratify the infantile wishes of the patient. Instead, he points out the inappropriateness of the attitudes and feelings. He analyzes the transference phenomena, pointing out their infantile and defensive nature in the hope that the patient will come voluntarily to relinquish the behavior in favor of more appropriate, realistic action. Rather than impeding or stopping this process, the analyst encourages it through an implied or explicit channeling of the emotions and the structuring of an atmosphere which has none of the inhibitions usually accompanying socially unacceptable expressions. In time the transference relationship is worked through to a resolution in which the patient sees situations "as they really are." The entire working-through moves along on the basis of interpretations to the patient of the full and often hidden meanings of his attitudes and behavior.

Many workers believe that by restricting his approach to *reflection* and therefore avoiding transference and interpretation, Rogers has severely limited the full potential of the process. Rogers has said, however, that ". . . it would be correct to say that *strong* attitudes of a transference nature occur in a relatively *small minority* of cases, but that such attitudes occur in *some* degree in the majority of cases" (Rogers, 1951, p. 200). He further states:

[It is the] . . . possibility of therapy without a deep transference relationship which deserves close attention. The possibility of effective brief psychotherapy seems to hinge on the possibility of therapy without the transference relationship, since the resolution of the transference situation appears to be uniformly slow and time consuming (Rogers, 1951, p. 200).

Rogers re-emphasizes that the client-centered counselor's attitude toward transference is consistent; he tries to under-

stand and accept. This acceptance will lead to realization
by the client that the feelings are his, not the clinician's.
The counselor has not judged, evaluated, approved, or dis-
approved—he has tried only to accept and to understand.
Transference attitudes are not displaced or sublimated;
". . . they simply disappear because experience has made
them meaningless" (Rogers, 1951, p. 211). The whole issue
of transference, interpretation, and resistance is a vast one.
The reader wishing a more detailed treatment of the inter-
pretation-reflection debate will find Mowrer's critique of the
Rogerian view provocative (Mowrer, 1954, pp. 564–72).

Some Evaluation. In relation to the methodological weaknesses cited, almost exactly the same reactions can be made
to all other theories of therapy. The voluminous literature
of psychoanalysis, for example, is a testimonial to methodological lack. How many clinicians make complete diagnostic
evaluations of all their cases prior to beginning therapy?
How many experimental studies are available to us, comparing the efficacy of one therapeutic approach to another?
Precious few. How many clinicians validate their therapeutic procedures and findings by the collection of corrobora-
tive evidence? On this point, Rogers would maintain that
the only way to fully understand human behavior is by thor-
ough self-probing and self-reporting done in a totally acceptant atmosphere. At least he makes clear his inductive and
deductive therapy operation limits. Thus, he makes it possible to duplicate standard therapy formats or structures,
something less possible in most other treatment approaches.
Even Thorne's criticisms of client-centered therapy must be
regarded in the light of the fact that Thorne, himself, an
important representative of the "eclectic" school of counseling, finds neither methodological or explicitly systematized
frameworks available on eclectic theory nor definitive comparisons made concerning the relative therapeutic efficiency
between eclectic and other approaches. The most difficult,
though most crucial, kind of research is that which compares
relative successes of various therapeutic approaches. This is

why there is such a dearth of literature on this subject. Equating therapeutic variables and maintaining necessary experimental controls are tremendously challenging tasks.

In recent years, an increasing amount of research on client-centered therapy has been evident. Analyses of the process itself, studies of relationships between client and counselor, research on personality changes occurring during therapy, experimentation relating Rogerian to learning theory, and even comparisons of client-centered counseling methods with other therapies have become available (Hall and Lindzey, 1957; Rogers, 1957, 1958; Rogers and Dymond, 1954). It is probably safe to say that within the next decade, more research will be done in the area of client-centered methodology than in most of the other therapeutic approaches combined. The current criticism of client-centered beliefs is a natural and welcome reaction to a young and vigorous discipline. Fifty years, not only of criticism, but of slander, have not dulled the edge of the Freudian sword. Client-centered theory, being far less geared to the level of basic impulses postulated in psychoanalysis, has proved more acceptable to the general public and for similar reasons may appeal to an increasingly larger number of professional workers in the future. However, its emphasis upon *client* rather than *counselor* may be a block to acceptance of the client-centered process for some workers.

It must be admitted that all theories of human behavior available to us today leave something to be desired; for, again, what is a "good" theory? It is a set of hypotheses or relevant assumptions chosen to represent certain dimensions of human behavior of interest to the proponent. Ideally, its usage leads to further hypotheses and increasingly accurate specifications through the derivation of all pertinent variables from operational analyses. None available approaches this ideal. Rogers would be the first to admit that the client-centered approach *is* a theory, not yet fully substantiated. Its ultimate value will be judged by the utility it reveals in helping troubled persons to live happier lives. Finally, it must be appreciated that Carl Rogers' philosophy is essentially an idealistic (some think naïve), optimistic one, a theory of human behavior imbued very deeply with the personality and faith of a man who has been cognitive of his theory's deficiencies and who has at the same time been far more tolerant of the views of others than many of those same individuals have been of Rogers' own beliefs.

Perhaps some would describe Rogers' philosophy as essentially "passive." And it is true he does not "read into" therapy. That is, he cannot be accused of false inferences in therapy, for he makes none; he cannot be accused of "selectively perceiving" only those case data which support preconceived notions, for theoretically he neither selects nor holds such notions. Although the approach is a purely clinical one, having little appeal to hard-core experimentalists, it has had tremendous appeal for a large body of workers. Time, thought, and research will help to decree its ultimate worth.

Additional Considerations. Highly intellectualized stutterers, those operating on lofty semantic levels, often do so as a reaction formation to the unacceptable wish to express very basic feelings (especially in the sexual or hostility spheres). The higher the verbal intelligence, the more esoteric or obstruse the verbal defensive may become, and of course *this* symptom must be dealt with therapeutically if oral communication is to become healthy in all its aspects. Many stuttering persons verbalize partial insight that would make the casual observer optimistic. Such stutterers have partial understandings, but for the most part they have not come to accept them emotionally. For example, here is one 17-year-old talking:

Well, my mother is quite nervous, so that it permeates her life I would say. I can recall that, even as a youngster, she would shower me with love one day, and cloud me with yelling the next. She would simply explode, evidently with no provocation. It made me feel—well, unwanted. I'd do everything in my power to satisfy her, but she merely got increasingly angry. Perhaps this accounts for my inability to get along with my teachers—my women teachers. And now as I regard this thing, I find myself disliking girls also—though not actually—something makes me—mistrust them. And so I—well, I make it difficult sometimes—I make remarks about them to their face, you see—joking, but I don't know. I seem to be taking it out on them. They're my scapegoats you see (laughs).

In this instance the person actually did have partial understanding of some of the underlying dynamics, but it was really a case of a small amount of knowledge about many of the interrelationships plus a good deal of intellectualization. As counseling progressed, the level of verbal behavior became more concrete, more affectual, and the abstract consideration of many discrete incidents gave way to deeper considerations and extensive understandings of his important basic attitudinal and feeling structure.

Rogers has stated that although some clients may need auxiliary help (drug therapy, hospitalization, and other medical aids), client-centered counseling is applicable to just about any category of emotionally troubled people. Although it has been used very little with psychotics, it has been successful with most categories of personality disorders, including severe anxiety and even hysteria cases. Like other counseling methods, it, too, has experienced failure in every category. If we assume that individual stutterers may present us with any degree of severity of emotional disorder, from very mildly involved to severely disturbed, the reasonability of using client-centered methods with some of them seems evident. Perhaps it is not unreasonable here to mention that it is quite possible that client-centered therapy may hold extra appeal to a few *clinicians* who are basically passive, for it is the one method which allows a passive clinician to cater to his infantile passivity needs completely—*though incorrectly,* from the point of view of proper client-centered procedure.

It needs to be emphasized that *passivity, lack of guiding, or indifference are not forms of Rogerian counseling.* Rather than an acceptance, they are a rejection of the client. The clinician in trying to "get" the person to become more independent may pull the therapeutic rug (support) out from under the dependent stutterer's feet. It is presumptuous to structure a therapy situation which forces or tries to force the stutterer into a completely independent role immediately.

The process has to be designed so as to allow the person to learn what his role and responsibilities are. The stutterer probably has not been independent; his problem quite often has been one of overdependency, and he cannot perform the acrobatic feat of shifting life-role horses in midstream without preparation. Just as he learned to become dependent over a long period of time, so must we allow him a long time to break down old, habitual adjustment modes and time to build up more desirable, independent behaviors. As clinicians, we must be very sensitive about propelling persons into a completely forced-independency situation immediately. Therapy is not a product for which the clinician is the dispenser; it is a process in which the clinician provides opportunities for the person to perceive his problems and to reach problem resolutions within the framework of a clinician-client relationship; a process in which the person comes to grips slowly but increasingly with the life forces motivating his stuttering behavior.

In conclusion, the stuttering person who is so severely blocked vocally that the production of one word or phrase is a victory will need more time to be helped by this technique than will those more verbally fluent. For success in the client-centered method, some emotional pliability certainly is necessary. A person whose defensive system is so rigid as to render it impossible to permeate his emotional fortress will not fare well in the client-centered framework. Finally, of course, the person should have some amount of personal motivation.

Thus far we have presented a picture of client-centered counseling in a comparatively "pure" form. This was done to help maintain clarity and ease of communication. The experienced worker will be aware of the many "exceptions to the rules" speech clinicians encounter during years of day-by-day work situations. The intent of this chapter is not to imply, much less explicitly state, that client-centered counseling can and should be used with *all* adolescents or adult stutterers. Rather, the purpose was to convey the idea that this approach has been and can be used very profitably with *many* stutterers by *experienced clinicians.*

GENERAL SPEECH COUNSELING

Murphy (1955) defined speech counseling as a process applicable to those individuals who have speech or hearing problems which are emotionally motivated or to those clients in whom the communication ability is disrupted primarily, or in part, by a "nonfunctional" factor such as organic or intellectual deficit, or foreign language influence, but which is complicated by psychological overlay. Below are some capsule case histories which show the general speech counselor in action (Murphy, 1955).

1. In making a referral to the Speech and Hearing Center, an instructor states that Ed N. doesn't participate in class discussions because of a "speech block." When Ed arrives he sits down and starts talking immediately. He says that sometimes he forgets what he wants to say or his thoughts go faster than his speech; also, his "mind goes blank." He has a moderate stuttering symptom but the speech counselor structures a client-centered setting and lets him do the speaking. He does so for 35 minutes on a highly intellectual level concerning various speaking-situation difficulties. He does not mention his stuttering. The counselor, without mentioning stuttering as such, implies the presence of repetitive speech. Ed reacts quickly, denying that he "stutters," insisting that he "just can't think of what to say" and his "mind goes blank, that's all." He insists also that as long as he is relaxed and slows down he has no problem and that "it's my responsibility." He feels that the difficulty is so mild there is really nothing to worry about and clearly is resentful at being referred to the Center. When asked if he would like to continue a discussion of the problem, he is basically resistant, but agrees to come in again. The counselor arranges to have a Rorschach and Thematic Apperception Test administered before considering further therapeutic arrangements.

2. Several instructors report that Arthur M. stutters and withdraws completely from all speaking situations. An informal note is sent to Arthur suggesting that he drop in to discuss his present educational situation. There is no response until a second suggestive note is sent. During the interview there is a paucity of verbalizing; answers are abrupt and innocuous; hands are clasped and eyes downcast. Arthur

says that he stutters but little more. He agrees to come in again but does not. The Guidance office in his department is notified and the director meets similar resistance but over a period of several weeks gets him to verbalize some of his feelings. Arthur expresses a wish for specific help for his stuttering, and he is referred back to the speech counselor, who places him in a client-centered therapy group composed of young adult male stutterers. In the supportive group setting, he is much more expressive, is beginning to achieve some insight concerning his problems, and is more active in class situations. Although the stuttering symptom is negligible during therapy, it is still severe in outside settings. He is scheduled for another year of similar group plus individual counseling.

3. William K. stutters severely. He has had a wide variety of "speech correction" in many cities. A Sentence Completion and Thematic Apperception Test are given. The TAT responses are used therapeutically as discussion stimuli for three sessions. Motivation is good and verbalization free but highly intellectual. He is placed in a client-centered therapy group of male and female adult stutterers. This group has been in process 15 hours and some basic feelings are being brought to the surface. William contributes intellectual responses that are mostly gleanings from basic psychology books or isolated facts given to him by his former, evidently directive, therapists. By the 6th hour of group work he becomes very quiet and when he does speak, the stuttering symptom is severe. At this time he requests an appointment with the counselor and states that he thinks he could get more from individual counseling. He also states that he "hates the guts" of one of the group members, but "you can't always say what you think, can you?" He says he gets so angry he can't talk. The counselor leaves the decision of his expressing or withholding basic feelings in the group up to him and suggests the possibility of continuing in the group and seeing the counselor individually when he feels the need; this is accepted. In the following group sessions, he verbalizes in a generally antagonistic fashion, especially toward "the guy." This intensifies the group interchanges and in following periods William releases more feelings. The stuttering symptom practically disappears in the group situation, although it continues outside. William has two school years to go, is still in therapy, and if necessary, will continue to receive therapy until he graduates.

4. Janet C. has a very mild stuttering symptom which is not noticeable in the majority of everyday speaking situations. However, she is highly anxious and individual counseling is given. She lives at home in a highly suppressive, formal atmosphere in which her basic strivings, such as her independency drives, clash constantly with her parents and younger sister. At one point in therapy, she insists on having her mother and father visit the therapist, who allows her to make the

decision of their visiting. They are seen, and some general implications are made concerning the effects of both rigid and more permissive attitudes. They react by allowing greater general freedom for Janet in the form of week-ends at the sorority house, more dates, etc., but their basic attitudes return with full force within a month, creating greater confusion for Janet. By the twenty-fifth therapeutic hour, conflict areas are being discussed on an increasingly deeper dynamic level. At this time her school assigns her to a practice nurse's-aide position. She flees from the hospital her first night on duty. After several additional meetings, she is referred to one of the University psychiatrists.

Conclusion. It will have been noticed that the general approach depicted in the above capsule histories, rather than being completely client-centered, was rather what might be considered as "dynamically eclectic." Evaluations were being made, advice was being given, outright counselor interpretations were not avoided. In addition, diagnostic tests were used as a general routine in many cases. Where there is no emotional subsoil basic to the speech symptom and where no other important observable personality problems exist, a direct, informational approach is efficacious. Where the speech symptom is psychogenically motivated, the two-way relationship of supported, reflected, and integrated communication-meaning is created. The focus is not on the speech as such, but upon the individual and the release of more positive adjustment through insight concerning the symptom-behavior-dynamics relationships. In most cases, the basic principles of client-centered therapy were being followed, or were serving as a basis upon which more directive and sometimes interpretative therapy occurred. Purist client-centered clinicians, then, would not refer to what was happening as client-centered counseling in any accurate sense. In some cases it was strictly client-centered, while, in others, more "depth-oriented" psychotherapy was indicated. The clinician in such a setting is not unlike a tennis player. He keeps changing his position in accordance with the needs of the situations. He must do this in order to meet the challenge. Perhaps, however, rather than saying that we have incorporated client-centered counseling into our working structure, it is just more accurate to say that, as working speech clinicians, we maintain attitudes of acceptance, respect, warmth, and support for these persons who come to us for help. An accepting and permissive atmosphere is a characteristic of *all* productive counseling relationships.

REFERENCES

ABT, L. E., and BELLAK, L. *Projective Psychology.* New York: Alfred A. Knopf, Inc., 1950.

CLARK, R. M. "Supplementary Techniques to Use with Secondary Stutterers," *J. Speech Hearing Disorders,* **13**: 131–34, 1948.

GREENSPOON, J. "The Reinforcing Effect of Two Spoken Sounds on the Frequency of Two Responses," *Amer. J. Psychol.,* **60**: 409–16, 1955.

HALL, C. S., and LINDZEY, G. *Theories of Personality.* New York: John Wiley & Sons, Inc., 1957.

HILGARD, E. R. *Theories of Learning,* 2d ed. New York: Appleton-Century-Crofts, Inc., 1956.

HORNEY, K. *Neuroses and Human Growth.* New York: W. W. Norton & Co., Inc., 1950.

JOHNSON, J. *People in Quandries.* New York: Harper & Bros., 1956.

MCGINNIES, E. "Emotionality and Perceptual Defense," *Psychol. Rev.,* **56**: 244–51, 1949.

MAY, R. "Historical and Philosophical Presuppositions for Understanding Therapy," in *Psychotherapy, Theory, and Research,* ed. O. H. Mowrer. New York: The Ronald Press Co., 1954, pp. 9–43.

MOWRER, O. H., *et al.* "Tension Changes During Psychotherapy, with Special References to Resistance," in *Psychotherapy, Theory, and Research,* ed. O. H. Mowrer. New York: The Ronald Press, Co., 1954, pp. 546–640.

MURPHY, A. T. "Counseling Students with Speech and Hearing Problems." *Personnel Guid. J.,* **33**: 260–64, 1955.

ROGERS, C. R. "A Process Conception of Psychotherapy," *Amer. Psychologist,* **13**: 142–49, 1958.

———. *Client-Centered Therapy: Its Current Practice, Implications, and Theory.* Boston: Houghton Mifflin Co., 1951.

———. "Conditions of Therapeutic Personality Change," *J. of Consult. Psychol.,* **21**: 95–103, 1957.

———. *Counseling and Psychotherapy.* Boston: Houghton Mifflin Co., 1942.

———. "Some Directions and End-Points in Therapy," in *Psychotherapy, Therapy, and Research,* ed. O. H. Mowrer. New York: The Ronald Press Co., 1954, pp. 44–68.

ROGERS, C. R. "The Development of Insight in a Counseling Relationship," *J. Consult. Psychol.*, 8: 331–41, 1944.

ROGERS, C. R., and DYMOND, R. F. (eds.). *Psychotherapy and Personality Change.* Chicago: Univ. of Chicago Press, 1954.

SCHULTZ, D. A. "A Study of Non-Directive Counseling as Applied to Adult Stutterers," *J. Speech Hearing Disorders*, 12: 421–27, 1947.

SEEMAN, J. "A Study of the Process of Nondirective Therapy," *J. Consult. Psychol.*, 13: 157–68, 1949.

———. *The Case of Jim.* Nashville, Tenn.: Educational Test Bureau, 1957.

SEEMAN, J., and RASKIN, N. J. "Research Perspectives in Client-centered Therapy," in *Psychotherapy*, ed. O. H. Mowrer. New York: The Ronald Press Co., 1953, pp. 205–34.

SMITH, M. B. "The Phenomenological Approach in Personality Theory: Some Critical Remarks," *J. Abnorm. Soc. Psychol.*, 45: 516–22, 1950.

SYNDER, W. M. "Client-Centered Therapy," in *An Introduction to Clinical Psychology*, 2d ed., eds. L. A. Pennington and I. A. Berg. New York: The Ronald Press Co., 1954.

SNYDER, W. M., *et al. Case Book of Nondirective Counseling.* Boston: Houghton Mifflin Company, 1947.

THORNE, F. C. "A Critique of Nondirective Methods of Psychotherapy," *J. Abnorm. Soc. Psychol.*, 39: 459–70, 1944.

———. "Further Critique of Nondirective Methods of Psychotherapy," *J. Clinical Psychol.*, Monograph Supp. No. 4, 32–39, July, 1948.

THORNE, K. "Client-Centered Therapy for Voice and Personality Cases," *J. Speech Hearing Disorders*, 12: 314–18, 1947.

Chapter 12

Counseling with Parents

*Take away the rust from silver, and there shall come forth
a most pure vessel.*——Proverbs 25:4.

It is impossible to overemphasize the importance of parental attitudes in the emotive and communicative development
of children. Parental attitudes can be the "primum mobile"
in the genesis of a child's stuttering problem as well as the
motivants for the child's positively or negatively charged
emotional responses to the presence of his stuttering speech,
to his speech ability, and to communication in general.
Kanner defined the optimal parental attitudes which can
presage for a child positive emotional adjustment. He wrote:

It is possible to state categorically that, just as there are ideal standards
of nutrition and other hygienic safeguards, so is there also, an ideal
attitudinal constellation which gives good promise of healthy emotional
adjustment to the environment. It can be formulated briefly as made
up of the three A's of affection, acceptance, and approval. Any child,
regardless of physical condition and intelligence quotient, who has
cause to sense, "They (my parents) like me; they want me; they think
I am all right," has a better chance to be comfortable and behave well
than one with the same state of bodily health and the same intellectual
endowment who cannot experience himself as liked, wanted, and approved as he is (Kanner, 1957, p. 39).

Parents, and to a lesser degree teachers, are the most
important adults in the child's life. Home and school environmental pressures which are incompatible with the child-
stutterer's basic needs tend to activate, precipitate, or accent
anxiety and maladaptive defenses. In child therapy, one

basic goal is to enhance and fortify the stutterer's self-concept, thereby reducing his need for stuttering. The primary goal in environmental modification by means of counseling with parents or teachers of children who stutter is to promote the child's maximal use of any gains which he has made in therapy. The auxiliary aims of parent and teacher counseling are the development of better understanding of the child's needs and the creation of home and school environments which rest upon positive mental health principles. Thus it is that in a total therapeutic program the broad purpose is the modification of the child's *internal* milieu as well as his *external* environments.

Our culture has assigned the task of child rearing primarily to the mother, who must accept the group's censure if things go wrong. Sometimes, the mother is "the home" while the father is merely a house guest. The child's association with his father may include little more than a quick glance across the table in the morning, and a few tired, paternal words delivered just before the child is put to bed for the night. The father as breadwinner, although legal head of the household, forms a vague conception in a young child's mind. The home relationship between father and child may be nil. The child may share none of the father's home activities of golfing, working in the den, or socializing with friends. Not until later childhood or adolescence does the father's presence assume more importance. Although many fathers may have spent much time with their children—playing, working, loving, helping—the unwritten law is that the mother is the responsible member.

The secondary role of the father may be judged by the nature of the literature on the effects of parent attitudes on child behavior. Ninety per cent of it concerns maternal attitudes. This bias in favor of the mother arises largely because of the inability of fathers, because of work schedules, to attend school programs, guidance sessions, or clinic conferences concerning their children. Fathers are not so accessible to children, wives, teachers, and clinicians because of

their job commitments. Thus the information we have concerning parental attitudes is based, per force, primarily on
maternal characteristics.

Recently, a slight shift in parental attitudes and roles has
been occurring. Many fathers are assuming a more active
participation in the care and management of the children.
Sometimes it happens that both father and mother will seek
help regarding their child's stuttering. In such a case, both
parents may be seen jointly for the initial interview or for a
series of interviews. When mother and father are seen jointly,
counseling becomes a shared experience.

PARENT COUNSELING AND ITS BASIS

To have a child whose speech is marred by stuttering can
be narcissistically traumatizing to parents who tend to view
their child as an extension of self. Being the parents of a
child who stutters can hold an intense emotional meaning,
causing parents to concentrate their efforts on eradication
and correction of the stuttering, which they may perceive as
stigmatic. They particularize their child's speech nonfluencies as they try to palliate the problem and their own feelings
as well.

Whether one considers the psychogenesis of stuttering to
lie in the "ears of the child's parents" (Bloodstein, 1952; Gold-
stein, 1957; Johnson, 1957) or the neuroticism of the child's
parents (Despert, 1946; Glauber, 1951; Moncur, 1951, 1952),
parent counseling is a vital portion of the total therapeutic
program. Are not neonate and child suspended in the
familial pattern as a paper mobile is suspended in air? A
child is set in psychic motion by the emotional drafts and
blasts of parental security or anxiety; by love, ambivalence,
or hate; by acceptance or rejection, much the same as the
mobile is set in action by the air currents which reach it.
It is the interaction between the child's physical growth and
his psychic learnings which determines a child's emotional
development. In order to meet the demands which growth
and maturation place upon the child, he needs to feel from

the beginning that he is *loved* by the most important people in his life, his parents; that he is *accepted* as the individual he is; and that he belongs in the family constellation. When these three needs go unrecognized or unmet, wholly or partially, the child is subject to emotional assaults or conflicts of raw anxiety, plaguing to the economy of his immature psychological structure.

The many episodes which make up a child's neonatal life become emotionally colored and shaded by one another. Evolving during a period of absolute dependence upon his parents for the satisfaction of basic physical and emotional needs, language is tuned in early to the child's emotional life and parental affective responses. Language's sensitivity to emotional impairment is unfailing. As heart murmurs may be symptoms of cardiac insufficiency, stuttering speech, with its verbal murmurings, may be the symptom that all is not well with the child's perceptions and esteem of both self and surroundings. Unhealthy self-esteem in a child implies the presence in the parental sphere of similar faults. Maladaptive functioning in a child reflects maladaptive parental attitudes and practices. It is this mutuality—a positive and negative giving and taking—which characterizes parent-child relationships. In the healthy parent-child relationship, love flows back and forth from parent to child. But, in an impaired relationship, a parent may be psychologically impotent in meeting adequately many of the emotional needs of the child.

Experience with parents of children who stutter demonstrates that such parents rarely present problems of deep psychological origin. Moncur (1951) suggested that there is a syndrome of environmental factors which fosters the development of stuttering, viz., parental domination through the use of discipline, oversupervision, negative criticism, and high levels of aspiration in relation to behavior and speech standards. An analogy may be drawn concerning sculpture and dominating parent attitudes toward a child. A child is to his parent as marble is to the sculptor. The child is measured by parental self-ideals as sculpture is measured by calipers. Parental drives and control are to the child as hammer and chisel are to the limestone. The child who rebels covertly or overtly to the "raps and taps" of parental domination may disintegrate emotionally much as marble responds to the faulty tap of the sculptor's hammer and chisel.

In his book *Love or Perish* (1956), Smiley Blanton, who has devoted much of his life to fruitful considerations of the stuttering phenomena, stated: "Suppression does not work! . . . [it] merely perpetuates the evils it hopes to abolish. It does not eliminate or even hold back the (destructive) . . . drives in human nature—it merely forces them into hidden recesses where, like steam under pressure, they must eventually explode" (Blanton, 1956, p. 104). Suppression, harsh discipline, and unrealistic demands upon a child are akin to spraying young flowers with a harsh insecticide—their growth and development inevitably become distorted or cease. Perhaps the (parental) spraying is not sufficiently intense to produce outwardly observable signs of trouble, although the delayed or fixed maturation may be inferred as we hear such phrases as "he isn't growing up like the others," and "he isn't doing as well as he should." The damage has been internal and unseen.

Time and again, one observes parents who have unrealistically high aspirational levels for their child in terms of his general behavior, and more specifically, in terms of his speech fluency. Some parents seem to live in perpetual fear of the future—the child's future and the satisfaction of their own (present and) future needs through the child's later experiences—his success or failure, health or illness, happiness or sorrow, fluency or stuttering. Studies are available which reveal that primitive peoples who have fears for their children's future welfare encounter more difficulties in their children than do tribes who have no such fears (Bateson and Mead, 1942). Some researchers have found that in cultures where there is little anxiety concerning children's speech patterns, there is no stuttering (Bullen, 1945; Johnson, 1944; Snidecor, 1947). Johnson has made the observation that parents of children who stutter are inclined to be perfectionists, holding the child to high standards in toilet habits, cleanliness, eating, and speech:

> The more anxious the parents become, the more they hound the child to "go slowly," to "stop and start over," to "make up his mind," to "breathe more deeply," etc., the more fearful and disheartened the child becomes, and the more hesitantly, frantically, and laboriously he speaks—so that the parents, teachers, and others become more worried, appeal more insistently to the child to "talk better" with the result that the child's own evaluations become still more disturbed and his outward speech behavior becomes more and more disordered (Johnson, 1946, p. 447).

Sometimes parental perfectionistic strivings are camouflaged by defensive allusion to "nonparental" reasons which are cited as being the cause of the child's speech difficulty. What better solace is there than the notion that the child's stuttering is due to heredity factors, for example? Anyone can find a family skeleton to use as a scapegoat. It is less disturbing than to face the fact that perfectionistic, suppressive, or inconsistent parental attitudes may be the roots of the stuttering evil. The child may be transported from one clinic to another in search of "the answer," which must have something to do with his glands, or his nervous system, or the fact that "he thinks too fast for his speech to keep up with his mind." Every visit to a specialist, indeed every parental reaction toward the child, is designed to "make him better or different from what he is." It is not uncommon for mothers of stutterers to have had a long history of obsessive compulsiveness (Despert, 1946).

Perfectionistic parents may have the best-kept home in the neighborhood; they may live by a rigid schedule and set routines. Books on child care and management are consumed, even memorized. The child of such parents must fit into a well-ordered "pattern," although "web" may be a more appropriate word to describe the resulting ensnarement. If the child varies from the prescribed developmental "norm," the parents become anxious, and they try to force him to behave in accordance with "the plan." Such dealings give the child a sense of dissatisfaction with himself. "I am not what my parents want me to be." "I do not speak the way they wish me to speak." If approval comes only when the child succeeds in reaching the desired high achievement levels, he has no recourse if he wants their love but to strive continually for "perfection." His goal in life becomes a series of quests to keep the parents from saying, "You are a naughty boy"; "We don't like naughty words"; "Can't you speak more slowly?" But he may pay a bitterly high price. Continuing frustrations in being unable to behave according to rigid parental expectations or demands soon lead to feelings of despair and to a lack of competence in regard to self and speaking ability. The child begins to doubt himself. He develops guilt feelings. He is on the treadmill of anxiety and discomfort, traveling toward unknown destinations of symptomatic behavior which can precipitate even more anxieties or symptoms.

Parental negative criticism approaches rejection the more chronic and severe it becomes. Derogation may be the most harsh of all psychological trauma which children can experience, for complete derogation signifies utter rejection. Although parents of stutterers may tend to overprotect more than to reject their children, the challenge of rejecting parents is experienced by the clinician from time to time. It is important for the clinician to be sensitive to the signs of such a relationship. Maternal overprotection, of course, can be a reaction-formation to an unconscious maternal attitude of rejection, i.e., the mother copes with her feelings of rejection by centering more and more of her thoughts and actions on the child. Some of the parental attitudes which have been discussed are brought out in a different light in Table 2, which is an adaptation of one formulated by Kanner (1950, p. 131).

The aim of parent counseling is to provide the parents with conditions in which they may find for themselves greater confidence, comfort, and competency. Most parents want to do right by their child. They want to be the *good* parent and to have good parent-child relationships—no matter how far removed their day-to-day course of interaction appears to take them from this aspiration. In counseling, we help the parent to move in the direction of his aspiration, i.e., to be the good parent. This does not happen in one interview. When it eventually does happen, the stuttering child becomes a self of greater personal and communicative adequacy.

TABLE 2

PARENTAL ATTITUDES—THEIR EFFECT ON THE CHILD

Attitude	Characteristic Verbalization	Handling of the Child	Reaction of the Child
Acceptance	"It's the child that makes the home interesting."	Fondling; play; patience	Security; normalcy
Overt rejection	"I hate him." "I won't bother with him."	Neglect; harshness; severe punishment	Aggressiveness
Perfectionism	"I don't want him as he is; I must make him over. He must not stutter."	Disapproval; fault-finding; coercion; excessive correction	Frustration; obsessiveness; lacks self-confidence
Overprotection	"How I sacrifice myself for him."	Spoiling; overindulgence; nagging	Delay in maturation; overdependency

THERAPEUTIC APPROACHES

Approaches to the treatment of the child who stutters may embrace therapy with one or both parents only, joint therapy with both the parents and child, or therapy with the child alone. With the young stuttering child who is three, four, or five years of age, counseling solely with the parents may be the indicated therapeutic program. This is especially the case where the parents are able and sense intuitively the need to establish an intensified relationship of closeness with the child, as has been described so well by Wyatt (1958). A child of such tender years is in a stage of emotional pliability. His feelings and attitudes are plastic and noncrystallized, thus more amenable to change. The child surveys his world and important people through the eyes of his parents. His feelings, attitudes, and apperceptions about himself and others are those which his parents have communicated covertly by feeling tone and overtly by words and actions. The child is but a thesaurus of parental attitudes, feelings, and responses.

When a parent experiences a period of therapy, he finds himself better able to work through some of the troubling feelings which have resulted in his oppressive demands upon the child for unrealistic achievement, including speech and language accomplishments. The parent finds that he is able to accept his child's nonfluency. He has faith that some of his child's repetitions are to be expected in the course of normal language development. He feels able to react to his child's communicative attempts with respect and understanding rather than with correction and criticism. The parent becomes able to use therapy to neutralize anxieties and effect needed changes in relations between himself and his child. He is able to create a relationship which rests upon acceptance, faith, love, respect, and understanding. When these conditions exist, the child's need for his tension-reducing symptom, stuttering, is reduced. The child becomes better able to cast off his fetter of nonfluency.

With a child who is in the period of latency (6 years through 11 years, approximately), the most common approach to the total treatment program is the involvement of both child and parent in counseling. The child is seen by one clinician while the parent is seen by another in either individual or group therapy situations. Although oftentimes the speech clinician is forced to be counselor to both child and parent, experience indicates that therapy carried on concomitantly by two clinicians is the most efficacious approach. When the same clinician works with both child and parent, there is always the danger that the child may perceive the clinician as his parents' ally with a resultant bridling effect on his freedom and use of the therapy periods. Another risk lies in the dichotomy which such a condition imposes upon a clinician-client relationship which requires one clinician to work with two clients who are so emotionally dependent and so emotionally intermeshed. However, if limitations in staff number or training preclude the possibility of counseling on a divided basis, and the alternatives are no parent counseling or counseling of both child and parent by the same clinician, parent counseling should not be abandoned. In such a case, however, certain precautions may be in order. The clinicians must be alert to any emotional bias toward either the child or parent. He will need to work through such feelings in order to avoid any obstruction to therapy with the child or the parent. Through joint therapy, child and parent grow, evolving for themselves a relationship which becomes more mutually rewarding and satisfying.

Sometimes it is an impossibility to work with the child's parent or parental surrogate. The parent may be unable to involve himself in counseling because of physical, emotional, or environmental factors. Resistant parents may refuse to consign themselves to counseling over the weeks. To such parents, the contemplation of continuous counseling over a number of months, with its potential abrasion of their defensive layers, may be a threatening, turmoil-producing situation. Such parents may seek to ward off therapy. They will exercise their inventiveness, especially their unconscious wiles, in order to find reasons for cutting themselves off from counseling. Whatever the defense is, it is usually a form of resistance in which the parents try to deflect the focus of therapy from themselves to their child. With such cases, the clinician leaves the "latch" off the door of therapy so that the parents may reactivate their contacts when and if they decide to do so. Therapy may have to focus upon the child alone. Axline (1947) proposed that it is not necessary for the adults in a child's life to be helped in order to ensure successful play therapy results with problem children. The following excerpts are examples of defensive resistance in which the parents withdrew early from speech counseling sessions.

MRS. ABBOTT: (Employing overreaction and idealization) "You have been so wonderful. I've really received so much help from our talk. I know just what I should do now, and I don't need to come every week. It has been so good to talk with you."

MRS. BROWN: (Employing rationalization) "I'm disappointed. I'd like to come, but I'm taking an adult education class in typing. I want to brush up on my typing so I can get back to work. My typing class is the same time that you have the meetings. Maybe, when I finish my class, I can come. Can't do two things at once—it's too bad."

MRS. CONNOR: (Employing denial) "My husband says that I am making too much of Bobby's stuttering and that I am getting myself too upset. He doesn't want me to come any more. He thinks that if we don't make so much of it, we'll all be much better off, and I think he's right."

Parent counseling may be on an individual or group basis. It may embrace many approaches and many levels of intensity from supportive to reconstructive therapy. Treatment may be authoritarian or directive, concerning itself with the intellectual imparting of information concerning the child, his speech symptom, and the best methods of coping with the stuttering problem. Or counseling may be client-centered, focusing upon feelings, attitudes, insights, and the parent's inner capability to find emotional growth (Rogers, 1942, 1951).

CONTRA-INDICATIONS FOR ADVICE GIVING

Self-adequate parents beget secure, self-adequate children. Such parents are able to perceive parenthood, from its earliest beginning, as an experience in which they as well as their child learn, err, and develop. They are able to maintain a resiliency, a "give and take," with which to withstand the wear and tear of daily family life. Such parents may be exposed to the ever-present abundance of conflicting opinions presented by popular magazine articles, "expert" speakers, and books on speech and child development, but because of their genuinely fond feelings for their children, their personal relationships are not threatened by such disclosures. Emotionally insecure parents, however, are more apt to misinterpret, be bothered by, or misuse such information. They are more liable to manipulate the information in accordance with their own infantile needs. Usually an assessment of the intensity of the parental misperception can be obtained in several interviews. The deeper the parent's psychic prejudices are, the more a permissive counseling therapy is needed.

Immature parents may be consumed with doubts and anxieties concerning their roles as parents, their aspirations for themselves and their child, and the child's special problem or problems. When such parents seek help for their child, they bring their scourge of feelings with them. Their need is not for advice or corrections, though they may ask specifically for them—in fact, they derive very little value from formal methods. But they do need someone to talk with about their feelings. Their therapy should be at a time during which their thirst for catharsis is quenched rather than hours consumed by an advice-giving clinician. Similarly, the procedure of arranging talks or lectures by the staff or consultants is often interesting and bolstering to the ego of the speaker, but its effectiveness in developing parental understandings remains doubtful. It would be more productive to expose the parents to a technical background after they have reached the stage where they can talk without inhibition or defense about themselves, their child, and their interrelationships.

Directive advice-giving therapy involves several undesirable features.

1. The clinician assumes a probing authoritarian role (in a few cases this may happen because he needs the status and safety it affords).
2. The parent experiences emotionally dehabilitating effects, such as intensified guilt or inadequacy feelings. As the parent's mistakes in handling his child are sighted and offered as evidence by the clinician, the relationship be-

comes similar to certain unhappy parent-child relationships which the parent may have experienced with his own parents.

3. The clinician leads the way, instead of allowing the expressed needs of the client to indicate the therapeutic direction. Once again, the interaction becomes a re-enactment of earlier teacher-child or parent-child relationships.

4. The exchange is definitely an intellectual one, with little opportunity for emotional expression, release, or growth.

5. Feelings of ambivalence (which are likely to be ignored in a directive setting) concerning the clinician's advice develop as the parent listens to the directions and instructions. In such a setting, the clinician, giving a ticket of remediation, is comparable to a policeman who hands out the ticket which describes a traffic violation. The parent plays the submissive role of offender.

6. The clinician's words of advice may be used as one more dividing wedge between husband and wife if a conflict regarding methods of child management exists.

The needs system of the regulative clinician motivates mandatory, clinician-centered action, and these familiar statements characterize such parent-clinician interaction: "I advise you not to mention his speech"; "I urge you to just let the speech situation wait and rest"; "You know, stuttering is emotional in character"; "I recommend that you adopt a relaxed, patient approach to his speaking." Such clinician feelings, thinkings, and functionings result in the interjection throughout the interview of such similar nontherapeutic phrases as: "I urge you," "I recommend," "I want you," "I advise you," "I suggest," "I advocate that you," or "I propose."

FOCUSING ON PARENTAL FEELINGS

Provision for the discharge and realignment of parental feelings and attitudes rather than the parceling out of advice helps to develop and nurture a more productive working relationship between the parent and clinician. The counseling sessions may be far from pleasant for the parent, for he must face basic, and perhaps hitherto unconscious, feelings and urges, a task which can be one of life's most difficult experiences. But through such counseling, the parent is able to find for himself insights and attitudes which he is able to translate into more mature behavior.

To have a child with such an attention-arousing and tenacious handicap as stuttering may be a severe blow, wounding to the parent's self-esteem. Indeed, it may be the effects of the disorder on the parent, rather than on the child, that stirs the parent to seek professional help. Thus the parent will consult the family doctor, the pediatrician, the university speech and hearing clinic, the child guidance clinic, or the speech and hearing department of the local school system. This is how one parent, in retrospect, described her feelings as she approached her initial interview in relation to her eight-year-old son (whose stuttering speech was marked with severe disruptions and associated symptoms):

> At the time, when I sought help for Danny, I felt I was taking him. Little did I realize I was taking *us*—me, my husband, our entire family. I felt I was seeking help for Danny's stuttering which was so distressingly pitiful. I found out that it was not just Danny's problem, rather, it was my problem and my husband's. Danny's whole world was making problems for him and all of *our* problems were mirrored in his stuttering.

This attitude, recalled and expressed so well by this mother, is one felt by many parents who have sought out professional help for their child and his special problem—be it a speech, behavioral, or learning difficulty. The problem which is perceived by the parents as deleterious is centered, as the parents see it, within their child. The parents seek help in order to eliminate this abomination. The stuttering is regarded as some demon residing within their child which must be removed. At a first interview it is common for parents to show little conscious realization of the possibility that they may have created and sustained the stuttering symptom. The verbal paradigm for this situation runs as follows: "One of our children stutters but the others are well adjusted. Why cite family attitudes as villains? The problem must be within the child or due to influences outside the family—it is 'his' problem and I'll wait outside until you are through. Anyway, what about heredity factors? My husband had a cousin who. . . ." However, the hard fact is that parents do not have the same attitudes toward each of their children. It is true that there are fundamental similarities in attitudes, but there are also specific variations in degree and directions. Attitudes change, and this is fortunate from the viewpoint of therapeutic considerations, although occasionally parental attitudes are so firmly entrenched that they defy a therapeutic breakthrough. At the beginning of counseling, parental guilt and hostility can be set into motion very easily. The parent comes with the impression that the problem is the child's problem. The implication that the child's problem may be related to impaired family relationships can be very threatening and anxiety-producing. Benedek (1952, p. 104) observed that to be the good, loving mother is the ego ideal of every normal woman. A mother's failure to achieve this role can cause her to experience punishing feelings which are as great or greater than those which the mother experienced from punishment by her own parents. The clinician's skill is called upon to handle parental feelings as they arise, enabling the parents to transpose them into meaningful insights. How these feelings of guilt are handled and worked through with a parent can be a determining factor in the success or failure in the total counseling process involving child and parent.

Younger children who stutter seldom come for help on their own initiative. They are brought by a parent or teacher, sometimes by some other adult. The child's difficulty as presented by the bearer is not merely a statement of the child's problem; it is an indication of the adult's perception of the child and an indication of the adult's attitude toward him. A complaint statement is the important opening in a vital story. Kanner has discussed this situation cogently:

If the symptom is compared to an admission ticket, the complaint statement may be looked upon as representing Act I, Scene 1, of the play itself. It introduces the players and gives enough of the background to make one aware of the "setting."

The . . . first task is therefore one of listening. To listen is more than merely to hear. A good listener, by his general demeanor, encourages the speaker to speak freely. He does not cut the speaker short, does not show impatience, and uses more than his ears in the process of "listening." The complaining mother tells him many things besides those expressed in her verbal account. Her gestural behavior is not less expressive. It gives an indication of ease or tension, fond acceptance or resentment of the child, fear of the . . . "examiner" or confidence in him. Sometimes a seemingly casual side remark gives a more telling clue to the essential nature of the problem than a most detailed description of the symptom or symptoms. Parenthetically interpolated questions or explanations may disclose attitudes, beliefs, and assumptions of cause-and-effect connections not otherwise indicated by the complainant. . . . Some parents try to make their complaints sound like dispassionately objective enumerations of facts. Example: "Nervousness. He is always on the go, cannot sit still a minute. When you have him sit on a chair for punishment, he wiggles all the time and, as soon as you turn your back, he moves to another chair. (Pause.) The teacher has sent me a note and complained about his restlessness. (Long pause. Then, responding to "yes?" as an invitation to continue.) That's all (Kanner, 1950, pp. 181–82).

Of course that was not all! Even this brief introduction, seemingly intended to produce a report without commentary, contains an indication of a punitive parental attitude.

When parents seek help for their child's stuttering, they bring anxieties, hopes, and doubts with them. They are uncertain as to how they will be received as persons. They have to cope with trying to relate to the clinician; trying to deal with their troubling feelings; and trying to reveal the aspects of their child's problem which they believe consciously to be pertinent information. They need acceptance deeply and completely—no matter how unrealistic and incongruous their reactions, wants, needs, or even demands may seem to the clinician.

Often, in routine speech evaluations, lack of time and space dictate that the parent and child be seen together by the same clinician. Thus case history information is obtained in the presence of the child, who hears something about his early speech and possibly his eating habits and social behavior, as well as much he does not understand. He may even learn something about the illnesses in his family background. What may be neglected in such a setting is a consideration of the effects of such discussions or verbal mysteries on the child. He hears, he understands some; he is apt to misinterpret what he doesn't understand; and he wonders about all this and himself. He may even hear the clinician say a few words about the prognosis for his type of stuttering. By the same token, getting a child to imitate words, name pictures, read, or speak spontaneously while the mother is present is likely to produce quite a different oral behavior from that obtained when the mother is out of the room. Situational stuttering is commonly observed, and its analysis can have great meaning. An extension of this type of practice occurs in some clinical or training settings when the child and/or mother are interviewed before a group of training clinicians or students. Here, again, lack of time, space, or one-way observation facilities may force the situation. However, it is still an undesirable setting for both mother and child. An adept interviewer will be able to establish rapport with the child even under such working conditions, but some parents, less pliable and more defensive, will present another problem. The mother, reasonably enough, does not feel free to tell the family secrets to a group of staring strangers. The instances in which mothers give false information during such a session and a quite different history at later private interviews may be few, but they illustrate the importance of structuring the process with the interviewee's feelings in mind. Incidentally, the mother is also apt to give false answers if her child is present. In the familial background, there may be information which the child's parents do not wish him to hear.

The parent who is emotionally immature may be unable or unwilling to change attitudes and modes of behavior. Such a parent offers a poor prognosis in counseling. To a similar degree, this poor prognosis may be extended to this parent's child. A parent who is chronically rigid, defensive, and aggressive is in need of deep and continued psychotherapy. The necessity for continued counseling or referral depends on the individual clinician or treatment situation. To cite an example, the mother of a child in therapy had stuttered herself. This mother was seen in both individual and group counseling sessions. Although she rarely revealed a non-fluency, her general attitude is implied in the following excerpt, which was taken from a transcription of an individual counseling session:

Everyone here is analyzing, and I'm doing some myself. . . . I'm afraid of high places and I get nervous with sweat when I come down an escalator. But Joe, he doesn't fear anything, not even his father. I always thought that children should have some fear of their mothers and fathers. Perhaps Mrs. Green put her finger on the cause when she told me I was too critical of Joe. But why is Mrs. Green coming here, then? I don't know. Maybe I'm a better mother since coming here. I have hit Joe only once since coming here, so maybe the meetings are worth while. They are better than sitting outside anyway . . . Joe stuttered so completely the other night that I couldn't listen to him. Even when I'm not busy I can't listen to him. Of course I know he stutters more when he's with me, and I also know that I am the cause of Joe's stuttering, but I don't need to have somebody tell me that. He gets along with everybody but me. He even threatened to leave home, and I have told him to go ahead. One day I said to him, "I thought you were going to leave home . . ." and I thought I would throw some money away on a psychiatrist with Joe one day. I took him to a psychiatrist, and all he did was ask Joe three questions. I felt that *I* was being analyzed . . . I would like to have you tell me why my son stutters. I've gone through all this with the person at the B— guidance clinic, and he couldn't tell me what the answer is . . . and I've certainly told you everything. I don't know of any more which will be of help.

This mother was referred back to a child guidance center offering psychiatric services to both parent and child, but she failed to keep the appointment. We assume that not only has the mother been unable to accept help, but the boy has received no additional aid for his stuttering problem.

TRANSCRIPTS OF INDIVIDUAL COUNSELING SESSIONS

An Initial Interview with Both Mother and Father. Mr. and Mrs. Johnson sought help for their 6½-year-old son, whose present problem is that of stuttering with many secondary or associated symptoms. The stuttering is severe in the home environment, although it is almost absent in school. Both of the parents have consistently high levels of aspiration for themselves and their children. Both reveal extreme perfectionistic strivings. Both have perpetuated unwittingly their son's submissive behavior by their praise and acceptance of any docile behavior. Thus they have reinforced submissiveness, at the expense of their boy's spontaneity, self-expression, and verbal functioning. The mother is an attractive person of medium height and weight. She appears to have high normal intelligence. She is inclined to be quick in her actions and speech. The father is a tall, dark, tense man of approximately 40. He wears a drawn expression, keeping his lips compressed tightly in a taut, straight line. He appears to function at a high normal level of intelligence also. A transcript of the initial interview follows:

CL.: Won't you sit down over here? . . . The purpose of our getting together is to explore the problem of Richard's stuttering and the problems which center around it. I would like to make a tape recording as we go along so I can take notes later on. Will that be all right with you?

MOTHER (M.): That's all right. It would be impossible to remember everything that everyone tells you.

CL.: Keeping a record is helpful, and of course everything we discuss here is held in complete confidence.

FATHER (F.): That's good to know; it's hard to talk about your own son.

CL.: Talking about problems can be hard, but it can make things easier, too. You are concerned about Richard's stuttering.

M.: We are—but for different reasons. I never worried too much about his stuttering before—until we moved into our new neighborhood. I never liked his stuttering, but it never bothered me. You see, there is a man who lives a few houses down from us in the same development. He is a terrible stutterer; he can't get a word to come out. He just stands there, and his face flames. He sticks his tongue out, and he bulges his eyes—but nothing happens. It is terrible to watch, and terrible to listen to. He must be 30. People have said to me, "Don't worry about Richard's stuttering, he'll outgrow it." But I don't buy that any more. If he were to get to be a severe stutterer like that, I'd die. His stuttering isn't too bad. But he's only six. If he ever gets like our neighbor, I don't know what I'd do. I seem to be worrying more and more about his stuttering. I'm afraid he won't get over it. I'd do anything—just as long as his stuttering never gets to the point where it's like that fellow's. (This mother's intense anxiety about the problem is a positive indication of high motivation for therapy. When motivation is high, the prognosis becomes more positive.)

CL.: Richard's stuttering is becoming more upsetting to you, and you're more worried about it now.

F.: Worry—it seems that's all Kay does now. When she hears his stuttering, she really gets alarmed. Now the thing that bothers me is that it's holding him back at school. His teacher says that he should repeat the first grade next year. I know that he knows the answers, but he just doesn't talk much. Just sits there. We don't want him to repeat the grade. I know what a repetition can do to a person. It can trouble a person's whole life. When I was a boy, we moved to New England. I was in the fifth grade, and I was put back. I know what it can do to a person. I know what it did to me. I left school—didn't graduate because I was so much bigger than the other kids were. I don't want that to happen to Richard. If he can lose his stuttering, he won't be as afraid to give the answer. I know that he's a smart boy. Why, when he was only a little fellow, he knew every flower that was in a nature book. You couldn't mix him up on them. He was only a little shaver then, about three. I thought that we had a genius on our hands. Not that I want a genius— just a normal, little boy who gets along with people. His teacher said that if he stays back, he'll be at the top of his class next year, but I don't want that, I just want him to go along normally. They gave him an I.Q. test in school the other day. The teacher told me that the woman who gave him the test said that Richard said "I don't know" to a lot of the questions. She said he was very quiet and wouldn't talk much. Even at that, he came out normal. They wouldn't tell me what his I.Q. was—just that he came out normal.

I think that his stuttering held him back in that test, too. In school, his stuttering doesn't show up much because he just doesn't talk much.

CL.: In school Richard's stuttering is a lot less severe. And you feel that this is because he doesn't talk.

M.: He's afraid to talk in school—whenever he has to do something special involving talking he just doesn't want to do it. Other than that, he likes school. Earlier in the year, his class put on a play for the mothers and the other children in the auditorium. Richard almost died. When he walked on the stage, even though he had three other children with him, I thought he would wilt—he looked so scared.

CL.: Being in a play was a frightening experience for him.

M.: He's afraid of doing the wrong thing—he holds back.

CL.: Doing something wrong is upsetting and uncomfortable for him. He doesn't want to be found lacking.

M.: I feel so bad when he acts that way. He's a good little boy, but I never can understand why he acts as he does. It makes him appear stupid, and he's not stupid.

CL.: When he holds back, you feel uncomfortable too.

M.: It's contagious. I think when he acts so scared and tied up, I find myself feeling tied up too. We always tell him what a good boy he is when we take him out to visit. He is always so good, and we tell him the nice things people say about his behavior. We can always be proud of him because he's always well behaved.

CL.: Of course some children regard adults as judges you might say. They are afraid they won't measure up to what they think the adults expect—that they may be unable to merit approval from others.

M.: We always tell him when he's good or for that matter when he's bad.

CL.: Uh-huh.

F.: Richard is a sensitive youngster. He cries very easily. His eyes fill up just like that. He cries a lot; wouldn't you say so, Kay?

M.: Yes, he is sensitive. He'll fill up, and then he goes to his room. But he'll come right out. He gets over it quickly.

F.: He can be full of the devil too. When his sister and he get together they really whoop it up. She is different—as different as night is from day. She's affectionate and loving—

a real sunny disposition. But Richard is cool—very much on the reserved side.

M.: Even as a baby he didn't like to be cuddled.

CL.: Richard keeps his distance with people. But he and his sister get into mischief you say?

M.: What one doesn't think of the other does. When you punish one, the other one will try to make him laugh. We never punish the children by hitting them—we just make them sit in a chair. Each tries to get the other one to laugh. They make funny faces and try to make each other laugh. They think the world of each other. They're generous, and each worries when the other one is sick. (Sibling rivalry camouflaged by overreaction is a possibility that would be too threatening to discuss at present with these parents. Such a possibility is allowed to remain dormant for this interview.)

CL.: You discipline the children by isolating them—not by corporal punishment.

F.: Once in a while I will hit them. But usually we send them to the chair to sit and to think by themselves. This makes them think about what they did that was wrong.

CL.: You feel that he thinks about what he did or—

M.: Well, Richard is a serious boy. He wants to do everything right.

CL.: Do you mean that he feels that he must be perfect, that no one must criticize him, that no one must know that he is the inadequate little boy that he feels he is—that sort of thing?

M.: For that matter we're like that too ourselves. We want everything to be just right—as right as we can have it; our house, the yard, and even our children (grins weakly).

CL.: When things are right, you feel more comfortable. So you try to make everything as right as possible.

M.: I don't want anyone to have anything on me. When we have company, everything must be perfect. When things are right, people can't criticize. Criticism is something that I can't take. I'm thin-skinned. Criticism—well it can make my stomach buckle. When I was a child one of my older sisters was always so critical. She's 16 years older than me. She made me feel that I wasn't, well—really capable of even breathing in the right way. I always thought that I would fail. You're the same way, too, you know, Fred. Maybe that's what attracted me to you at first (laughs). He always was so correct. We always went to the best places. We do want Richard and Marilyn to be perfect or as good as can be. We're pleased when someone compliments us on the children's behavior. Then at home when they start cutting up, well, we correct them because we want them to do us proud I guess.

CL.: I suppose there is always a consideration of how much a child has to pay to stay good and to do right always.

M.: Well, I haven't thought of it like that. Of course you can't expect them to be perfect in everything.

CL.: It seems this would include perfection in speaking too.

M.: Yes, of course. He's far from perfect there. And certainly it's a strain for him.

CL.: It's very difficult for him to speak well or to speak the right way—the best way.

M.: Yes, and it's true—that's what we hope for, the best way—I don't know.

CL.: Could be that this burden Richard's carrying—I mean—his feeling he has to always do the right thing—speak the right way—could be that's what we see, the speech breaking down under the strain, his fear of speaking, his withdrawal from people.

M.: I keep thinking of the way my sister used to talk to me about Richard's speech. Got so I hated to see her come to visit. Guess she's told me a thousand times that I should *do* something for it. I got so nervous—just like I'm nervous now every time he stutters. Well, anyway, here we are.

CL.: (Smiles) You feel that reducing Richard's stuttering will give you greater peace of mind. (Pause) We do find that a stuttering problem usually calls for a kind of family effort—everybody pitching in—and it is hard work—very hard work to identify and change all the conditions which affect Richard and his speech. The fact that his stuttering varies usually according to the way he feels or the situation he is in, for example, is an indication to us that some factors in environment, the attitudes and reactions of different people, for instance, may be pretty important.

F.: We've never been mean to the boy. But we have corrected him—made him do things our way—the way that we felt was the best way. If he didn't, we'd punish him—have him sit on a chair and think about what he had done wrong.

M.: Marilyn is hardy. She can shake things off. But Richard, being so sensitive, he probably broods over what we say to him.

CL.: He takes your corrections and criticisms inwardly you mean. When you correct him you mean it one way, but he may put in more meaning and different meanings. And I suppose criticism is troubling to him, preventing him from feeling confident.

F.: He does lack confidence. That's something we'll have to work on.

CL.: You feel that it is important for Richard to feel really more self-confident.

F.: I suppose we'll just have to cut out expecting too much from him, go easy on him—let him alone more.

CL.: Mmm.

M.: Maybe if we let up on him, he won't be so scared through. Goodness knows, there is never anything that should scare him.

CL.: You mean that, while you plan to go easier with him, at the same time you're a little confused as to why he should be fearful and lack confidence.

M.: We were never mean—why, we love him. Anything we said or did was just to get him to be a better boy so that he could be proud of himself and so we could be proud of him.

CL.: You've always felt that you were doing the right thing.

M.: I feel bad that Richard feels as he does because we certainly didn't mean it that way. But there is no need of crying over spilled milk. We'll just have to see what we can do. We'll just, well, we'll have to.

CL.: Some changes may be necessary you mean.

F.: When I correct him, you tell me (to his wife). And when you start, I'll tell you. We'll check on each other.

M.: (Laughing) Team work.

CL.: (Smiling) Your sharing the same feeling is important—and wanting to change is a good sign.

M.: What should we do about it when Richard stutters? We've heard so many theories—correct him, don't pay any attention, and so on. What should we do?

CL.: (Avoiding the giving of advice in response to the question but supplying the requested information.) We do have some pamphlets for parents about stuttering. You may have a copy of several if you wish. Next week, if you like, we can go over your feelings and reactions as to what you read.

M.: I'd like that. Say, Fred, do you remember last week when you got breakfast? You were pulling out a cereal that Richard usually doesn't eat for breakfast, and he said to you that he wanted sh- sh- sh- sh- sh- sh *Sugar Jets,* not the kind of cereal that you were giving him. He was stuttering unmercifully. You repeated *Sugar Jets* with a decided accent on the "sh" sound. And he said to you, "I say it my way. I'm not a big boy yet. When I get bigger, I'll say it your way. I'll pour it myself." Pouring his own cereal into the bowl is something Richard never does for himself. Now that I look back I can see that he was telling us that maybe we do expect too much of him.

F.: Out of the mouths of babes—.

CL.: You feel that he was telling you that the demands for grown-up behavior were too much for him and he was sort of crying out against these demands.

M.: He always seemed to go along with us. I mean he does everything we want him to do—everyone remarks on it.

F.: You know I'm in business for myself and sometimes I take him around with me. He is always very good. He'd speak when people would speak to him, but otherwise he'd just sit and watch. He'd never get into anything, and everyone always remarked about how well behaved he was.

CL.: Richard's perfect behavior and the comments it causes always pleased you.

F.: Yeah—but we were always so pleased that we, well I guess we never considered Richard in it—only the way we felt. You know—how good it was to have people admire him.

M.: It made me feel successful as a mother; other people admiring him and the way he behaved. He never made a fuss; so I guess we didn't consider his feelings—maybe only our own.

CL.: He's kept his feelings to himself, so maybe you never realized how he felt—unsure and maybe unhappy. It's true that stuttering is one way of announcing that all is not well with the child's inner feelings.

F.: We've had Richard on display now that I think of it—just the way a dog is at an obedience class. When people talked about his good manners and behavior we felt good. But maybe we've kept him too much in check. I can think of lots of times when we'd say to him, "You're not going to act silly, are you? People won't like it if you do." We couldn't let him be silly, it's funny . . .

CL.: It's hard to let go of something which, though satisfying to ourselves, may be not good for somebody else.

M.: I think we'll have to let up a little and not keep after him quite as much. Gee, I don't think I'll ever forget that remark he made—when he was trying to tell us.

CL.: You're beginning more to think about the way he feels about these things and the way he feels about himself.

M.: I think we'll have to think about him and how to help, instead of about what people say and what people may think about us.

F.: I guess we've had the wrong slant. Certainly it will have to be Richard and not what people say.

CL.: You both really want to help him. Strong feelings about wanting to help will be a big factor for both of you and for Richard too. (pause) Well, Mr. and Mrs. Johnson, the time is about up. Here are the pamphlets that we mentioned earlier, and I'll see you next week at the same time. O.K.?

M.: Thanks. Good-bye.

F.: We'll see you next week. Thanks a lot—good-bye.

CL.: 'Bye.

During an initial interview, the development of a positive relationship is in an embryonic state. Rapport flourishes in the therapeutic atmosphere of acceptance, respect, permissiveness, and understanding. In an initial interview, it is imperative that a parent's self-concept is not left vulnerable to assaults from guilt. In this initial counseling session above, the design for future therapy was established, enabling these parents to comprehend that counseling is concerned with the exploration of feelings, attitudes, and the nurturing of insights. A strong motivation for a change within the parents indicates a favorable prognosis. Mr. and Mrs. Johnson may be a cut above the intelligence and emotional adjustment level of the average parents of stutterers. They show a good potential for insight-development. Although they want to place themselves in the hands of the clinician, it is clear that they are not so rigid as many in their demands for specific help. (It is more common to deal with parents who hope the clinician can present them with a list of suggestions and rules to follow; procedures which will not require of them the responsibility of working through with their problems.)

The Johnsons have good reasoning powers and common sense but do not deal with Richard on the basis of the child's reality; rather they tend to deal with him primarily as a means of unknowingly satisfying their own emotional needs. In such an instance, the child truly becomes the parents' symptom, a signal that all is not emotionally harmonious. The Johnsons are honest people, direct and frank with Richard, but their interactions with the boy are intellectual exchanges rather than sensitivities to Richard's feelings. They do not sense his feelings at all times, and they do not know his thoughts. Thoughts and actions which are not "good" are rejected. In short, they do not accept Richard quite as he is, and Richard senses that he will receive full acceptance and love only if he is what they think he *should* be. In terms of his speech, it means that he feels that he will be liked only to the extent that he speaks the way they expect him to and want him to speak. Anything less than the best (fluent speech) is unsatisfactory. But Mr. and Mrs. Johnson have other *positive* attitudes. They do want their child to grow up and become independent. They sense the necessity of allowing a child to express himself, his individuality, and his rights. Their married life is basically a happy one. If they have a glaring fault, it is that their demands, soft-spoken or implied as they are, are a little too difficult for Richard to meet. He is a little too docile, a little too gentlemanly, a little bit too well behaved—too early in his life. Richard is rather inhibited, uncertain, and lacks both general and verbal spontaneity. He is in the grip of a too-strong conscience. He has introjected his parents fully. Were the situation to continue, he probably would become, among other things, an overdependent youngster.

When parents make all the decisions, set all the rules and limits, and establish the (parentally) "desired" goals, children tend to lose their ability to think through and to make an adequate adjustment to problems which they encounter. They will do what they are told, or they will become very uncomfortable in the trying. Initiative will wane. It is very much like the classroom situation in which an authoritarian, rigid teacher will soon condition many of the pupils to a passive acceptance of the prescribed learnings, methods, and materials. Decrease in creativity and spontaneity will result. The stutterer who realizes that displeasure is being experienced by his parents because of his speech inaptitudes, his stumblings, and his withdrawals will develop into a chronically unhappy individual. Many adult stutterers are known to be depressive in character, with powerful feelings of inferiority and inadequacy which are based primarily in inadequate early emotional relationships of childhood.

An Initial Interview with a Mother. This excerpt from an individual "eclectic" counseling session shows how a beginning emphasis upon a child and his stuttering symptom may become diffused so that the counseling embraces parental attitudes and feelings without the activation of excessive resistance within the mother. This client is a 33-year-old mother of three. Her socioeconomic status is middle class. Her intelligence level is superior. Her perfectionistic strivings are evident in her careful grooming and exact, almost pedagogical, speech.

CL.: You are concerned about Billy's stuttering.

M.: It's something which has bothered me for a long time. But his stuttering is so much more severe just now. It appears to be increasingly more difficult for him to even speak. At present, it is pathetic (sigh). He struggles and struggles, but his words refuse to come out. When he talks, people are really, well, they are taken aback.

CL.: Listening to Billy's stuttering is painful, and it makes you feel tense and uncomfortable.

M.: It's excruciatingly difficult for him to speak. The more difficult it is, the more I find that I just hate to hear him talk. It's a terrible thing to say, but I can't stand to listen to him sometimes—standing there—almost idiotic . . .

CL.: It really affects you.

M.: It bothers me so I find myself clenching my fists and actually digging my nails into my hands. If I'm out of the room, I bite my hand.

CL.: You're really distressed.

M.: Much worse (with a deep sigh and a pained facial expression). That is the reason I decided Billy needed help. I do hope that you can do something for him. He just can't go on the way he has been. You know, his stuttering is affecting his schoolwork. He's failing. They marked his report card "Promotion in danger."

CL.: Billy is unsuccessful in two areas that are important to you—speech and school.

M.: Well, in order to get along in this world, one has to be a good forceful speaker and to have at least a Bachelor's degree. His grandmother has set aside a trust fund for college for him and the other two children. But at the rate he's going, he'll wind up digging ditches. Speech and education are so important (shaking her head—followed by a short sigh).

CL.: And Billy's feelings about these difficulties—how do you feel about those?

M.: He doesn't seem to care—one way or the other. I talk, talk, talk. I tell him to speak more slowly and take his time when he speaks. I help him every night with his schoolwork. But he seems to go on his merry way—stuttering and failing (stated with strong feelings).

CL.: Your actions have little effect on him, you mean.

M.: If he cared enough, if he would try to change. Well, if he cared enough, he would change. He's the funniest child (pause). When he doesn't do things right, and I correct him, his face gets stonylike, and he'll just walk out of the room. Then he'll come back and act O.K., as if I'd never said a word.

CL.: Would you like to tell me more about this?

M.: Well it makes me annoyed—very cross, in fact. And then again it makes me feel sad. He ought to know that what I do, I do for his own good. If I didn't care, I wouldn't correct him. You'd think he would know that I want only what is the best for him.

CL.: You think he doesn't see your point of view.

M.: I suppose he thinks that he has failed, and that I am disappointed in him.

CL.: You think he has this feeling of failure or inadequacy—that he's failed you and that he is disappointed; is that it?

M.: His indifferent attitude—it's always infuriated me. But of course that may be a cover-up.

CL.: M-hm.

M.: I always get cross when he acts indifferent. Then I take away his privileges: TV, his bike, special treats. I try to get him to care enough so he'll try to change. Never thought that he cared—that he would really like to change, but maybe his indifference is a cover-up and maybe he really does care.

CL.: You mean that inwardly he may be deeply bothered. So bothered and troubled that he hides his true feelings by a cover-up, appearing indifferent.

M.: I always become so annoyed that I never thought about that. But I always felt the sense of desperation in terms of those times.

CL.: (Waits.)

M.: The more I urge him, the more he seems to fail (pause). The more he fails, the more disappointed I get (pause), and when I get more disappointed I seem to urge him more—it's like a trap.

CL.: So that these urgings have not helped, and you're really wondering about—oh—how wise it is to act like that.

M.: I see the futility of talking to him about the way he acts. Both his feelings and mine . . .

The accepting, permissive climate of this initial counseling interview enabled this mother to achieve an initial release regarding her pressing problems as she perceives and deals with them. In the process of putting feelings into words, her verbal productions enable her to begin to see relationships that heretofore have escaped her. This mother reveals positive prognostic evidence that she will be able to use the experience of therapy as an aid in releasing and integrating her potentiality as Billy's parent. She indicates some of the areas which will need working through. She regards the stuttering problem as one centered within her child, and she has thought little of the possibility that the problem is related to parental or environmental stresses or anxieties. We may assume that the exasperation and tension that she reveals in the initial interview are typical modes of reaction to Billy when he stutters. Again, there is a concern with school achievement. Also, she reveals suppressive behavior toward Billy, as she suggests, advises, or pleads with him to "slow down." As parent counseling progresses, we may well expect more obvious manifestations of guilt feelings concerning her own ability to "make" him a more capable person. These are some of the problem areas about which this mother needs to talk and to achieve insight. The analysis of her own feelings, with a gradual clearing of vision as she works through the therapeutic process of sweeping away the emotional cobwebs dimming her view of Billy, his true needs, and herself in relation to the entire problem, can occur only in a speech counseling atmosphere which is psychodynamically therapeutic.

A Fifth Counseling Session with a Mother. Mrs. Allen is a woman of 35 whose social-economic status is lower middle class. She is the mother of two, a 13-year-old son and a 9-year-old son who is a stutterer with no secondary symptoms. She has been divorced for three years and works in a textile mill. She is of average intelligence and appears to be quite tense. She tends to be authoritarian in her relationship with her children. In previous sessions, the hostility she feels toward her divorced spouse had been displaced onto her stuttering son, Tommy, who is very similar to his father in physical attributes. All sessions were of a half-hour duration.

During the first and second counseling periods, Mrs. Allen persistently had questioned the clinician concerning the causes and cures of stuttering. She had come to the speech counselor expecting a prescription of some sort, with advice and information concerning what "she could do to Tommy's speech and breathing." She is not a severely emotionally disturbed individual. She is not ridden by anxieties or complex defensive processes. She is able to derive help from a counseling structure which gives her a chance to release her aggressions and to receive continued support. The speech counselor's role has been primarily client-centered. In this transcription of the fifth counseling session we see that Mrs. Allen has moved away from a highly specific focus on her child's stuttering symptom to a focus on self-attitudes, reactions, and needs as they relate to and affect Tommy. The transcript reveals how the symptom of referral, i.e., her son's stuttering, has become de-emphasized in the course of therapy to the point where the underlying causes for the stuttering behavior are being considered. There is a steady progression of the sessions' verbal content away from the child's stuttering toward the consideration and discussion of *self*. Between the fourth and fifth speech counseling sessions, Mrs. Allen has received a single, diagnostic interview by a middle-aged, male psychiatrist.

CL.: Hello, Mrs. Allen. Won't you sit over here so we can talk.

M.: Yes, thank you. Well, we saw Dr. T. last Saturday. I dropped Eddie at the barber shop, and Tommy and I went on to Dr. T's. It's rush, rush, rush all of the time. I have so much to do—(sigh and pause) and so little time to do it.

CL.: You're very busy.

M.: You know, Tommy—he just loved it. But the doctor said some things that made me do a lot of thinking.

CL.: Uh-huh.

M.: When I went into his office he said, "You must be very unhappy—you never smile." I don't know why he said that. Why should I be smiling? It was something serious that I went for. I have enough on my mind to make me serious so why—just tell me why—should I be smiling? I felt like telling him that, but I didn't.

CL.: You didn't feel like mentioning it then.

M.: Well, I don't like to assert myself with people. I've always been like that. Lord knows, I have enough on my mind to be serious about.

CL.: You've never been able to say what you think?

M.: I've always been like that, even when I was a kid. My father had a violent temper. He would hit us if we stood up to him. Even my mother was afraid of him. Mine was a home where nobody cared; nobody cares even now. My mother never cared what happened to us—to any of us. Even today, my brothers and sisters don't care about each other. All for themselves. Do you know that when I telephoned my sister long distance to tell her Walter and I had split up, she didn't care. She didn't want to talk about it. I have no one to talk to.

CL.: You feel alone you mean.

M.: That's it. Alone—all alone—except for Eddie and Tommy. But I can't talk things over with them. Once I had a person that I could talk to, an older woman, a neighbor of mine. She was an older woman—almost 60—old enough to be my mother. I used to talk things over with her after Walter left —after we broke up. It was good to have someone to talk to.

CL.: Made you feel better to talk things out.

M.: But not for long! (pause) I thought that she liked me—that she was sincere, but all she was doing was repeating everything to the neighbors. And I was the laughing stock.

CL.: Umm.

M.: I was at the store, and two women were talking and laughing about what I had told my so-called friend. They were talking about my problems. From that time on, well, I just keep still. I don't tell anybody nothing. That's why it seems good to be able to talk things over here.

CL.: You feel like talking things over—it's helpful, but you don't want to tell your confidences to anyone who might treat them lightly.

M.: Never again! I was made a fool of once, but never again. Dr. T. said something else that made me think. He told me about a boy who at the age of 19 ran off and got married. He left his mother who had worked and slaved all her life bringing him up. The doctor said everybody criticized the boy for leaving his mother, but that he understood why the boy had left home—his home was never a happy one, so he left just as soon as he was able.

CL.: And you have thought about this?

M.: It made me realize that I am like that mother. Our home isn't a very happy place. I think all the time that when the children get working, things will be easier. I'm always tired, and I'm always crabbing and nagging about something or other, especially to Tommy. It made me think that I am taking care of the children—food, clothing, and things like that—but that I'm not making things happy at home.

CL.: You mean you thought of the importance of a happy home, that other things are not so important as a happy home—let's say, a place free from bickering and criticism.

M.: I know that I'm always picking on Tommy when he wets the bed each night. I get so cross. It means so much extra work. I've taken him to three different doctors, and each one says there is nothing wrong with him. But I get so cross when he wets; sometimes I even threaten to tie a tin can on him.

Cl.: You get really exasperated—.

M.: Uh-huh. I know that I should accept the bed wetting just the way I should accept his stuttering without a mention. I know the more I talk about it, the more it will happen.

Cl.: But it's hard not to do something when he wets or stutters.

M.: Yes, knowing and doing it, they are not the same thing. It's one thing to know what you're supposed to do and it's another thing to—well—to do what you know you should do.

Cl.: Certain things make it hard to do what you know is better, you mean.

M.: Oh, I get mad, and then after, I know I only make things worse. But I have decided to make things better. To get on the right track. I've decided to use the little money that I have saved—I'm going to buy an old used car. In that way we can go places together on week ends. We can have a little fun and happy times as a family. I decided it's better to spend the money that way than it is to pay doctor's bills. Sometimes I think that's what I'll be doing if things don't get better. Sometimes lately I feel that I am going crazy. Gosh, I've changed! I swear all the time now. You know I never used to swear, but now I'm always swearing. I hate to hear profanity, but I swear all the time now.

Cl.: Your swearing bothers you, but something makes you do it.

M.: Well, I'm mad—mad at the whole world and everyone in it, I guess. When I swear I feel better afterwards.

Cl.: You get rid of your angry feelings that way.

M.: And another thing, I don't trust people the way I did.

Cl.: (Nodding.)

M.: From now on, I'm not going to concern myself with other people. I'm going to try to build a home that's a little happier for the three of us.

Cl.: You really want to change things at home, and you've started to think of ways in which you can start. Well, I see that our time is up—see you next week?

M.: That's fine. I'll see you next Wednesday. Good-bye.

GROUP COUNSELING WITH PARENTS

Group therapy has its roots in social experiences. It is a closer duplication of social relationships than is individual therapy. Much of what holds true concerning group work with adult stutterers applies in principle and often in method to group procedures employed with parents, just as the principles and techniques utilized in individual therapy with other stutterers may approximate closely those applied in individual parents counseling sessions. Group therapy approximates individual therapy in many aspects; however, there are differences. Hobbs stated:

The similarities arise from a common purpose and from a shared conception of the nature of human personality and how it changes. The differences arise from the important fact that in individual therapy only two people are immediately involved, whereas in group therapy five or six or seven persons interact in the process of therapy (Hobbs, 1951, p. 278).

The counseling of parents of children with problems is unique because the persons involved at the outset are not participating in the therapeutic process for purposes of self-improvement, increased insight, and comfort. Their interaction is in consideration of an important person, their stuttering child, who is the reason for their seeking help in the first place. Because of this differentiating element, group speech counseling with parents may embrace any number of the following goals: (1) awareness of the existence of stutterers' and other children's problems; (2) understanding of the child's stuttering problem and the relationship of his emotional needs and deprivations to that problem; (3) the recognition of one's own needs and attitudes (increased self-awareness); (4) the receiving of emotional support from the group and the group leader; (5) the provision of an outlet for parental attitudes and feelings; (6) the clarification of confusions or doubt regarding the causes and treatments of stuttering; (7) increased ability to react on a positive emotional rather than an intellectual level with the child; and (8) increased appreciation of social, vocational, and religious values, pursuits and family activity in the life-adjustment of the stutterer. Often we find that the group therapy structure, with its group interaction and duplication of a family constellation, is threatening and anxiety provoking to some parents. In severe cases of such stress, group therapy may be contraindicated, and individual therapy may be the therapeutic mode needed. Other parents may find that the group structure provides them with a feeling that "I am not alone" or that "others have greater problems than I." Such feelings may, in fact, become the basic motivation for continuing attendance at the parent-counseling sessions.

Group therapy with parents often goes beyond the confines of the therapy hour itself. Parents ruminate about the specific problems of the other group members in the time which elapses between one session and another. The parent is able to respond with greater objectivity in his evaluation of problems which are not bound closely to self. In so doing, he often is able to arrive at insights into his own problem areas. Group therapy encourages the acquisition of new insights and learnings under an accepting structure. The group structure provides experiences which extend the boundaries of understanding in relation to others and self. It extends the bounds of conscious awareness. The attitudes and verbalizations of each parent act as therapeutic activants. The societal setting of the group may actually place each group member in the role of group "clinician" at one time or another.

In parent counseling, factors of parenthood itself usually hold the parental age range within workable boundaries. At the same time, age divergencies promote role-taking possibilities among participants. Various group members may view the oldest member as maternal, the youngest as the young sibling surrogate, or the person similar in age as a sibling substitute. In regard to the size of each group, perusal of the literature shows the range to be from 5 to 15 members. Seven persons have proven to be an optimum working number, in the authors' experience.

The role of counselor in either individual or group therapy

remains essentially the same as in other forms of therapy which have been discussed previously. The concern is with feelings and attitudes. Acceptance, permissiveness, and respect characterize the clinician in both individual and group parent therapy. The clinician holds the belief that, under appropriate therapeutic conditions, each parent has the inner faculty to find for himself, in his own way, in his own time, his own needed changes in attitude and reaction tendencies toward his child.

Hobbs pointed out the added demands which group therapy places upon the counselor. He suggested:

> He now must respond sensitively to six people instead of to one; he must be able to recognize and handle objectively the cross currents of feeling that develop within the group; he must clarify his own feelings towards the several members of the group, in order that he may respond to each member with consistent understanding (Hobbs, 1951, p. 305).

Transcript of an Initial Counseling Session. The initial therapeutic session of group or individual therapy may be the most critical interview of all. The success of future therapy depends much on the successful structuring of the initial session. The excerpt of the group parent-therapy session to follow includes the clinician's opening remarks, in addition to the major portion of the entire counseling session, which lasted about one hour. Seven mothers of stutterers comprised the group.

MRS. A.: Is an attractive woman of superior intellect. She has some psychological sophistication which she acquired mainly through involvement for a six-month period in a case-work relationship at a child guidance clinic where her son received treatment for a learning problem and severe stuttering. She has supplemented her case-work therapy with reading and much thinking. This mother has a history of a negative relationship with her own authoritarian, controlling mother. Her 12-year-old son is emerging from a long siege of severe stuttering with associated symptoms. Although he received six months of psychiatric treatment, his stuttering did not change and remained for three years after the termination of psychiatric help. Deep sensitivity to her own needs and to those of her family have developed within this mother. She speaks of her experience as the mother of a severe stutterer as "soul sensitizing." This mother is a positive growth factor in the group, a stimulating and a synthesizing agent.

Mrs. B.: Is an attractive, efficient, determined mother of two boys. Her relationship with her mother also was impaired. She is incapable of giving complete love, or even of showing her feelings of love. She copes with anxiety by means of a character defense of perfectionism with a compulsion towards cleanliness and order. Her nine-year-old son is a stutterer with associated symptoms. The staff feels that Mrs. B. displaces her feelings of hostility toward her parents onto her stuttering son.

Mrs. C.: Is an obese woman, 32 years old. She is the mother of one son, a nine-year-old child who is a stutterer with associated symptoms. She says she is "highly nervous and under the doctor's care for my nerves." She has a mother-son relaitonship which is built on authority and demands for conformity.

Mrs. D.: Is a frail, tense, shy woman of 37 whose life style is one of deep feelings of inferiority and inadequacy. She is the mother of three, two girls, 17 and 14 years of age, and a 12-year-old son who is a severe stutterer with associated symptoms. Her daughters are successful academically, while her son, who is of high average intelligence, possesses problems in learning, in addition to the speech behavior. This mother married at an early age to escape the unhappiness of her own home life.

Mrs. E.: Is an attractive woman of about 34. Her socioeconomic level is upper middle class. She places high value on this. Her social ease hides irritability and aggression. She uses the mechanism of denial in order to cope with anxiety and existing negative realities. Her 6½-year-old son is a stutterer, seemingly untroubled by the stuttering, while having in addition a pronounced lingual-protrusion lisp.

Mrs. F.: Is a 25-year-old mother of two girls and a boy. Her eldest child, a girl, is a severe stutterer with no associated symptoms. Mrs. F. herself had experienced intense sibling rivalry with her older sister. Her self-ideal is to be a good wife and a faultless mother of well-behaved, academically

successful, attractive children whom others can admire and
of whom she can feel proud.

Mrs.G.: Is a large, uncommunicative woman of 39 who relates
poorly to others. She is the mother of two; a married daughter of 21 who lives in her parents' home and a nine-year-old
son who is a severe stutterer with associated symptoms. She
adjusts through overcompensation, substituting overprotection for rejection. She represses her rejecting feelings by
binding her son to her by means of anxious oversolicitude and
restriction.

The following common denominators were represented
by all members of this group therapy constellation: (1) a fractured relationship between the mother and her own mother;
(2) an incapacity to give complete, true love based on acceptance, respect, and understanding; (3) the need to be assertive,
authoritarian, and demanding in the role of parent; (4) a high
level of aspiration set for the child in all areas, especially in
speech behavior.

The therapy session was held in a large, airy room. The
group sat in straight-backed chairs around an oblong table.
Ash trays were available. (Although smoking appears to reduce tensions, there is some question in group therapy as to
whether the oral activity detracts from or dilutes the oral
activity of speaking. However, smoking usually occurs in
group sessions unless the group decides otherwise.) The
clinician sat at the side of the table, avoiding either the head
or the end of the table in order to lessen the possibility of
parental association of the "head" of the table with the "head"
of the family or the authoritarian group leader. Although
one or more individual meetings may precede entrance of a
parent into group therapy, all these group members were
participating in their first counseling session.

After the group members introduced themselves around
the table, the clinician opened the session with a lead statement designed to set the general structure of the meetings.
The particular form which the clinician's words took at this
session may differ according to the working setting. In a
public school setting, parents have become accustomed to

parent-teacher conferences, and they may think of their first meeting with the clinician as another such conference. Their motivation may be low. In a clinic, parents usually have sought out help. They have traveled to the clinic while paying a baby sitter to mind the house. They are not likely to associate school with clinic activities. They are apt to be highly motivated. Such considerations will affect the level and form of communication used by the clinician in his introductory statements. The following introduction has been used in both clinic and school settings.* The transcript follows:

CL.: I'd like to say a few words before we get started. We'll be meeting each week at this same hour and in this room. The time is available to you. If you decide not to come, this is your decision. We want to keep this on a voluntary basis. The group as it stands is now at its maximum size, and this is the size we'll maintain. If anyone has to leave us, we'll probably have a new person take her place, but that decision will be up to you, the group. From time to time, some of you may feel the need to do some talking to me outside the group situation. I hope you'll feel free to let me know if you want to do this. Of course everything we'll say here is completely confidential. I hope you will feel free to say what is on your mind, no matter how trivial or irrelevant you may think it is. Group discussion may be helpful as we try to find out more about our common problems. (Pause)

A.: Well, I've found out from my own experience that talking yourself out always helps. (Looks around the table.)

B.: Even when you talk to a friend over a cup of coffee, things seem better, if only for a little while.

CL.: Talking out our feelings can be helpful. Talking about your children, their stuttering, and your reactions to them—these are the kinds of things we'll be talking about (continuing to structure the situation).

---

* Once again, the initials Cl. refer to the clinician, while the initials A, B, C, etc., refer to Mrs. A., B., C., etc., respectively. For ease of communication, the first letter of each child's name has been made to correspond with the letter designating his parent; thus, for Mrs. A., the child's name is Allen.

E.: This is my first time in a clinic—or getting any kind of help. Can you give me an idea as to how long it will take?

CL.: This is something most of you have been wondering about. (Pause) After we come to know the situation well, we may be able to give a better idea of that.

A.: Take it from me, it's no picnic—I've been at it for a long time —too long—but I think it's worth a struggle.

G.: Oh, you've been here before.

A.: No, not here. Another clinic.

C.: Well, I do want to talk to you about Carl's stuttering; I mean when he starts to stutter. It makes me feel so nervous. I know it shouldn't, but I hate to hear it. I'm a nervous person anyway—everything bothers me.

CL.: Carl's stuttering really upsets you.

C.: Every time he stutters, I could scream.

F.: Oh, come, I've felt like that a dozen times!

CL.: (Nodding)

F.: I mean exasperated when Frances fumbles her words—it gets me all keyed up. I'm tense until she stops. (Pause)

CL.: This kind of feeling is pretty common with everybody. (General group nodding of affirmation)

A.: I used to be like that until I found out that this made Allen worse. The more keyed up I became, the worse he seemed to get. When he was younger I'd keep right after him to slow down. Right after him. He must have felt awfully hounded. But I think I've changed now—for the better, I hope.

E.: Well, I'll admit I'm like that even now—I keep reminding Eddie to relax and try to help him along and so on, but you have to do something.

CL.: There is always the question of just what is the best way to react to a youngster's stuttering. I suppose the two opposite approaches would be either to prod him or to leave him alone.

B.: Leaving Ben alone just seems to get things from bad to worse. Every so often I'll just forget his stuttering—without mentioning it to him even—but it hasn't made any difference as far as I can see. No matter what I've tried, it doesn't work. I hope I can find the answer to his problem here.

F.: Sometimes I think that I'd jump out the window if Frances would just stop stuttering. I honestly would do anything— wouldn't you? (Looks at Mrs. G. sitting beside her.) (Silence.)

G.: Well, I've been wondering if we could talk about how to get a child not to be so shy. Every time we have company, George hides. What can you do in that situation?

CL.: He's afraid of new people in general.

G.: Well, no, mostly his uncles. With his aunts, he's fine, but he won't go near his uncles.

CL.: It's just with men that he acts that way.

G.: Well, yes, it seems so. I don't know why he should. They are all good men, you know. They treat him nicely.

B.: My Ben is like that—always clinging right by my side. But he isn't even very friendly with his own father, I'm sorry to say.

A.: I think a boy who doesn't get along well with his father is automatically going to have a little trouble with men in general later. (Silence.)

CL.: You mean the kind of relationship a boy or girl has with parents is likely to affect the way they get along with other adults.

A.: I believe that.

E.: Well, maybe I'm lucky, but Eddie adores his father. Can't leave him alone when he comes home from work and on week ends. Of course my husband isn't home very much; you know how traveling salesmen are (laughs). We really don't get to see much of him. But when he's home, Eddie is right there. I might as well not exist when his father is home.

G.: But George—well, he doesn't stutter more when his father's around, but now that I think of it, he has an awful time when Margaret's—that's his sister—when her husband—they are living in our home just now—when her husband is around, he just has an awful time.

A.: Maybe he doesn't like the—his sister's husband (smiles).

G.: Oh! no, he's very nice to George, and George likes him I'm sure—nothing like that. Although I can't spend the time with him that I'd like to—with Margaret and her husband and the baby around you know—but you know George's speech has been kind of bad ever since they came to live with us—I don't know—

B.: He might resent it.

G.: Yes, he might resent it (ponders).

C.: Well I did want to mention to you that when Carl starts to stutter it makes me feel so nervous. I hate to hear him. I'm a very nervous person anyway—everything bothers me. When he's going through a bad stuttering scene I feel so tense and nervous that I could scream.

F.: Frances goes through those phases—it probably is a phase. She's got good days and bad days. She'll go along for several days with little or no stuttering then the stuttering comes back just as bad as ever.

CL.: It's difficult to account for why there's little stuttering one day and maybe a lot the next you mean.

A.: I've found that if Allen feels good, his stuttering is less, haven't you? (She looks around. General nods of affirmation.)

CL.: You mean his stuttering is tied in with his feelings.

F.: When Frances feels happy about herself and things around her, her stuttering certainly is not as bad.

E.: My Eddie has nothing to feel unhappy about. He's a very happy child. There is nothing to make him unhappy that I know of. He just stutters any time—when he's telling about anything. He's an easy boy to handle—you can always reason with him.

CL.: As you talk and explain things with Eddie, he always comes around to your way of thinking, you mean. When he does these things that you want, is he releasing his true feelings, do you think?

A.: I don't think you can always use a logical approach with children.

E.: Well, he's a very intelligent child, and so logic and reason make sense to him. He knows if we explain things.

A.: Well, I've found that when Allen feels happy about himself, his stuttering is less or it may go away completely. On the other hand, when he's unhappy about himself or other things, but most of all about himself, his stuttering is terrific—very intense. For instance, he was in one of his bad stuttering periods; then the other night he came home from dancing class, and all was right with the world. He was talking a blue streak—no stuttering—easiest boy in the world to live with that night. Everything was great. He mentioned that one of the little girls that he liked in his dancing class had asked him for a dance during the "girl-ask-boy" dance, and that she said, "I like to dance with you, Allen, because you're such a wonderful dancer." Of course the wonderful feeling didn't last, but it was plain to see that when he feels good, his stuttering is on the decrease. How he feels about himself, especially, influences everything he does.

C.: Well I don't know. When Carl had his accident he scarcely stuttered at all. The accident was a terrible experience, just terrible. We were all so upset—we were nearly crazy—we almost lost him you know; he was in the hospital for a month. We thought that his stuttering would be terrible but it wasn't —he didn't stutter much at all.

A.: I suppose because everyone showed a lot of interest in him— that probably helped a lot too.

F.: Frances has a habit that really is a habit. She plays with an old baby blanket which she has had since she was three years old. She won't do anything without that blanket. It's frayed, and almost in ribbons but she won't give it up. You can't take it away from her. It makes me so mad when I see her with that thing. She's much too big for it. If I take it away and hide it, she has a tantrum, and of course her stuttering is worse. It's a comfort to her, but it's certainly no comfort to me.

Cl.: Frances' use of her blanket seems similar to the comfort which some children get out of sucking their thumb. You feel that when she gets other kinds of satisfaction, she tends to give up the blanket.

F.: Well—if I don't break her of this habit, she'll never give it up. She's too old for it.

A.: That blanket seems to give her some emotional comfort.

F.: Yes. It's like a choice between blanket play or stuttering. Hmm—both are hard to take.

A.: No, we can't seem to get away from it—the tie-in between the stuttering and how they feel.

E.: I've found myself that if I just tell Eddie to take it easy that it usually helps.

B.: I read an article in the paper the other night that said you shouldn't call your child's attention to his stuttering, and that if you do, it only makes his stuttering worse.

E.: (Laughing in a patronizing manner) Well, when I speak to Eddie about it, I say it sweetly and nicely. He knows that I am only helping him with a little problem. We're very close you know. We just laugh, and he goes right on. A year ago, Eddie had a habit of blinking his eyes, and I took him to an eye specialist, who found nothing wrong. So I had a little talk with Eddie and told him there was nothing wrong with his eyes and that there was no need for him to blink. Then I asked him to try to stop. When you understand a child and he knows that what you do is for his own good, a mother and child can do anything together. Why, he really has nothing to be upset or to have any unhappy feelings about, as this lady says (gesturing to Mrs. A.). I would consider us a very happy family—we do everything together—Eddie dances, rides, swims, skiis, fishes, he can even pilot our cabin cruiser. He does very well in school too. There's nothing in his life, as far as I can see, or in the family which would have to make him unhappy. I think that it is just that his mind is so fast that he's—well, he just thinks too fast to speak. When I remind him to slow down and take it easy that's all he usually needs.

F.: How long has Eddie been stuttering?

E.: Since he was a little fellow. About 3 or 3½ years old. Even as an infant he was easy to manage.

CL.: He's never been a problem to you—never resisted you at all. (Mrs. E. shakes her head—no.)

B.: Maybe he does what you want him to do because he's afraid to do anything else—I mean not because he wants to be afraid but because he doesn't want to say what's on his mind—sometimes I think Ben is like that.

E.: (Becoming more defensive) Well, I think I know Eddie pretty well. You would have to see us together.

CL.: (This is a threatening situation for this client. If too much anxiety is provoked, Mrs. E. may remove herself from the group through verbal or physical distance. For this reason the next response of the clinician is supportive.) It is hard to convey to us your feelings and your relationship with Eddie. It's hard to get others to see just what the situation really is and to see how you've made every effort.

B.: I use to tell Ben how to slow down. I liked to think that he stuttered because he was advanced in his thinking and thinking faster than he was able to speak. It made me feel pretty good to tell him to slow down, but it made him stutter more and the more I mentioned it the worse the stuttering got.

CL.: You mean that mentioning Ben's stuttering helped your own feelings but that it made things worse for him. The cares and the kind of feelings that we, as adults, have seem to be pretty important—in terms of how we do things or how we react to the children. How do you feel about that Mrs. D.? (Mrs. D. has not spoken as yet and the clinician feels that it would be best if she were to be given a little extra encouragement in terms of being brought more actively into the situation.)

D.: Yes—well—stuttering is a thing that has always upset me. My younger brother was a very bad problem—stuttering, I mean. When I was a girl I had to take care of the family— we had a big family. And I had a lot of responsibility. My brother was a stutterer and I would get wild—angry you know. We never got along. Then when my own son began to stutter, I thought that I was getting paid back for being mean to my brother. I'd walk away when David would stutter—couldn't stand it. It kept getting worse.

A.: Allen used to do that, or rather I used to do that with Allen— but I've gotten over it. I'd get worse, and he'd get worse— I'd get upset, and he'd get more upset (pause).

CL.: The more upset he gets, the worse the stuttering gets usually.

F.: Gosh, a parent has to be perfect. When things go right, the children don't bother me. But, when I have a bad day, they get on my nerves and I'm always picking on them. The more I pick, the more Frances stutters. Even though I know it, I just go on picking like I'm driven to it—and Frances goes on stuttering. If I get mad, the whole family gets it in the neck, and they get mad, too.

CL.: You mean our feelings influence the people around us and makes them feel the same way. It affects how we behave, too.

G.: Well, I know that when I feel good, George's stuttering doesn't bother me so much.

CL.: M-hmm. I see that our time is drawing to a close. Well, we'll meet next week at the same time. I'll look forward to seeing you then. O.K.?

The clinician and parents bid each other good-night. The group members walk down the stairs, breaking into two groups of two, Mrs. A. and B., and Mrs. F. and D., and one group of three—Mrs. C., E., and G.

The focus of this initial session was in the exploration of the parent's feelings and attitudes. The role of the clinician as a nonauthoritarian, nondominating, and nonjudgmental figure was defined. The permissiveness of counseling was demonstrated—leading to verbalization or the freedom to listen. Acceptance and respect were communicated, creating a beginning and necessary working relationship which had as its basis the rapport which was established within the group. Clinician acceptance, permissiveness, understanding, respect, and faith in a parent's potential for change and interchange—these are the therapeutic agents upon which the parent draws during a counseling period. As she lives through her therapy, the parent finds that her feelings of inadequacy and her unrealistic attitudes become diluted. In some cases, ultimately they evaporate. The parent becomes equipped with a kind of "psychological montage"—wherein there is a fading away of former maladaptive attitudes and an unrolling of more positive ones. The parent becomes more able to recognize the inner motivations for her child's behavior—however unacceptable and unwelcome that behavior may be. The parental need to respond to the child's behavior in terms of her own emotional response becomes reduced.

Analyzing Parent Counseling Protocols. A complete description of the group parent counseling process, including full verbatim accounts with an appropriate discussion of the speech counseling rationale, the role of the clinician, and the evaluation of parental behavioral and attitudinal changes as well as the effects of such changes upon the stuttering child, is a prospect that is worthy of several volumes in itself. The present discussion is but a brief sample designed to indicate a child-centered counseling point of view with parents of children who stutter.

Most clinicians do not have time to perform detailed analyses of their sessions with parents. Instead, they make a running, subjective evaluation of "how the parents are doing." As the counseling process unfolds, the clinician is keyed to detect such factors as: (1) indicators of parental negative or positive attitudes toward the child, (2) attitudinal changes toward the therapy or the clinician in terms of how "successful" they feel the treatment of stuttering is, and

(3) the amount of parental insight or awareness regarding the dynamics of the stuttering constellation.

In trying to siphon off the most pertinent material and meaning from the counseling sessions, it is helpful to separate parental verbalizations into categories (those cited below have been found to be most useful by the present authors). By so doing, it is possible to define, in a general way, the lines of parental development or change as the counseling sessions move along. For example, such statements as the following may be classified as *neg. att. ch.* (negative attitude toward the child*):

1. John is sucking his thumb, but we are scolding him and trying to get him to stop.
2. We made Paul go to kindergarten this year even though he hasn't liked it at all. Sometimes he even comes home before his class is over.
3. The other day I threatened Jimmy, and he asked me to count to ten.
4. Gary stuttered so completely the other night that I couldn't listen to him.
5. Bobby wants a desk of his own. I got along well in school, and I never had a desk, so I don't see why he needs one.
6. He will probably outgrow this nail-biting habit when he gets old enough to be good and ashamed of it.
7. I've always believed that children should have some fear of their fathers.

A decrease in the number of such statements as speech counseling progressed would be taken as one indicator of counseling progress.

Another category, *pos. att. ch.* (positive attitude toward the child), embraces such verbalizations as those given below, and gives another check on the counseling progress, in accordance with whether or not the statements or attitudes are shifting in number from one counseling session to another:

1. I always give Dan some jobs which he does well. It makes him feel good.

* All parental statements given in this section are from actual parent counseling sessions.

2. I feel that I should praise him when he does something which he thinks is important, although my husband doesn't agree with this.
3. I'm trying more and more to get Teddy to do things by himself—to make him more independent.
4. The other day Peter broke a neighbor's window, but I told him not to worry too much about it because that's just a thing that children do some time or other.
5. My son doesn't like to receive help from others when he talks—he has said so—so I don't think that I should help him with any words.
6. I believe that my son will find a solution to his problem within himself as he matures.

A third category that can be used concerns the number of "insights" (I) which a parent expresses during a counseling process. Statements such as the following have been judged as revealing "insight" or increasing awareness:

1. My scolding may have had a lot to do with his stuttering.
2. Perhaps we shouldn't have forced him to go to kindergarten. He may not have been mature enough for it.
3. Perhaps I did the wrong thing in getting rid of Blackie, Jimmy's dog. He never completely recovered from the shock of losing Blackie. Even has a picture of Blackie in his room. Sometimes he looks at the picture and he cries. But I have promised to get him another dog just like Blackie. I see it's important now.

Other "scoring" variables could be mentioned, such as "number of allied problems brought up by the parents during therapy," but these methods of analysis are too exploratory to warrant more than a cursory discussion. Placement of these factors in a frequency distribution table which concerns itself with the number of times these various factors are expressed by each parent can help to determine trends in counseling. The accounting in Table 3 gives some idea as to how such data may give new therapeutic meaning to the counseling process.

TABLE 3

THERAPY CHANGES IN GROUP PARENT COUNSELING

	Number of Negative Attitudes	Number of Positive Attitudes	Number of Insights	Number of Allied Problems Mentioned
Abbot	29	15	13	15
Baker	12	11	12	11
Coleman	5	6	11	10
Drake	4	6	5	8

Such a tabular description shows only trends. For example, the parent who happens to be highly verbal is apt to score higher on a number of categories, whereas the parent who is very inhibited in discussion is apt to show a much smaller number of occurrences of the given factors. The importance of this variable in terms of the amount of verbalization produced is unknown but it is probably considerable. Obviously, there is a need to correlate such parental changes with changes in the stuttering child's behavior. There is also the question of determining whether the parent's "insights" are emotional and "true" or mere intellectual ones. However subjective and tentative such a quantitative approach is, it is presented as a matter of interest.

SUMMARY

Counseling with parents of children who stutter will proceed with greater clinical competence when the fundamental importance of the following therapeutic principles is recognized:

1. Counseling is a personalized relationship between clinician and parent.
2. Counseling has its rootings in the empathic communication of feeling between client and clinician.
3. The focus on the parental role in the etiology of the child's stuttering may be anxiety-provoking for the parents who are involved in counseling.

4. The initial interviews may be the most critical of all counseling sessions.
5. Resistances will spring up in the course of counseling.
6. The prognosis for counseling is brighter if the parent approaches counseling with a high degree of motivation.
7. The clinician has to find for himself a therapeutic orientation in which he believes and in which he has both clinical competency and experience.
8. Intellectual presentation of advice by the clinician has limited value for most parents of children who stutter.
9. Systematic record-keeping on the counseling sessions by means of tape recordings is helpful.
10. The clinician perceives the parents of the child who stutters with acceptance, empathy, and respect.
11. The clinician has faith in the parent's ability to use the counseling sessions productively.
12. The clinician avoids even a tincture of cynicism or censure from tainting the all-important counseling relationships, accepting and trying to understand fully the motivants for disturbed, disrupted parent-child interaction.

In counseling parents of children who stutter, the clinician holds to the aims which are offered in this age-old prayer of St. Francis of Assisi:

> Where there is hatred . . . let me sow love
> Where there is injury . . . pardon
> Where there is doubt . . . faith
> Where there is despair . . . hope.

REFERENCES

Axline, V. *Play Therapy*. Boston: Houghton Mifflin Co., 1947.

Bateson, G., and Mead, M. *Balinese Character*. New York: N. Y. Acad. of Sciences, 1942.

Benedek, T. "Personality Development," in *Dynamic Psychiatry*, eds. F. Alexander and H. Ross. Chicago: Univ. of Chicago Press, 1952, pp. 63–113.

Blanton, S. *Love or Perish*. New York: Simon & Schuster, Inc., 1956.

Bloodstein, O.; Jaeger, W.; and Tureen, J. "A Study of the Diagnosis of Stuttering by Parents of Stutterers and Nonstutterers," *J. Speech Disorders*, 3: 308–15, 1952.

BULLEN, A. "A Cross-Cultural Approach to the Problem of Stuttering," *Child Develpm.*, **16**: 1–88, 1945.

DESPERT, J. L. "A Psychosomatic Study of Fifty Stuttering Children," *Amer. J. Orthopsychiat.*, **16**: 100–16, 1946.

GLAUBER, I. P. "The Mother in the Etiology of Stuttering," abstract of a report in the *Psychoanalytic Quarterly*, **20**: 160–61, 1951.

GOODSTEIN, L., and DAHLSTROM, W. "MMPI Differences Between Parents of Stuttering and Nonstuttering Children," *J. consult. Psychol.*, **20**: 365–70, 1956.

HOBBS, N. "Group-Centered Psychotherapy," in *Client-Centered Therapy*, ed. C. Rogers. New York: Houghton Mifflin Co., 1951, pp. 278–319.

JOHNSON, W. *People in Quandaries.* New York: Harper & Bros., 1946.

———. "Perceptual Factors in Stuttering," in *Handbook of Speech Pathology*, ed. L. E. Travis. New York: Appleton-Century-Crofts, Inc., 1957, pp. 897–915.

———. "The Indians Have No Word for It," *Quarterly J. Speech*, **30**: 456–65, 1944.

KANNER, L. *A Word to Parents About Mental Hygiene.* Madison, Wisc.: Univ. of Wisconsin Press, 1957.

———. *Child Psychiatry*, 2d ed. Springfield, Ill.: Charles C Thomas, Publisher, 1950.

MONCUR, J. "Environmental Factors Differentiating Stuttering Children from Nonstuttering Children," *Speech Monogr.*, **18**: 312–25, 1951.

———. "Parental Domination in Stuttering," *J. Speech Hearing Disorders*, **17**: 155–65, 1952.

ROGERS, C. *Client-Centered Therapy.* Boston: Houghton Mifflin Co., 1951.

———. *Counseling and Psychotherapy.* Boston: Houghton Mifflin Co., 1942.

SNIDECOR, J. "Why the Indian Does Not Stutter," *Quarterly J. Speech*, **33**: 493–95, 1947.

WYATT, G. L. "A Developmental Crisis Theory of Stuttering," *Lang. and Speech*, **1**: 250–64, 1958.

Chapter 13

The Stutterer, the Teacher, and the Speech Clinician

How long a time lies in one little word.——Shakespeare

It is a truism that education is, after all, only another name for helping human beings to achieve maximum productivity and happiness through the release and development of their natural capacities. In this sense, the classroom teacher may be the best speech "field worker." She has the opportunity to observe and to draw upon the abundance of material which is enacted before her—day by day, week by week, month by month. She is able to watch the child during the course of his daily interaction in his educational, peer, and social environments. The majority of teachers do good jobs of sensing and satisfying the varied emotional needs of the 30 or 40 children in their charge. Indeed, in observing a child in the great variety of situations which the school offers, teachers would have to be emotionally myopic not to notice Mary, the quiet one; Johnny, the aggressive one; Billy, the day-dreaming one; Nancy, the lisping one; or Danny, the fearful one. Recognizing the more subtle behavior signs of children's emotional troubles as well as making discriminating analyses of the child's symptoms of inner tensions and conflicts requires experience and study. But, when all is said and done, the average teacher does meet a great many of the emotional needs of his many charges in addition to fulfilling his chief aim, instruction. Of course thousands of teachers experience daily frustrations in their sincere attempts to do what they honestly feel is best for a child's emotional growth. They are frustrated by the large classes they have to teach as well as by referral centers which are inadequate or non-existent. Sometimes the whole burden of satisfying the child's emotional needs is placed squarely on the shoulders of the teacher with but rare assistance from others.

THE TEACHER AND THE CHILD WHO STUTTERS

Infancy and childhood should supply a child with emotional and interpersonal relationships which yield satisfactions and security. Yet many children enter school with emotional and interpersonal voids which teachers and school administrators see reflected in symptomatic reading problems, learning difficulties, speech disorders of psychogenic origins, aggression, destructiveness, nail biting, jealousy, nervousness, thumb sucking, phobic reactions, temper tantrums, tics, and withdrawal—problems which children manifest in and out of the classroom (FitzSimons, 1960). When a child comes to school, he brings with him his past life; i.e., he reflects interjected parental attitudes, wisdoms, suppressions, kindnesses, inconsistencies, aspirations, and fears. Preschool learnings, especially the family experiences, have created a unique personality. The child is apt to think of new adults in accordance with the nature of his past experiences with adults, especially the parents. He is apt to assume attitudes toward and experience feelings about adults in relation to the kinds of attitudes and feelings he had developed about his parents. For example, Jimmy may be afraid of the teacher even before he meets her. He looks fearful and cries. His mother has to remain with him in the classroom the first morning—or perhaps even the entire first week. On the other hand, Mary may like the teacher immediately. She is comfortable and begins to participate in the group activity right away. Even before the teacher begins her association with the child, she may be helped or handicapped according to the child's ability to meet and adjust to any new situation.

Many children who stutter display their speech symptom for the first time upon entering the school situation. It is at this time that the teacher becomes, for the child, a substitute parent. To the child, the similarity of the classroom to the family situation may be great or little, depending primarily on the degree and kind of acceptance or rejection used by parents and teacher and the correlation between each's attitudes. If a stutterer has been exposed to a dominating, perfectionistic parent, and his first class teacher is of the same mold, the school becomes merely an extension of an unfortunate home setting. If the teacher is less authoritarian and a more pliable, affectionate person, the schoolroom may become the child's main safety valve by providing him with welcome relief from home. The teacher can be the key. If the attitude of the teacher is kindly, the suppressed child may overreact to the new-found freedom. He may test her to the limits. This can be a particularly crucial period in the child's personality readjustment. If the teacher is able to work through such a child's acting-out phase with him, if she can wait for the child to become certain that he is being accepted for what he really is, a great speech-feeling victory will have been won.

Sometimes the young stutterer is labeled immediately as a "problem" by the teacher. A reasonable question sometimes would be to ask oneself whether or not the "problem" is more the teacher's than the child's. For example, many teachers are themselves fearful of speaking in certain situations. They avoid making speeches before parents or allied professional groups; and when they must speak to such groups they may stumble and mumble in the process. Their difficulty here may be caused by anxiety or tension, lack of preparation, a feeling of inadequacy, or fear of adverse reaction from listening administrators and peers. Yet, we do not necessarily think of them as "problems." The teacher sometimes contributes to the child's speech problem in still other ways. A teacher or clinician may project his own speech anxieties onto the stutterer or even become more impatient or critical of this personification or mirror image of his own "weakness." Others, because of their own feelings, may empathize too completely with the stutterer, identifying with his attitudes toward speaking and thus be unable to help with his speech problem.

In the life of a child, the teacher's importance may be second only to that of the child's parents. School life ranks next to family life in its influence upon a child's development. In terms of the actual beginning of a child's emotional-speech problem, the teacher's role may be completely nonexistent. Yet, the teacher remains a key person who can regulate the emotional and the communicative comfort of children, especially children who stutter. It is the teacher who creates the emotional environment in which the child is called upon to formulate extrafamilial peer relationships. It is the teacher who structures the learning milieu in which the child must strive to attain academic achievements which are consistent with his intellectual capacity. It is the teacher who compounds feeling-learning relationships which contribute to the child's feelings of either self-acceptance or self-inadequacy. It is the teacher who establishes an emotionally comfortable classroom climate which can help children who have speech handicaps to reduce anxiety, and concomitantly, increase speech ease and fluency.

In all human relationships, projection is operant. The stuttering child can project hidden hostilities and feelings from parents to teachers, i.e., from significant adult onto significant adult. Many children who stutter have experienced early socialization conflicts which lead to covert feelings of hostility and self-concepts which are based on personal inadequacy feelings. Sometimes the early training and management interaction between mother and child fails to center on and nurture basic emotional needs. Such experiences can be the motivant for a flareup of speech and language problems such as stuttering, as well as the motivation behind feelings of hostility and personal inadequacy within the child. As the child grows older, his speech disturbance yields him even more instances in which his basic emotional and language needs are violated. The speech-handicapped child is corrected, compelled to exert more effort, or counseled to speak more slowly and more clearly. He may be made to feel ashamed of his speech attempts. In short, he and his speech are never accepted completely. The warmth and the understanding of an acceptant teacher can be counteractives for the negative projections and the feeling of personal and communicative inadequacy which the speech-handicapped pupil may bring with him to his classroom. Thus the teacher's importance in the creation of both a positive classroom atmosphere and a positive teacher-pupil relationship—based on acceptance, respect, and understanding—can never be overestimated (Johnson, 1956).

A positive learning climate, based upon child needs and sound mental hygiene principles, provides the kind of atmosphere essential to psychological and educational comfort and growth. The absence of such an atmosphere decreases the chances of the stuttering child's becoming a better organized, happier, and more fluent speaker.

School experiences probably seldom create a stuttering problem; however, the classroom situation can intensify or reduce the child's discomfort and his stuttering, depending upon the absence or presence of a warm, accepting teacher attitude and schoolroom atmosphere. Stutterers in the classroom situation often are unable or do not get the opportunity to verbalize or otherwise reveal their innermost thoughts, desires, and conflicts. The true thoughts of most stutterers about themselves in relation to the class setting and about their teachers seldom are aired directly, except perhaps in a confidential therapy situation, at which times such statements as the following are made: "Every time I stutter, she looks away, and that is the worst thing anybody can do to me"; "she makes me so angry whenever she says the word for me—doesn't she think I can get it out by myself—but I just take it"; "I like her all right, except every time she says to slow down or speak more slowly, I just about bust. God, wouldn't I speak slower if I only could—wouldn't I?"

A former stutterer has reported in an educational journal (Shapoff, 1954) how he might have been helped to live his school life more comfortably if his teacher had been more alert in fostering within him a greater sense of security as a stutterer. Shapoff discussed the ways in which one of his former teachers failed to meet his needs as a pupil who stuttered. He recounted his feeling of not belonging as he found himself consigned to the side lines by this teacher, after an initial encounter with his stuttering reactions in the course of classroom interpersonal communications. He recalled his craving for peer relationships and his teacher's failure to utilize his musical aptitude as a means to provide him with recognition which he needed so gravely. He contrasted this teacher's attitude with that of an understanding teacher who became a most positive life force for him. Shapoff stated that the understanding teacher is one who believes that the aims in guiding the personality development of the pupil who stutters are the same as those for any other child.

To be effective, school experiences should promote the mental health of the students as well as their academic achievement. There has been increasing recognition in recent decades of the importance of psychological principles in education. The concept of a positive psychological learning "climate," recognition of the importance of attitudes and feelings, and the impress of the emotions on learning efficiency are reflected in a wide range of literature which represents many disciplines such as psychiatry (Lippman, 1956; Wolberg, 1954), field-theory psychology (Lewin, Lippitt, and White, 1939), client-centered therapy (Arbuckle, 1957; Axline, 1947; Rogers, 1957), contemporary psychology and education (Burton, 1952; Cantor, 1953; Johnson, 1957; Leeper, 1948; Wiles, 1952). Of course the extent to which these psychological insights are implemented in daily teacher-pupil interaction depends primarily on the individual teacher. To some degree, as far as stuttering pupils are concerned, the extent to which the teacher incorporates such concepts may depend on the kind of working relationship there is between the child's speech clinician and his classroom teacher.

Each teacher reacts to his pupils in the light of his own individualized dynamisms, and he influences various dynamic responses within the pupils in his class in accordance with his own needs. Reactions of teachers to stutterers may range from complete acceptance to complete rejection. Optimal learning and adequate emotional comfort in the learning situation occur under the instructor who understands the child's needs. Less learning occurs when the class situation is geared primarily to a working through and a satisfaction of the teacher's own needs. The child who stutters has a problem that usually is tied in with feelings of anxiety. Anxiety, being a state of uneasiness or apprehension, tends to interfere with concentration on tasks. Thus the presence of anxiety in a child tends to disrupt his learning potential. Highly formal classroom and speech therapy settings are types of situations which provide little or no diminution of the stutterer's general emotional discomfort. Anxiety prevents any child from accomplishing in terms of work accuracy and output. A child's failures may meet with the teacher's criticism in the form of strong verbal or implied unspoken constraints. The more anxious the child is, the more he is apt to stutter, and the more lacking in concentration he will become. The more distracted or uneasy he becomes the less purposeful and accurate will be both his work production and his speaking efficiency. Anxiety can generate more anxiety, more stuttering, and more learning and work inadequacies.

Teachers are continually reminded of how to identify "problem children." While it takes no special training to identify a stutterer, identifying the personality dynamics of the individual stutterer often requires special training and abilities. Most teachers do their best in trying to clarify the causes of children's problems and attempting to uncover solutions to them. Sometimes merely taking a special interest in a stutterer will help reduce the stuttering—the extra attention, if it is not overpowering, may satisfy recognition needs sufficiently to reduce the child's inner discomforts. Increasingly, teachers make informal studies of challenging children. A passage from Stewart and Workman, whose book is highly recommended reading for all teachers and clinicians, gives an excellent sequence of events teachers may utilize in learning more about children with special problems:

. . . It may be helpful for the teacher to think of himself as a detective. He looks in the simplest way possible for clues which may explain whether or why the child is a "problem." Because he is not a specialist in making a case study and because he has many other things to do than spend an excessive amount of time studying a single individual, the teacher must begin his study at the easiest level. He can begin by thinking, as he drives to and from school, about such questions as these: Am I unfriendly or do I dislike this child not because of what he does but because of the way I feel about him and if so why? Are my teaching methods right for him? Am I expecting too much or too little? Does he need my help in finding friends and truly belonging in the classroom? Am I retaliatory when he does something "wrong?" In other words, the teacher tries to estimate how and why he reacts as he does to the child.

The teacher then makes a plan of operation from his analysis. He attempts to modify his own behavior on the basis of this self-analysis. He tries to become less punitive, more consistent, more patient, and more firmly strict, the course of his behavior being determined by his "rethinking" about the "problem child." If modification in his behavior does not prove beneficial, he will search the school record file to see whether anything helpful is to be found there. He examines the I.Q. to discover whether there are any discrepancies among the scores, or between the scores and his judgment of the child's intelligence. He does the same thing with achievement test scores. These test scores may show him that he has expected too much or too little of the child, or that the child's problem is connected with lack of opportunity to exercise special abilities, among other reasons. He particularly notes what other teachers have thought of the child as indicated by their comments or the marks that they give him. He may find that things went well until a certain year. What happened in that year to the child? He may find a certain kind of teacher got along better with the child than another. "Why?" he asks himself.

With all this information in his mind, the teacher continues to think. Like the detective, he is formulating new hypotheses from the number of easily accessible sources.

. . . If the problem persists after these preliminary steps, he begins to make more organized observations of the child's behavior. This does not mean that the teacher need scout around the classroom with a notebook in hand, jotting down everything the child does. But he can look and listen more closely than he did before. Looking takes on new meaning and purpose for him. He looks now to compare the child's behavior by himself with that in small groups and in large groups; with members of his own or the opposite sex; with adults as well as with children; in the playground and in more formal work environments.

Whether the teacher writes his observations down or not is dependent upon the time he has. The important thing . . . is that he sees as accurately as possible what the child is really doing. In brief, he may find that he has developed preconceptions of the child's behavior which careful observations invalidated.

. . . These observations may give a whole new picture of the child and may lead him to the root of the problem. Discrepancies, unexpected insecurities or facade aggressiveness may be revealing to the teacher in his search for the way of the child's behavior.

There are other steps the teacher may take in studying a problem child. He can talk over the child's behavior with his principal, supervisor, and other concerned teachers. In some cases, parent conferences are in order, and in some systems the services of various specialists are available (Stewart and Workman, 1956, pp. 217–19).

TEACHER-CLINICIAN RELATIONS

Just as parents and teachers react to the child in terms of their own dynamic motivants, such motivants characterize the interaction between the teacher and clinician. Ideally, the teacher-clinician relationship is one based upon mutual professional respect. For each is a needed professional who shares the common goal of working with the stutterer so that he may reach his maximal potential. However, it is the psychological need structure of both teacher and clinician which will be the determining factor in whether or not an attitude most conducive to a stutterer's growth prevails. Sometimes misunderstandings and defensive behavior creep into the relationship, distorting it so that little of the desired professional interaction is apparent. Although most teachers are receptive and cooperative, it is not unusual for speech clinicians to meet resistance from a teacher concerning the clinician's procedures, philosophy, and scheduling of case load. This condition is more likely to occur (1) if a speech therapy program is just beginning within the system; (2) if the speech clinician is a young, inexperienced person; (3) if the prevailing general administrative or school policies concerning special services are not defined clearly; (4) if the teacher's own general philosophy and personality are rigid and resistive; or (5) if the clinician himself is inconsistent, anxious, disorganized, or inept. (In the latter case even the best adjusted teacher may rightfully "resist" the general speech therapy program, including the suggested procedure of dealing with the stutterer in the classroom.)

But even an impaired teacher-clinician relationship is not a hopeless, static thing. Resistances can be worked through by means of an awareness of the dynamic motivants which are at work, by a counseling attitude and approach by the clinician, and by adherence to the best in current educational leadership practices. Acceptance, permissiveness, and respect are the vehicles by which resistances are brought to the fore for clarification and interpretation. In keeping with this principle, a clinician aims at fostering a democratic, nonauthoritarian, permissive relationship with the speech-handicapped child's teacher. Conferences between the teacher and the clinician can be scheduled on a permissive basis.

One method for the implementation of a teacher's scheduling of conferences is the placement of a "clinician to teacher letter" and a "teacher-clinician conference sheet" upon the school's bulletin board. On page one of the sheet appear the directions for its use. On page two are the following headings: the teacher's name, the child's initials, the date of the conference, the time of the conference. The teacher fills out the card before the clinician arrives at the school. The clinician checks the card upon his arrival so that he may arrange his work according to the conferences on schedule. Teacher-clinician conferences are of necessity brief, ranging from 5 to 15 minutes. On occasion, when a longer conference is in order, an after-school meeting may be arranged.

Teacher counseling concerning stuttering differs from parent counseling. The parent is attached intimately and emotionally to his child. Seldom do teachers have such a strong, close emotional attachment to a pupil. Most certainly, a positive teacher-pupil relationship is warm and friendly, but it does not have the deep emotional bond of the parent-child relationship. Thus a teacher usually is more able to view and appraise the child with greater objectivity than are many stutterers' parents.

The teacher should be able to regard the clinician as a consultant on whom she may call for suggestions and help. In counseling with the teachers of stuttering children, imparting information on an intellectual basis has only limited usefulness, although bibliotherapy or suggested reading in response to a teacher request for information may have some value in chosen cases. Sometimes a teacher will have unreasonable expectations of the speech clinician. Having referred the child to the clinician, she may shrug off further responsibilities for his problem or she may even be on the alert for therapy failure as a compensation for her own sense of failure with the stutterer. And, of course, weeks and even months of speech therapy may pass without any visible signs of improvement. The teacher and clinician who are aware of this possibility from the beginning will increase their chances of a more harmonious and comfortable working relationship.

Speech clinicians themselves may set up blocks to successful counseling if they have an exaggerated conception of the importance of their role or if they feel inadequate and defensive because they are fearful of not being able to help or cure every stutterer. The teacher-clinician counseling relationship, and thus the child, may suffer as a consequence. In addition, just as a rigid, uncompromising, intellect-bound teacher may impede the establishment of a productive counseling relationship by the speech clinician, so can a rigid, uncompromising speech clinician hinder the establishment of a good teacher-clinician counseling relationship. In the case of the uncompromising teacher, the clinician may find it difficult to change basic attitudes, and the stutterer will continue to suffer from the exposure to the teacher and the learning climate in which the instruction is given. In the case of the uncompromising clinician, the accepting teacher, in accordance with her own best dictates, will continue to act as the principal therapist for the child, regardless of what specific advice or rules may be offered by a rigid clinician.

In teacher counseling, as in the counseling of parents, the clinician feels deeply an acceptance of and respect for the teacher. The experience of the relationship which is built upon the needed deep acceptance and respect enables the teacher to better extend these to the stutterer. Acceptance, empathy, permissiveness, and respect on the part of the clinician are the sparks which may detonate attitudinal changes within the teacher, and eventually, positive changes within the stutterer.

The viewpoints within this chapter should not be construed to mean that the average teacher can develop a systematic, psychotherapeutic, speech-rehabilitation program within her classroom for the stutterer who may be more emotionally disturbed. With severely involved stutterers, the role that the teacher can play in working through, analyzing, and re-developing feelings and attitudes becomes quite limited, even though her warm and receptive relationship with the stutterer is therapeutic. The more disturbed the stutterer, the more necessary it becomes for him to have the services of specialists who are highly skilled in the diagnosis and treatment of a stuttering behavior disorder. Admittedly, the teacher's chief goal is instructional; however, in order to be successful here, the teacher must become a communicator of more than the subjects in the school's curriculum. When the classroom teacher communicates the psychological necessities of acceptance, respect, and understanding as well as subject matter knowledge, all pupils, including the pupil who stutters, will find optimal educational placement.

The basic aims of the speech clinician who counsels teachers regarding the therapeutic activity and classroom behavior of stutterers are: (1) to help maintain or develop teacher attitudes which are more accepting, democratic, and oriented to the stutterer's *feelings;* (2) to help decrease or erase teacher attitudes which are suppressive, rejecting, autocratic, and oriented chiefly to the stutterer's intellectual or speech behavior; (3) to explain (when necessary), interpret, and present the rationale and goals of the speech therapeutic relationship with the stutterer. These goals attest to the necessity of helping teachers to understand that stuttering is a problem which is linked closely with the child's attitudes and feelings toward self, others, and changing environments. The focus of these goals is the belief that the stutterer's speech instability as well as his general behavior is only the surface manifestation of troubled feelings and that it is not something which can be handled or molded into a more desirable form by suppression, pity, criticism, or sheer intellectual control. The allied aims are to develop a practical and realistic degree of permissiveness within the classroom setting in order to help free the stutterer's repressed behavior; and to create an atmosphere in which both the stutterer's and the teacher's feelings can be accepted and clarified whenever possible.

TRANSCRIPTS OF TEACHER-CLINICIAN COUNSELING SESSIONS

Some teachers are preoccupied with academic achievement, conformity, and the surface implications of the child's maladaptive behavior. Other teachers may possess a deep sensitivity to the full meaning which a satisfying personal relationship can have for their pupils as well as for themselves. In either case, teacher counseling during teacher-clinician conferences concerns itself with the attitudes and feelings of the teacher as she interacts with the pupil who stutters. Most of the excerpts of teacher-clinician discussions in this chapter are accounts of actual situations, recorded as accurately as possible by clinicians immediately following the incidents. The selection represents some of the different types of counseling relationships a speech clinician can experience in a public school setting. The selections, although excerpts of complete sessions, will indicate the directions that teacher counseling often takes as the clinician works to keep or obtain an emotionally healthful classroom climate for stuttering pupils. In all accounts "T" refers to the teacher and "Cl" refers to the clinician.

The Suppressive, Intellectual Classroom Teacher. (As the clinician walks by Gary's second-grade classroom, the teacher is standing by the open door.)

T. 1: What do you think of a boy who doesn't finish his work day after day—a boy who just sits and does nothing but write his name on his papers. You know whom I'm talking about, don't you Gary? (Gary, with a hurt look in his eyes, fails to respond verbally. The teacher is alert in her response to Gary's silence but indifferent to the emotional reactions which a public condemnation produced. The teacher's manner brings forth a "y-y-yes, M-M-M-Mrs. North." Gary appears constricted and consumed by the teacher's verbal cuff to his self esteem.)

Cl. 1: There are a lot of reasons I suppose for Gary's not getting his work done, eh? (This statement conveys no condemnation but rather attempts to give some support to Gary in his moment of need. The clinician moves from the doorway and the conference continues in the corridor. During his speech-therapy period Gary will have an opportunity to rid himself of any troubling feelings which this situation may have provoked.)

T. 2: He never finishes a thing. He just sits there. Takes him an hour to move. I keep after him. I take away his privileges. But I can't get any work out of him. He really annoys me.

Cl. 2: You really have strong feelings about this situation with Gary.

T. 3: Well, he's such a problem. When I stand over him and prod him, he'll get busy. But on his own, he does nothing. I have too large a class to work with him constantly.

Cl. 3: The large class and Gary—both are real problems.

T. 4: A problem—he's so different to have in a room. You can't reach him. Even his own mother says the same thing. He's a problem to her. She finds him just the way I do.

CL. 4: Gary is a problem at school and at home. In counseling Gary's mother, by the way, my goal just now is a reduction in punishment and disciplinary action.

T. 5: Does Mrs. D. punish him a lot?

CL. 5: She's very concerned about his lack of work. She checks on him every day and when his papers aren't finished, she punishes him by sending him to bed at 6 o'clock—right after dinner.

T. 6: Hmm. I didn't know that. He's really getting an overdose.

CL. 6: Too much punishment.

T. 7: You know, she's probably wrong there—in a way I've been doing here what he's getting at home.

CL. 7: (Waits.)

T. 8: Getting it at both ends.

CL. 8: Everything pinpointed right at him—all his faults—his troubles.

T. 9: Going to bed at 6 o'clock. That's too much. Well, probably I'll ease up on him and see what happens.

CL. 9: Try a new approach, you mean?

T. 10: Well, I'll close my eyes and see what happens. Maybe what I don't see won't hurt—him or me.

CL. 10: You've got a real challenge all right—large class and all. But less pressure on him should pay big dividends.

In this situation, the teacher was hoping that the speech clinician would support her own attitude by agreeing with her. The clinician avoided this (Cl2) by reflecting the teacher's first statement in a manner which was supportive for Gary and continued to reflect the teacher's feelings, allowing an opportunity for the ventilation of those feelings. (Cl2, 3, 4). The teacher has become aware as to how she may serve a more positive role in Gary's school adjustment. The clinician is supportive toward the teacher and gives a more direct statement of agreement concerning the new attitude to be adopted.

It will be helpful here to alter the above transcription to show how the conversation would have sounded if the speech clinician had taken a more formal and intellectual approach to Gary's problem.

The Formal, Intellectual Clinician and the Classroom Teacher

T. 1: What do you think of a boy who doesn't finish his work day after day—a boy who just sits and writes his name on his papers. You know who I'm talking about, don't you Gary?

CL. 1: I'm sorry to hear that.

T. 2: He never finishes a thing. Just sits there. Takes him an hour to move. I keep after him. I take away his privileges. But I can't get any work out of him. He really annoys me.

CL. 2: I can't understand it. He's such a pleasant boy when I work with him.

T. 3: He's such a problem. When I stand over him and prod him, he'll get busy. But on his own, he does nothing. I have too large a class to work on him constantly.

CL. 3: Well, he does need to concentrate in order to do well. I can see that in his speaking. If he concentrates on slowing down and relaxing, then he speaks more fluently.

T. 4: A problem—he's so difficult to have in the room. You can't reach him. Even his own mother says the same thing. He's a problem to her. She finds him just the way I do.

CL. 4: Have you been able to give him successful speaking experiences? That may help. Giving him assignments that will give him some recognition.

This intellectual interchange reveals little concern for the child's feelings. In fact, the two adults are hardly communicating. In Cl1 the clinician shows disappointment in the stutterer and implicitly sides with the teacher. In Cl2 the clinician does not try to help the teacher to determine causes for Gary's behavior, nor does the clinician allow the teacher to give vent to her feelings. Instead, the clinician gives a personal reaction which implies that if Gary is a pleasant boy in the speech-therapy situation and not in the classroom, it is probably because the teacher is less adept at handling him. (Even though unintended by the clinician, it may well be the inference drawn by the teacher.) In Cl3, in siding with the teacher's suppressive techniques, the clinician reveals something of his own methods with the stutterer. In Cl4 the clinician moves directively toward a more positive speech structure but misses the crucial need by failing to react to the teacher's feelings in a way that would be more informative and more developmental for all persons concerned.

The Moralistic, Judgmental Classroom Teacher. This conference follows Don's first speech-therapy session in a new school semester. Rapport between Don and his clinician was positive, having been built upon a six-month period of previous therapy. Don had stormed into the therapy room saying, "I hate her. I hate her. I hate her" (in reference to his new sixth-grade teacher). The teacher-clinician conference follows:

CL. 1: I notice that Don's speech is quite hesitant just now. How are things going?

T. 1: Well, his stuttering has increased since the first week of school. He's a very difficult child to have in the room. Can't reach him. He erects a wall of surliness. This morning he annoyed me so much. I asked a question about his spelling test, and he answered my question with "yeh." He didn't even mention my name. I reminded him that I did have a name, but he refused to say it. He claimed that he forgot what my name was. I never had such a boy—very annoying.

CL. 2: You feel that Don is a difficult pupil to reach and to handle.

T. 2: In my experience I've met many children, but no one ever was so *fresh*, and that is the only word for him, fresh as a boy can be. I cannot find a way to approach him. When I correct him, he acts as though I weren't there. Bad for the other children, too. Frankly, I wish he weren't in the room. It's a battle. He does something he shouldn't—I correct him—he pays no attention to me.

CL. 3: His behavior is very disturbing to you.

T. 3: I feel lost. I can't reach him. I find that I—well he's not the most likeable boy.

CL. 4: He's a problem to you and most of all to himself.

T. 4: He's a problem all right. No teacher can really deal very easily with a boy like that. He's so disrespectful.

CL. 5: He doesn't show you any respect.

T. 5: Just ignores me. I can correct him and rebuke him, but I may as well not be here. I don't exist for him.

CL. 6: His relationships with all his teachers, from the first grade, have been negative. His surliness probably is not directed against you personally because it has actually been directed against all the teachers whom he has ever met. I'm pretty certain that he feels that all teachers don't like him, and he has come to the point where he doesn't like teachers. So he's a problem for teachers, but he's the greatest problem for himself. He's had authority rammed down his throat at home and elsewhere, so now he gags on it, resisting it every inch of the way.

The negative attitude of the teacher is revealed in her first statement (T1). Instead of a positive rapport between teacher and pupil, there is only a constant skirmish of aggression and counteraggression on the part of both teacher and stutterer. The clinician in Cl2, 3, and 4 is not interjecting, advising, or disagreeing. Rather he is listening acceptingly, reflecting back the teacher's outpourings and encouraging the teacher to release her feelings about the boy. The teacher is self-righteous and moralistic with the stutterer's adjustment problem. Obedience to the laws of the classroom, and respect for one's elders and those in authority, constitute the philosophy here. There is no concession, no meeting halfway. Whatever a child does is either all right or all wrong. In this setting, the stutterer stands little chance of improvement, of developing realistic aspiration levels, of being able to express his ideas and feelings, and of being able to see that adults can make mistakes too. The clinician will try to work with the teacher, but he realizes that the task in attitude changing in this instance may be arduous or even impossible.

The next excerpt reveals the clinician working with a teacher who is sensitive to the stutterer's basic, driving, life forces. This teacher is competent in meeting her pupils' psychological and instructional needs. She has a good academic background and she vitalizes her work with a philosophy structured upon a sincere belief in the potent influence of personality dynamics in all of life's achievements and failures.

The Well-Adjusted Classroom Teacher.

T. 1: Roger's reading is not up to grade level just yet. I've had him read with two groups, Group B and Group C, or as the children decided to call them, the Buicks and the Cadillacs. When Roger is reading in Group C, he doesn't stutter, but in Group B, he stutters a good deal. He looks so uncomfortable. He keeps his head down and sometimes he bites his nails. I think it would be to his advantage to take him out of Group B, but I don't want to make him conscious of his shortcomings, to make something too "special" out of him. So I asked him which group he'd rather read in, and he picked Group B. I'm a little in doubt as to what to do if anything at this point.

CL. 1: You really want to do the best thing for him, but getting the best answer isn't always easy.

T. 2: He's smart, and I think he's aware of that. Group B is a higher reading group.

CL. 2: He sets a high level of achievement for himself in just about everything he does. That's especially true in speaking. In fact, that's one of his main difficulties. He can't settle for anything less than perfection—can't settle for something less than that—less fluent speech in that case, less proficient reading in this case. I think we've both been trying to help him break up these strong perfectionistic strivings. Changing that attitude is going to take plenty of time and effort on our part, as you well know.

T. 3: Perhaps I'll mention casually to him that he no longer needs the extra practice of reading with two groups. After all, that's true—he has improved very nicely.

CL. 3: That's a possibility. Ease him over that way.

T. 4: I'll mention his improvement, and then I'll tell him that he may come up with either group. In that way, he may choose his own group.

CL. 4: Giving Roger a part in his own self-direction, letting him make the decision, that will be important to him.

In the preceding protocol, the clinician's role is more direct. The discussion is actually a factual exchange. The more intellectual discussion is more properly indicated here for several reasons. This teacher is not an anxious, defensive person. She is sensitive to emotional needs, objective, and accurate in her appraisal of human behavior, including her own. She sees things as they really are. There is no need for the clinician to structure a "permissive" or nondirective climate. The important points of the matter are gone to directly. With such a teacher, the prognosis for the stutterer becomes decidedly more optimistic. (Incidentally, Roger selected Group C, the lower reading group, and his behavior during subsequent reading periods was marked by greater comfort, more confidence, and less stuttering.)

The Oversolicitous Classroom Teacher. Occasionally a teacher worries excessively about a stutterer. She is shaken by his every discomfort and speech disruption. She sees the stutterer as needing special care, but she intensifies the situation beyond reality's requirements. She frets as he blocks in class, shakes her head, and spends a great deal of energy in helping the stutterer—except that the help, being excessive, is actually a form of perpetual and inept supervision.

T. 1: I'm so glad to see you. Eddie's been awful this week—can't get a word out. I can just cry when I look at that boy. Pitiful.

CL. 1: What's been happening?

T. 2: Well, he's just drawn into a shell more. I've given him every chance. I skip over him and over his reports. I cover up for him before the pupils if he stutters. I explain what he's trying to get out, you know.

CL. 2: Doing everything you can for him.

T. 3: Well, not exactly, but trying to make things easier. Keep telling him to take it easy, but he's all tied up in knots—can't relax.

CL. 3: He does need chances to get rid of some of that energy, those bottled up feelings.

T. 4: Isn't there something I can do? Anything at all. He never stutters when he's singing—you know that. I've been wondering if he could speak sort of singsong. I've heard that's helped people. I could try that.

CL. 4: Well, as you say, he's tied up in knots. He keeps all his feelings to himself. It must be pretty uncomfortable and I suppose the real problem is to relieve him of some of his discomfort. If we can do that, he'll relax more. You've seen how he speaks better when he's relaxed. Of course, it has to be a natural kind of relaxation.

T. 5: You know, I keep telling him to relax; we're all his friends here, but he can't relax.

CL. 5: I can see you spend a lot of time thinking about it.

T. 6: After all, he's my responsibility. It's so uncomfortable in here when he goes into one of those—spasms. You feel you have to do something. Tuesday I tried something new. Maybe you'll say I did the wrong thing. I had him rest his head on his desk for a few minutes before giving his talk on what they did during vacation week. But, it didn't help. I had to interrupt his talk. He was stuttering so badly. I told him that he could try with the next group. . . .

Eddie is being suffocated by well-meant but ineffective attention. He is set up as the "different" one. He is catered to, but there is little concern about his discomfort or his reactions to such oversolicitude. If he doesn't already, eventually Eddie will see himself as a special person requiring special methods, special attention, and special supervision in order to be what people want him to be. He may even come to use these "reasons" to justify his failures. The teacher's overtures to "make him better" are created by her own discomforts or projections about the situation. The pupil who stutters becomes overconcerned, chronically overconcerned, more anxious about his inadequacies and his lack of ability to do "better" when the teacher is "good enough to do all these special things to help me." The child's classmates are daily witnesses to his teacher-induced failures. Under such conditions, Eddie's stuttering becomes worse, and nobody can understand why.

A NOTE ABOUT THE "STUTTEROPHOBIC" CLASSROOM TEACHER

Some teachers are afraid of stutterers. A stutterer can be regarded as a threat (a previously unknown challenge) or as a symbol of defeat—"doesn't improve in my classroom." People who are uncomfortable with stutterers are able to cope with the distress quite simply enough—they merely withdraw from the stutterer. The teacher cannot elect this mode of adjustment, however. Usually, when the class assignments are made, Johnny is in a teacher's room for the rest of the year. A teacher who is fearful or anxious with the stuttering child is very probably most anxious about her own inadequacy in working with him. The more fearful she is, the better are the chances that exaggerations will creep into the situation. Adults usually are fairly capable of camouflaging overt fear reactions, but it is the covert elements (the skeletal and visceral components of the fear-reaction) which comprise the anxiety and lead to the use of faulty adjustive techniques with stutterers. The teacher who avoids the stutterer by not calling on him, who never speaks to him, or who is dictatorial or aggressive toward a stutterer, by way of a defensive retaliation to the "feared object," may be thought of as "stutterophobic." The clinician will need to be alert to the possibility that a few teachers' faulty relationships with stutterers may be based partially on a true fear of them. This type of situation is more likely to appear with teachers of teen-agers and adults, since older pupils tend to be, in general, more threatening to anxious teachers.

CONCLUDING REMARKS

Teachers want and need to meet the personal, special needs of stuttering pupils. But they must be prepared emotionally and cognitively for the demands involved. Thus, goals for attitudinal-behavioral-cognitive changes toward children who stutter can be achieved with classroom teachers through counseling and the use of bibliotherapy (Murphy, FitzSimons, and Pronovost, 1956). A teacher's past experiences or the lack of experience with stuttering pupils consciously or unconsciously influence her handling of stuttering individuals. The success or the lack of success which a given teacher achieves with a given speech-handicapped child will become generalized, influencing her attitude and behavior with other stuttering children with whom she will come in contact during subsequent teaching. Therefore it becomes important for the optimal psychological and communicative well-being of children who stutter that information concerning these children be presented within a counseling frame of reference with an emphasis upon support, acceptance, and clarification of the teacher's feelings concerning the information given, rather than with an accentuation upon the information per se. To summarize, it may be said:

1. The teacher is a crucial figure in the life of a stuttering pupil. She may provide a therapeutic experience along with educational growth or she may accentuate the stuttering problem. Her own basic attitudes and philosophy indicate the direction that her pupil relationships will take.
2. The teacher's ability to help a given stutterer varies not only in relation to her own personality but in relation to the availability, type, and philosophy of allied special services.
3. Stuttering pupils are not "made" in a classroom. Stutterers bring personality tendencies and traits with them from their preschool experiences. But the school may alleviate or accentuate the problem depending upon teacher attitudes and classroom climates.
4. Speech clinicians serve teachers and stuttering pupils best by structuring counseling relationships in a manner which is geared to the feelings, attitudes, and reaction patterns of both teachers and stutterers.

The teacher's concern must be on both the subject matter and the child. The stuttering pupil, or any other pupil, can drink deeply and fully at the academic fount only when and if he feels psychologically secure and adequate. The pupil who stutters will attain his optimal academic functioning only when and if he is emotionally and communicatively free to do so. Teacher-pupil practices which are based on acceptance, respect, and understanding can help the stuttering pupil to accomplish the fullest measure from his learning experiences, whether he is the fledgling in kindergarten or the senior in high school (FitzSimons, 1960).

REFERENCES

ARBUCKLE, D. S. *Guidance and Counseling in the Classroom.* Engle-wood Cliffs, N. J.: Allyn & Bacon, Inc., 1957.

AXLINE, V. M. *Play Therapy.* Boston: Houghton Mifflin Co., 1947.

BURTON, W. H. *The Guidance of Learning Activities.* New York: Appleton-Century-Crofts, Inc., 1952.

CANTOR, N. *The Teaching-Learning Process.* New York: The Dry-den Press, Inc., 1953.

FITZSIMONS, R. M. "Speech Handicapped Children and the Class-room Teacher," *Educational Administration and Supervision,* 1960.

JOHNSON, O. G. "The Teacher's Role in Providing a Climate to Grow In," *J. Nat. Educ. Assn.,* **46:** 233–36, 1957.

JOHNSON, W. (ed.). *Speech Handicapped School Children.* New York: Harper & Bros., 1956.

LEEPER, R. W. "A Motivational Theory of Emotion to Replace Emo-tion as Disorganized Response," *Psychol. Rev.,* **55:** 5–21, 1948.

LEWIN, K.; LIPPIT, R.; and WHITE, R. K. "Patterns of Aggressive Behavior in Experimentally Created Social Climates," *J. Soc. Psy-chol.,* **10:** 271–79, 1939.

LIPPMAN, H. S. *Treatment of the Child in Emotional Conflict.* New York: Blakiston Division, McGraw-Hill Book Co., Inc., 1956.

MURPHY, A. T.; FITZSIMONS, R.; and PRONOVOST, W. *Does Your Pupil Stutter?* Boston: Boston Univ. Speech and Hearing Center, 1956.

ROGERS, C. R. "The Necessary and Sufficient Conditions of Thera-peutic Personality Change," *J. Counsel. Psychol.,* **21:** 95–103, 1957.

SHAPOFF, I. "A Stutterer Writes to a Former Teacher," *J. Nat. Educ. Assn.,* **43:** 348, 1954.

STEWART, R. S., and WORKMAN, A. D. *Children and Other People: Achieving Maturity Through Learning.* New York: The Dryden Press, Inc., 1956.

WILES, K. *Teaching for Better Schools.* Englewood Cliffs, N. J.: Prentice-Hall, Inc., 1952.

WOLBERG, L. R. *The Technique of Psychotherapy.* New York: Grune & Stratton, Inc., 1954.

Appendix

Photographs
of Play and Projective
Therapy Productions
of Stutterers

Photographs by
R. K. Smith

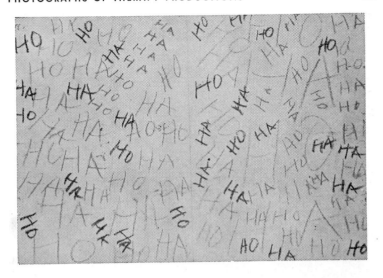

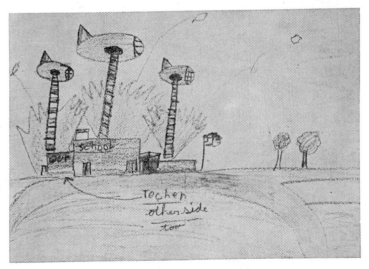

Fig. 1. Overt Expression of Covert Feelings. Feeling of hostility toward the school and the teacher are revealed in the spontaneous drawings of Lonnie (Chapter 8, p. 243).

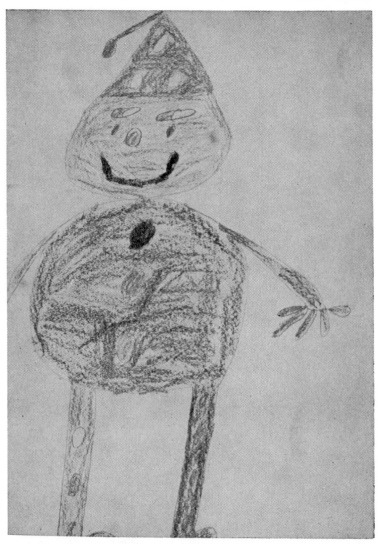

Fig. 2. Misery Is My Milieu. Eight-year-old Jonathan draws this sad-faced clown figure with large tears falling from its eyes. His stuttering, articulation problems, and learning difficulties have intensified feelings of complete rejection and isolation by parents, older siblings, and the world in general. In the words of a popular song of some time ago, "Bewitched, bothered, and bewildered am I" (Chapter 8, p. 257).

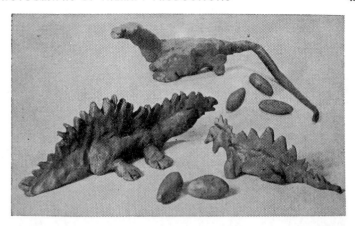

Fig. 3. **Benny's Fantasy Land of Dinosaurs.** Escaping to a world far-removed from his painful contemporary one, Benny strives for self-enhancement by verbalizing his knowledge of dinosaurs (Chapter 10, p. 319).

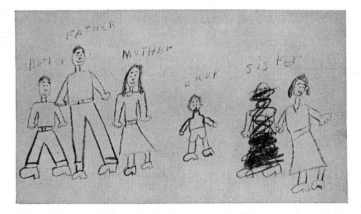

Fig. 4. **Paul's Family Constellation and His Self-portrait of Inadequacy.** Paul, age eight, first draws his own picture, then blocks it out with black crayon before drawing another picture of himself, smaller than the first. Note the spelling of "brother" (Chapter 10, p. 326).

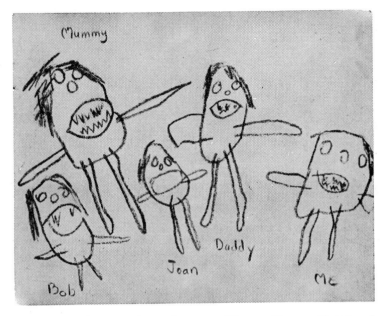

Fig. 5. Frankie's Family: Orality Is His Theme. Six-year-old stutterer's drawing emphasizes oral sphere. Mouths are magnified with large, sharp teeth, suggesting oral aggression or sadism. Similar attribution of prominence to the oral zone is seen commonly among stutterers (Chapter 10, p. 327).

Fig. 6. (Right.) Ours Is an Oral World. Orally centered and orally dominated (Drawings of 6-, 7-, and 12-year-old stutterers). Children tend to exaggerate those body parts or processes which have special meaning for them in terms of their own personality dynamics. The element common to each of these drawings is the accentuation of the primary zone of stuttering, the mouth (Chapter 10, p. 328).

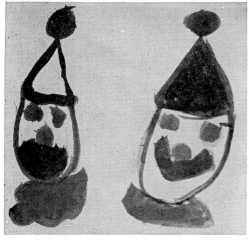

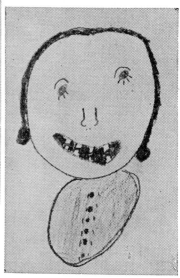

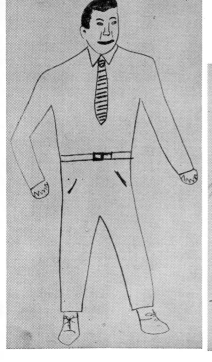

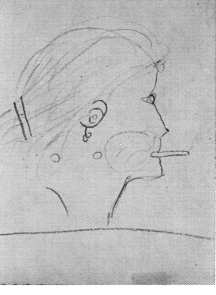

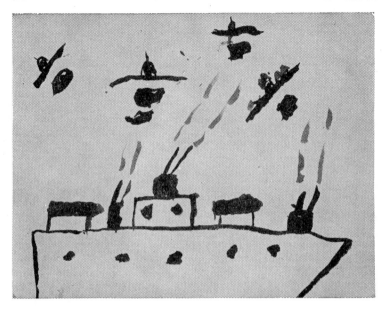

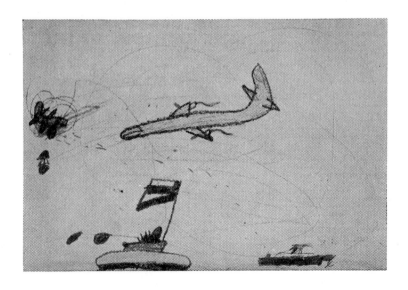

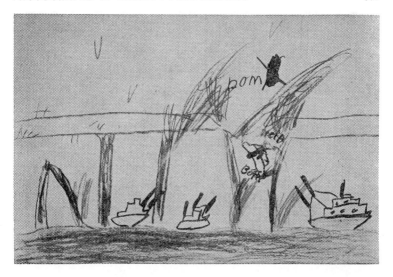

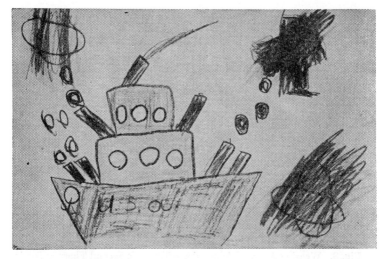

Fig. 7. (Left and right.) Our Words Explode into Stuttering, Our Feelings into Aggression. These drawings by young stutterers are indicative of their releases of aggression through depictions of bombing and fire scenes (Chapter 10, p. 328).

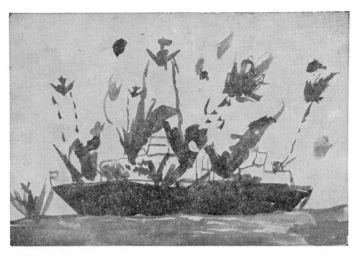

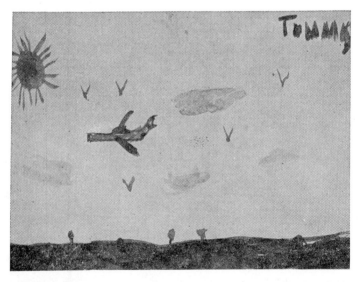

Fig. 8. **Wearing Away of Aggression—Tommy's Second Therapy Session Drawing and His Next-to-the-last Session Drawing.** Eight-year-old stutterer with strong feelings of being rejected and strong hostility toward people in general. Hate and aggression pour out in gunfire, bombings, and explosions in his first drawing. In his last drawing, made 18 months later, bluebirds fly, an airplane cruises, and the sun shines (Chapter 10, p. 328).

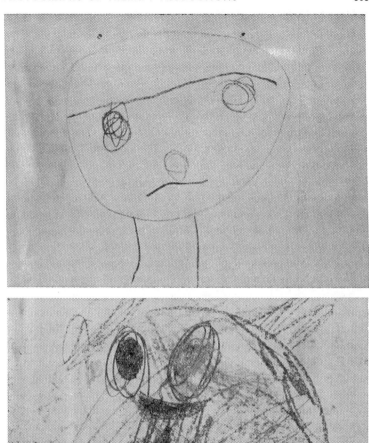

Fig. 9. **Beverly's Emerging Self.** This eight-year-old drew the forlorn self-portrait (*top*) in her first therapy session. At the eighth session, the rudiments of a total body sprouted out of a general bodily confusion (*bottom*).

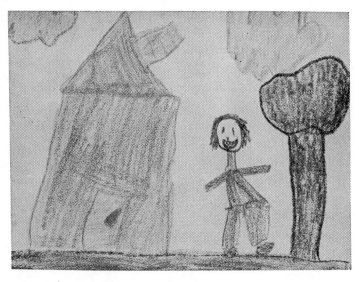

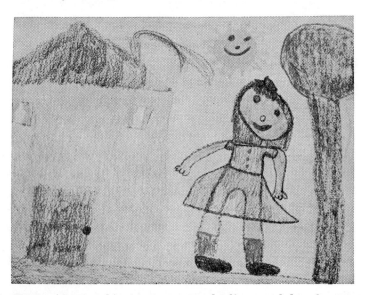

Fig. 9. (*Continued.*) A more integrated self is revealed in the picture drawn during the fifteenth session (*top*). At therapy termination, Beverly draws a colorful house-tree-person picture which reveals increased feelings of self-acceptance and personal worth (*bottom*). Her stuttering had been resolved (Chapter 10, pp. 329-30).

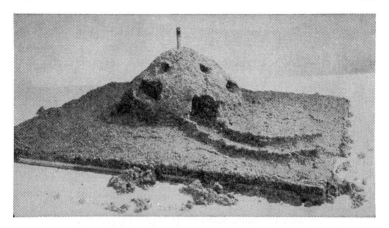

Fig. 10. Going Back—Regression, Reliving, and Regrowth. Modeling with sand offers many expressional opportunities. It is less threatening to the compulsively neat child than finger paint, etc. (Chapter 10, p. 337).

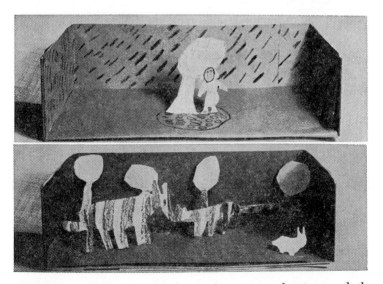

Fig. 11. Symbolic Projection. A shoebox, cutout drawings, and the needs and creativity of a child may produce dioramas representative of conflicts. Peggy draws a little girl standing all alone near a tree in the rain and puddles, projecting the isolation she feels in her family situation. Martin has two tigers, one larger than the other, and a small rabbit over to one corner. He projects a feeling of helplessness experienced during repeated and extremely aggressive parental quarrels (Chapter 10, p. 339).

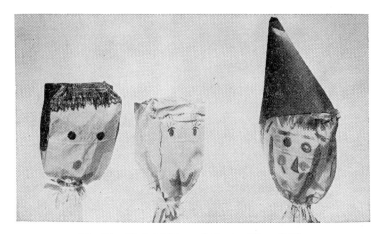

Fig. 12. Mask Making. (Chapter 10, p. 339).

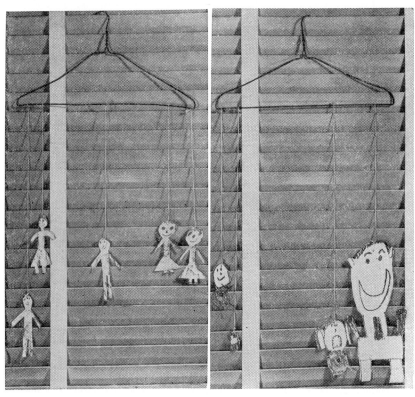

Fig. 13. Mobiles. (Chapter 10, p. 341).

Name Index

Subject Index